ROYAL ARMY MEDICAL CORPS TRAINING.

United Kingdom War Office

Fredonia Books
Amsterdam, The Netherlands

Royal Army Medical Corps Training

by
United Kingdom War Office

ISBN: 1-4101-0838-4

Reprinted from the 1911 edition

Fredonia Books
Amsterdam, The Netherlands
http://www.fredoniabooks.com

In order to make original editions of historical works available to scholars at an economical price, this facsimile of the original edition of 1911 is reproduced from the best available copy and has been digitally enhanced to improve legibility, but the text remains unaltered to retain historical authenticity.

ABBREVIATIONS.

A.M.O.	...	...	.	Administrative Medical Officer.
C.O.	...	.		Commanding Officer.
D.D.M.S.	...	...	.	Deputy Director of Medical Services.
D.M.S.	...	...	...	Director of Medical Services.
G.O.C.	...	...	...	General Officer Commanding.
G.O.C.-in-C.		...	...	„ „ „ in-Chief.
G.S.	...	...	...	General Staff.
I.G.C.	...	...	...	Inspector-General of Communications.
L. of C.	...	...	...	Line of Communications.
M.O.	...	...	...	Medical Officer.
N.C.O.	...	...	...	Non-Commissioned Officer.
O.C.	...	...	...	Officer Commanding.
P.M.O.	...	...	...	Principal Medical Officer.
Q.M.G.	...	...	...	Quartermaster-General.
R.A.M.C.	...	...	...	Royal Army Medical Corps.

This Manual is issued by Command of the Army Council for the guidance of all concerned.

WAR OFFICE,
14th July, 1911.

CONTENTS.

PART I.—MILITARY TRAINING.

PART II.—TRAINING IN TECHNICAL DUTIES IN THE FIELD.

SANITATION OR THE PREVENTION OF DISEASE.

PART III.—TRAINING IN TECHNICAL DUTIES IN THE FIELD.

THE CARE OF THE SICK AND WOUNDED.

PART IV.—R.A.M.C. DRILLS AND EXERCISES.

PART V.—TRAINING IN FIRST AID, NURSING, COOKING, &c.

DEFINITIONS.

Collecting Post.—A movable post formed by a detachment of a cavalry field ambulance, to which wounded are brought by the regimental medical establishments of cavalry engaged in operations involving dispersion.

Divisional Collecting Station.—A place formed by a tent subdivision or other detachment of an ambulance, where slightly wounded men able to walk to it are collected before further evacuation or return to their units.

Dressing Station, or Advanced Dressing Station.—A place for medical assistance formed by the tent division, sub-division, or other portion of an ambulance where the wounded are collected and cared for prior to removal.

Regimental Aid Post.—A place formed by the regimental medical establishment of a unit, at which wounded are collected with a view to being taken over by an ambulance.

Rest Station.—A place formed by a detachment of a clearing hospital or other medical unit on the L. of C., where sick and wounded are halted on their way down the L. of C.

Note.—The term "ambulance" means a field unit. The wagons for removal of sick and wounded are termed "ambulance wagons."

KEY TO FIGURES.
PART IV.

Commanding Officer.

Major.

Captain.

Lieutenant.

Quartermaster.

Serjeant-Major.

Serjeant or Staff-Serjeant.

Bugler.

Bugler in Cavalry Field Ambulance.

Cyclist Orderly.

6-Horsed (heavy) Ambulance Wagon (1 Wagon Orderly to each). (Length, with team, 16 yards.)

4-Horsed Ambulance Wagon (1 Wagon Orderly to each). (Length, with team, 10 yards.)

2-Horsed (light) Ambulance Wagon (2 Wagon Orderlies to each). (Length, with horses, 7 yards.)

Water-Cart. (Length, with horses, 4 yards.)

General Service Wagon. (Length, with team, 10 yards.)

Forage-Cart. (Length, with horses, 4⅔ yards.)

Bearer Sub-Division.

Tent Sub-Division.

ROYAL ARMY MEDICAL CORPS TRAINING.

1911.

PART I.—MILITARY TRAINING.

CHAPTER I.

GENERAL INSTRUCTIONS.

1. **Objects of Military Training.**—The Royal Army Medical Corps is maintained firstly, with a view to the prevention of disease, and secondly, for the care and treatment of the sick and wounded.

The efficient performance of these duties demands a thorough knowledge of medical science which must be acquired and kept up by deep and continuous study, and any instruction in purely military questions, beyond what is required for the performance of his proper functions, must be regarded as superfluous for an officer of that corps.

2. It is necessary, however, to remember that while these are the objects with which he is maintained, the interests of the Army require something even more than professional scientific knowledge from an officer of the R.A.M.C., because it is impossible for him to carry out his duties efficiently without a certain general knowledge of military science, especially as regards the administration of an army in the field.

For example, the work of officers of the R.A.M.C. includes the professional supervision of sanitary precautions, the collection of the sick and wounded, the compilation of records (general and professional) regarding them, certain arrangements in connection with the transportation of sick and wounded from the front, the discipline and maintenance of combatants under their charge, and the replenishment of medical and surgical requirements. Such duties bring the officers of the R.A.M.C. into close touch with the general work of the Army. Moreover, in addition to their professional work, they have executive duties to perform, in their capacity as officers of the R.A.M.C. units forming part of the Army. For example, they are as much concerned as officers of other units in the provision of food, clothing and other requirements to their men, in the care and management of transport allotted to them, in arranging their camps and movements, and fitting their units into their allotted places on the line of march, and, generally, in exercising the same functions as officers of other units, with the sole exception of actual combatant work.

As regards actual tactics, while officers of the R.A.M.C. are not charged with combatant duties, they are very intimately concerned in the combatant work of the other branches, and the efficient performance of their duties on the battlefield demands some knowledge of the general principles on which military operations are conducted. They must, for example, be capable of understanding from an operation order what is likely to be required of them.

3. **Responsibility for Training.**—In accordance with directions issued to the Commandants by the War Office from time to time, officers, on entering the service, are instructed in the principles of general and medical organization at the Royal Army Medical College and the Royal Army Medical Corps School of Instruction, at the latter of which recruits are also trained. Instruction in the principles of staff duties in the field is also included in the senior course at the Royal Army Medical College.

4. Under the authority of G.Os.C.-in-C., P.M.Os. of Commands, A.M.Os., and Os.C. companies and detachments, are responsible for the training of junior officers in the interior economy and administration of military hospitals, and for the further progressive instruction of all officers serving under them, during the subsequent years of their service, in the organization and administration of the medical service, as well as for the supervision of the technical military training of all ranks.

5. Under the same authority, and entrusted to the General Staff (with such assistance from other branches of the staff as may be required), is the instruction of Officers of the Corps in the principles of military science, and the giving of advice and assistance to P.M.Os. in matters bearing on the applicability of technical training to the purposes for which it is intended.

6. **General System of Training.**—General instructions regarding the training of all ranks of the Army are contained in Training and Manœuvre Regulations. Following the general system therein laid down as to the various means of training, the training of officers, R.A.M.C., in military subjects, and the training of N.C.Os. and men in the duties of the Corps is divided into (i) individual Training, (ii) Collective Training.

CHAPTER II.

INDIVIDUAL TRAINING.

OFFICERS.

7. Means of Individual Training.—The individual training of officers is effected by means of staff tours, war games, lectures, regimental exercises and indoor schemes, and essays.

8. Staff Tours.—The attendance of officers of the R.A.M.C. at staff tours may be considered conveniently under two heads—attendance at those primarily intended for the study of strategical and tactical problems, and at those specially designed for the instruction of medical officers.

9. As regards the former, it must be remembered that the best results are not obtained if more work is thrown on the directing staff than it is possible to do thoroughly in the time available, and it is difficult for a directing staff to supervise the work of both the fighting and the administrative services. It is often possible, however, for a few officers, R.A.M.C., to attend such exercises, to receive information as to what is going on, and to work out the necessary medical arrangements on their own account. They can gain valuable experience in this way, and, without seriously increasing the work of the directing staff, they can bring to notice any undue strain thrown on the medical service by the operations undertaken, and the probable consequences thereof. The resulting consideration of the bearing of administrative questions on the tactical and strategical problems to be solved, is of undoubted advantage to all officers taking part in the exercise. It will also be of advantage when problems connected with the administrative services are to be specially studied, to place a selected medical officer on the directing staff, in order to criticise the work of the medical officers taking part in the tour, and to bring to the notice of the director questions in connection with the arrangements for the medical service.

10. Staff tours for the instruction of officers, R.A.M.C., will be carried out on the following principles :—It is important that medical officers should, in peace time, be practised in adapting their arrangements to military requirements based on definite situations, and also that staff officers should become fully acquainted with the possibilities and limitations of the authorized medical organization. Officers of the General Staff should draw up strategical and tactical schemes, with subsequent situations developed therefrom, on which the medical arrangements should be based.

Medical officers taking part will carry out the work of their service under the direction of the P.M.O., who should be given every assistance by the general staff officers, working in close touch with him, and studying the organization and work of his service.

Such special staff tours afford scope for a detailed study of medical problems in the field, such as the actual disposition and movement of medical units, and the work in detail of the various lines of medical assistance, based on definite tactical situations.

11. Should circumstances permit, every officer of the rank of captain and upwards will attend at least one special staff tour annually, and field officers will, in addition, attend at least one staff tour each year.

12. **War Games.**—As in the case of staff tours, the attendance of officers, R.A.M.C., at war games comes under two heads :—

(a) Attendance at war games designed for the study of strategical and tactical problems.

(b) Attendance at war games specially designed for the instruction of officers, R.A.M.C., in their own duties.

13. Attendance at war games designed for the study of strategical or tactical problems usually afford but limited opportunities of working out in any detail the medical arrangements necessitated by the operations carried on. But, even relatively as spectators, it is of use to medical officers to see practical illustrations of time and space problems, and of march and battle formations, especially if arrangements are made to enable them to consider and discuss the duties which would fall to them in connection with such operations. As far as possible, therefore, opportunity should be afforded to medical officers, in connection with such war games, to work out and submit for discussion the salient features of the medical arrangements. This would not only afford useful instruction to the medical officers concerned, but would serve to remind combatant officers of the administrative requirements that have to be attended to.

14. War games specially designed for the instruction of officers, R.A.M.C., are similar in their objects to special staff tours for medical officers, and should be conducted on similar principles.

15. Attendance at war games may be supplementary or alternative to attendance at staff tours, as opportunity may offer.

16. **Lectures.**—In each Command, lectures will be arranged for the further instruction of officers of the Corps in the organization and administration of the medical service, and also upon the principles of staff duties in the field.

17. The lectures on the organization and administration of the medical service will be given under the arrangement of P.M.Os. by officers of the Corps. The subjects should be selected from any question of interest in military medical organization and administration, and the number of lectures will be not less than four annually. The period during which they should be given will usually be during the winter months, at such times and at such stations as may be convenient.

Among subjects considered suitable are the following :—

(a) The mobilization and formation of medical units, and all matters connected therewith.

(b) The duties of the R.A.M.C. in the field.

(c) The duties of the R.A.M.C. on the line of communication and at the base.

(d) The sanitary and medical problems of an army in war.

18. The lectures on the principles of staff duties in the field should include the various duties of the General Staff, Adjutant-General's Staff, and Quartermaster-General's Staff, and will be given, under the orders of G.Os.C.-in-C., by officers of the General Staff. The subjects, and the general scope of the instruction in each subject, should be on the following lines :—

(a) The organization of an army in the field, and the working of its various departments, etc., especially as regards the services of maintenance.

Under this head, broad general principles should be explained, showing the interdependence of the various departments, and their relation to the fighting troops. It should also be shown how and whence a R.A.M.C. unit obtains what it requires, e.g. in personnel, matériel, horses, etc. The broad general principles of the chain in command, and of staff duties, should be explained of amplification of Field Service Regulations so that a medical officer may know with whom he has to deal on the various matters affecting his duties.

(b) Such a general outline of strategical and tactical operations as will enable a medical officer to formulate the most suitable medical arrangements in connection with such operations.

It is probable that the best way to convey the required instruction under this head would be by giving brief sketches of various campaigns, showing the different kinds of operations which may take place. In connection with such sketches, opportunities should be taken to explain the characteristics and methods of work of the different arms, the meaning of technical military terms, marching and fighting formations, including simple time and space calculations and the essential points to be remembered in arranging movements, so that a medical officer may be capable of fitting his unit into its allotted place on the line of march, or elsewhere.

In connection with the above it should be explained how the medical service must be regarded as part of an organization which is maintained for the special purpose of fighting, and how this special purpose must be kept constantly in view by officers of the R.A.M.C. in carrying out their work in the field.

(o) The working of the lines of communication, with special reference to the evacuation of wounded, provision of hospitals, etc., selection of routes for evacuation of sick and wounded, and the general principles which regulate their choice.

(d) The system of intercommunication, and of writing field messages, reports, etc., in order that medical officers may be capable of communicating with other branches of the army in the field when required. The principles regulating the communication of orders, the different kinds of orders issued, and the points to be attended to in writing them, should also be explained sufficiently to enable medical officers to understand any orders they receive, and to frame such orders as they may have to issue.

(e) Map reading and simple field sketching, especially as regards the use of scales, conventional signs, and the use of the compass; the object in view being to enable an officer to reach a point indicated by reference to a map, to describe the proposed site of a hospital, etc., or to send in a rough sketch of such things as a dressing station, a hospital site, or a building with its surroundings and approaches, according to the accepted methods.

The instruction in map reading and field sketching should as far as possible be practical.

Each lecture should be followed by discussion, if possible. The lectures will be arranged so as to cover the necessary ground in a period of three years; not less than four lectures will be given annually.

As conditions vary in different Commands, the number of lectures in each subject, the stations at which they are to be given, and the period of the year most convenient, is left to the discretion of the Command authorities.

19. Regimental Exercises and Indoor Schemes.—In lieu of, or in addition to, lectures on medical organization and administration, regimental exercises or indoor schemes may be arranged, for the study of medical problems in the field.

20. Essays.—The writing of essays is voluntary, but P.M.Os. should encourage officers to write essays on any subject of military medical interest; such subject or subjects to be selected each year.

Non-Commissioned Officers and Men.

21. Training in the Special Duties of the Corps.—The courses of instruction for N.C.Os. and men in the special duties of the Corps will be in accordance with the various syllabuses laid down in Standing Orders, R.A.M.C.

22. Training in Semaphore Signalling.—The numbers of rank and file in field units trained in semaphore signalling are detailed in War Establishments. The standard of efficiency required is that laid down for semaphore signalling in the Training Manual—Signalling, and the annual inspection will be carried out as laid down for other branches. The numbers to be trained in each company (see Standing Orders, R.A.M.C.) need not be limited to those who will actually be required on mobilization, and encouragement should be given to officers and other ranks of the Corps to learn semaphore signalling sufficiently well to send and read proficiently, without necessarily acquiring the ordinary routine of message work.

CHAPTER III.

COLLECTIVE TRAINING.

23. Periods of Collective Training.—The field training of the R.A.M.C. is divided into (i) Regimental Training, (ii) Divisional and Command Training and Army Manœuvres.

REGIMENTAL TRAINING.

24. Practice Mobilizations of Medical Units.—In Commands where facilities exist, means should be adopted to give all ranks opportunities for examining, packing, and loading the equipment, and practising the formation and field work of medical units. The personnel of units so mobilized may be supplemented, if necessary, by men of other corps for the less technical duties.

25. Camps of Instruction.—Camps of instruction in each Command, or combined camps of instruction from two or more Commands, will be formed each year, at a suitable period during the summer months, and as many officers and other ranks as can be spared will attend. An instructor will be appointed. Each class of instruction should attend for at least two weeks, and the number of classes, and the size of each class, will be arranged as may be suitable.

The training will be upon the following lines :—

(i.) If the most is to be made of the training at camps of instruction, it is necessary that as much preliminary work as possible in the way of Corps exercises, first aid, etc., should have been done before the camp begins. For this purpose it must be borne in mind that one of the duties of an officer of the Corps is to direct and instruct his men, and every advantage should be taken at C.O's. parades to give instruction not only in the drills and exercises of the Corps, but also, according to the means available, to carry out such progressive training as will, by developing the initiative and self-reliance of the N.C.Os. and men, best fit them for the performance of their various duties in war. At small stations there may be difficulties in the way of giving adequate preliminary instruction, mainly on account of the small number of men present, but at very few should it be impossible to afford N.C.Os. and men sound instruction in first aid, including the carriage of wounded men. If this preliminary instruction is sufficiently thorough, a short period should suffice for Corps exercises, etc., when the camp is formed, and this should be followed by a definite scheme of progressive work.

(ii.) The syllabus at the end of this chapter is recommended as a guide in drawing up programmes for camps of instruction, or camps of units of the R.A.M.C.

(iii.) Where facilities offer, it would be to the advantage of the medical units if men of other troops could be detailed to act as patients, thus enabling the whole personnel of the medical unit to take part in the practical exercises. It would also be advantageous to the R.A.M.C., during the final stages of the training, if field days could be arranged, even on a small scale, for the purpose of practising regimental medical establishments and medical units in their duties ; the operations being planned with the object of illustrating, for example, not only the collection and reception of wounded men in field ambulances, but their removal to, and evacuation from, medical units on the line of communication. For this purpose, advantage could be taken of any means of transport by road, rail, or water which may exist in the Command.

26. Special Exercises.—In commands where arrangements can be made, special exercises will be conducted upon a larger scale, at which, with the assistance of other troops, the more important problems of medical organization and work in the field, and on the line of communication, may be studied practically.

27. Training in Field Sanitation.—Opportunity will also be taken, during the camps of other troops, to train the N.C.Os. and men of the Corps in the duties of sanitary sections and sanitary squads, as well as to train the N.C.Os. and men of the regimental sanitary detachments of the units in camp. The training will be supervised by sanitary officers of commands, divisions, etc.

DIVISIONAL, COMMAND, AND ARMY MANŒUVRES.

28. Wherever possible, the medical service will be represented as completely as circumstances permit, and the sanitary and medical arrangements and organization will be based upon those of an army in the field. Manœuvres afford special opportunities, of which every advantage should be taken, of training all ranks in field sanitary duties.

During divisional and command training, officers, by interchange where possible, will be given opportunities of practising the duties of the various lines of assistance ; while, during army manœuvres, all ranks, where circumstances permit, will be appointed to the duties that would fall to them on mobilization.

29. Regimental Medical Establishments.—The N.C.Os. and men of regimental medical establishments will also be exercised in their duties during manœuvres or other suitable period of training, both as regards sanitation and as stretcher bearers, according to their classification.

Careful practical instruction will be given by M.Os. to the regimental sanitary detachments in their duties in the field ; not only in sanitary methods, but also in the precautionary measures to be taken on the line of march, in camps and billets, and when temporarily occupying a village or town during military operations.

The regimental stretcher bearers will also be exercised in rendering first aid and carrying casualties on stretchers, in taking up positions for regimental aid posts under the instructions of the M.O., in noting ground suitable for moving wounded to or over, and in keeping in communication with field ambulance bearers.

30. Field Medical Units.—To obtain the best advantage from the training afforded by manœuvres, it is necessary that ambulances be exercised as divisional troops under the command of the A.M.O., as they are in war.

But the exigencies of peace training occasionally require that ambulances or sections be attached to cavalry or infantry brigades which are not necessarily acting independently at the time. They may also occasionally impose upon ambulances the duty of acting temporarily in the capacity of clearing hospitals.

However necessary such deviations from war organization may be in view of the limitations imposed by manœuvres more especially designed for the training of the fighting troops, the value of the training afforded to the R.A.M.C., both in administrative and executive duties, is much less than when the medical arrangements are based upon the organization of the medical service in war.

SYLLABUS OF TRAINING IN CAMP.

For the guidance of officers in preparing programmes for camps of instruction in the Regular Royal Army Medical Corps, and for annual camps of field medical units in the Territorial Force. This syllabus may be adapted to camps of varying duration by repeating or omitting such stages or items as may be suitable. As a rule not more than two days should be occupied by Preliminary Training, which in suitable cases may be omitted or shortened. If the instruction would thereby be rendered more efficient, the stages may be transposed and the various items interchanged or varied.

Every opportunity should be taken of giving instruction in general and medical organization; methods of field sanitation and the prevention of disease; general rules for marches, camps, and bivouacs; orders, messages, and reports; interior economy of units in the field; methods of field cooking; reports, returns, and indents; and in horsemastership. Map reading, simple field sketching, and semaphore signalling should be practised as occasion may offer.

The Transport Section of the Royal Army Medical Corps (Territorial Force) will attend such of the Preliminary and Intermediate Training as are applicable, and in addition will be instructed in riding, driving, fitting harness and saddlery, and in the care of horses.

	PRELIMINARY TRAINING.			INTERMEDIATE TRAINING.	
	Stage A. One working day.	Stage B. One working day.	Stage C. One working day.	Stage D. One working day.	Stage E. One working day.
Morning—1 hour..	Squad and company drill.	Squad and company drill, or stretcher exercises.	Hand-seats and improvised carriage of patients.	Preparing operating tent and tents for sick. Preparing G.S. wagons and vehicles of various types for carriage of wounded.	Field ambulance or cavalry field ambulance formations and movements.

	PRELIMINARY TRAINING.		INTERMEDIATE TRAINING.		
	Stage A. One working day.	Stage B. One working day.	Stage C. One working day.	Stage D. One working day.	Stage E. One working day.
Forenoon—1 hour...	Stretcher exercises ...	Equipping, loading, and unloading ambulance wagons.	Lecture on Geneva Convention and the system of removal of sick and wounded from front to base.	Preparing G.S. wagons and vehicles of various types* for carriage of wounded, and practice in loading and unloading wounded. *including motor-lorries, railway wagons, boats, and barges if available.	Collecting wounded, including improvised carriage, formation of dressing station of field ambulance or collecting post and dressing station of cavalry field ambulance; laying out field ambulance or cavalry field ambulance encampment, and reception of wounded. Preparation of divisional collecting station. Preparation of bivouacs and shelters.
2 hours...	Checking equipment and examining contents.	Packing and loading field ambulance or cavalry field ambulance equipment.	First aid and removal of wounded according to injuries and carriage required.	Practical instruction in making field kitchens and latrines, and in methods of refuse disposal.	Coupling horses: mounting and dismounting wounded men. Demonstration in stable management in horse-lines
Afternoon—Number of hours as required.	N.C.Os. and men—Tent pitching.—During these exercises opportunity should be taken to give N.C.Os. such instructions as may be necessary in guard and piquet duties in camps of medical units. Officers—Lecture on field medical organization and the rôles of medical units.	N.C.Os. and men—Tent pitching and preparing tents for patients. Officers—Lecture on duties in camp, on the line of march, and in the field, including the duties of regimental medical establishments in action, and the tactical use of field medical units.	N.C.Os. and men—Demonstrations of water purification and explanation of sanitary methods in the field. Officers—Selection of sites for encampments, billets, hospitals, &c., including study of ground, mapreading, and simple field sketching with a view to the above.	N.C.Os and men—Packing and loading field ambulance or cavalry field ambulance equipment. Forms and returns in the field. Officers—Selection of sites for dressing stations with reference to the ordinary danger zones for rifle and shell fire, including study of ground, map reading, and simple field sketching with a view to the above. Selection of sites for divisional collecting stations.	

ADVANCED TRAINING.

Stage F. (Number of working days as available.)	Stage G. (Number of working days as available.)
Exercises as a unit in the field.	Exercises as a unit in the field with other troops.
Large numbers of "wounded" to be collected, treated, and classified for disposal, reports and returns to be prepared.	(1.) It will be to the advantage of the medical units under training if field days, with a small number of troops representing larger formations, can be arranged for the special purpose of affording them practice in their duties, and of illustrating the work of medical units of various types.
Field Ambulances.	(2.) When special field days cannot be arranged, or in addition to special field days, medical units under training should be afforded such opportunities as may occur of taking part in tactical field days, if of a nature suitable for their instruction.
The above to be practised under varying conditions, *e.g.*, under the conditions of (1) a force holding a defensive position; (2) a force carrying out a deliberate attack on a position, (3) an encounter battle requiring arrangements to be carried out unexpectedly from the line of march; (4) a retirement.	
Cavalry Field Ambulances.	
The exercises to be practised (1) as if with cavalry engaged in operations involving concentration, under conditions similar to those enumerated under field ambulances; (2) as if with cavalry engaged in operations involving dispersion.	

PART II.—TRAINING IN TECHNICAL DUTIES IN THE FIELD.

SANITATION OR THE PREVENTION OF DISEASE.

CHAPTER IV.

THE EXTENT TO WHICH SICKNESS PREVAILS IN THE ARMY.

31. Every soldier knows that the efficiency of an army, as a fighting organization, depends largely upon the health of the individuals which compose it ; therefore, a knowledge of the causes and conditions which contribute to sickness, as a means of military inefficiency, and also of the principles and methods by which disease may be prevented is essential to every soldier.

It will readily be understood that the amount of sickness among soldiers will, and does, vary from year to year, but the prevalence of disease is chiefly influenced by such conditions as age and length of service, place where serving, and whether the conditions be those of peace or war. It is desirable that every one should have some idea of the main facts.

32. Influence of Age and Length of Service.—In our army, where men serve all over the world, the effects of both age and length of service are striking. In the garrisons at home, the sick admission rate is highest among the men between 20 and 25 years of age, and lowest among men of 40 years and over. The number of deaths is lowest among those under 20 years of age, but steadily rises in each five-year period. The most marked effects of age are shown, however, in the prevalence of enteric fever ; this disease occurs most frequently among young men, more particularly those of the age from 20 to 25 years. As the men get older, they become less liable to it. The influence of length of service is similar to that of age. For many years the greatest numbers of admissions to hospital for sickness has been among men with less than one year's service, and the lowest number among men with eight years' service or more.

33. Locality as affecting the Health of Troops.—It will readily be understood that this is largely a matter of climate. In the home garrisons, this influence is not apparent, but it is interesting to note that the smallest number of men constantly sick is found in

the Channel Islands, the Scottish and Western commands. When we look to the various garrisons abroad we see at once how diverse climatic conditions affect the health of the soldier. The general effect of foreign service is to increase the numbers of those who are constantly sick, of invalids, and of deaths. Roughly, the total loss by death is trebled by foreign service, the increase being due mostly to the more acute forms of disease, such as enteric fever in India, malarial fever in Mauritius, the Straits Settlements, and West Africa. The most healthy garrisons are in South Africa ; while as regards the average number constantly sick in hospital, Jamaica gives the highest figure.

34. **Health of Troops during Peace.**—The general extent to which sickness prevails in the army during ordinary times of peace will be apparent from the accompanying table. We are justified in considering the figures, as a whole, distinctly satisfactory. Further, if we compare these returns, which relate to the year 1909, with those of say twenty or more years ago we realize how great has been the progress made. But bearing in mind that the army represents a picked male population, and that those unable to maintain the required physical standard are rapidly discharged, we are hardly justified in accepting these returns as the high-water mark of sanitary efficiency. Looked at in this light, we see every reason for further effort being made towards a reduction of total admissions to hospital for sickness and of those dying from sickness.

European Troops.	Ratio per 1,000 of Strength.							
	Admissions for Sickness.		Average number constantly sick in hospital.		Invalided for Sickness.		Deaths.	
	1860.	1909.	1860.	1909.	1860.	1909.	1860.	1909.
All troops at home and abroad	1,335·8	504·8	57·08	28·86	13·71	8·65	19·42	4·10
United Kingdom	1,052·7	378·4	54·72	21·72	17·72	10·51	9·95	2·92
Gibraltar	825·3	370·3	40·55	25·44	9·68	9·03	11·06	2·46
Malta	983·0	373·6	47·40	24·47	6·05	8·29	10·59	2·97
Crete	—	584·1	—	25·52	—	5·90	—	5·90
Cyprus	—	586·5	—	16·54	—	—	—	—
Egypt	—	672·9	—	40·61	—	9·71	—	4·21
Canada	613·5	—	8·51	—	13·95	—	29·86	—
Bermuda	751·9	127·3	39·01	9·52	6·65	4·10	8·55	·82
Barbados	1,057·4	—	—	—	—	—	5·58	—
Jamaica	816·5	813·1	23·95	50·92	3·53	14·56	20·20	16·99
St. Helena	835·2	—	36·12	—	—	—	10·85	—
West Africa	—	1,026·1	—	47·89	—	11·19	—	—
South Africa	850·1	331·2	49·13	19·29	12·26	5·18	13·16	3·73
Mauritius	1,118·8	586·5	44·83	43·99	11·13	13·46	23·86	4·81
Ceylon	1,671·6	560·1	79·81	35·28	1·09	9·49	19·65	3·16
India	1,917·7	716·9	71·35	40·26	9·96	6·05	35·23	6·87
North China	—	643·8	—	40·80	—	2·94	—	3·91
South China	2,652·6	636·6	—	42·09	—	7·72	52·04	6·18
Straits Settlements	—	955·9	—	43·08	—	6·84	—	4·56

Of the various diseases which, taken together, determine the sanitary condition of our army in time of peace, it is found that venereal affections, malarial fevers, and digestive troubles (mainly diarrhœa), give the highest admission rates for sickness, but the deaths from these causes are few. Enteric fever causes the greatest number of deaths, the next most fatal form of disease being pneumonia and other kinds of respiratory trouble. Among causes of invaliding from the service, the first place is taken by various affections of the heart, while a variety of other ailments, such as tuberculosis, bronchitis, debility, and nervous diseases, contribute in a marked but lesser degree. Judged by the numbers constantly sick, the chief contributing causes of non-efficiency are venereal diseases, digestive troubles, lung troubles, enteric and other fevers, rheumatism, and injuries.

85. **Health of Troops in Time of War.**—The extent to which sickness prevails in an army during war varies greatly as do also the losses sustained from the acts of the enemy. This is not to be wondered at, considering the diversity of conditions under which wars are conducted. The most striking feature of all wars is the marked excess of the sickness admission rates over those for injuries received in action. Roughly, it may be said that for each man admitted to hospital for some wound or injury there are twenty-five admitted for some form of disease. The disparity is less marked in the corresponding death-rates, but even then it is the exception for the deaths from wounds to be in excess of those from disease. The usual ratio is five deaths from disease for one from wounds or injury.

Although most of the diseases occurring commonly among soldiers during peace are met with in war-time, still there is a tendency for some to predominate, notably those dependent upon such influences as exposure to climate, pollution of soil or water, and indifferent food. The influence of hostilities shows itself mainly in increased incidence and mortality from respiratory and digestive troubles, malaria, diarrhœa, dysentery, enteric fever, and cholera. The precise degree of increased prevalence which these diseases display naturally varies with the climate and other circumstances in which any particular campaign is prosecuted. This is particularly the case in our own army, which serves all the world over ; but in general terms it may be said that war conditions usually mean a sixfold increase of such diseases as diarrhœa, dysentery, and enteric fever, as compared with peace time : malarial fevers are increased about one-fifth, venereal diseases in camp life drop to about one-fourth of the number in ordinary garrisons ; respiratory and digestive affections generally show a slight increase ; while injuries, other than those received in action, together with other common disabilities, do not as a rule prevail more than in circumstances of peace.

CHAPTER V.

THE CAUSES OF DISEASE.

36. The prevention of disease depends largely on a knowledge of its causes. If we look closely into the nature of the chief diseases we find that they can be divided, roughly, into the following groups: (1) diseases which are the result of some inherited defect or fault in the make of the body ; (2) diseases which are the result of accident or injury ; (3) diseases which are the effect or result of climate ; (4) diseases which are due to either foolish habits or faulty modes of life ; and (5) diseases which are due to some cause or causes introduced into the body from without.

So far as soldiers are concerned, we may say that the first group does not apply, as all soldiers are medically examined before they enlist, and no men become soldiers who have bodily defects likely to give rise to sickness or disease. The second group we may dismiss as largely non-preventable ; accidents and injuries are bound to occur occasionally, even in a well-regulated army. Of the diseases caused by climate or weather, it is doubtful whether there are many, the chief one occurring among soldiers being sunstroke or heatstroke. In the fourth group are such diseases as the various venereal affections, alcoholism, and those forms of sickness, the result of the abuse of both drink and food. In the last or fifth group are diseases like enteric fever, cholera, dysentery, smallpox, plague, malaria, and a number of others, all of which are caused by the entering into the body from without of the cause, which is a living thing or germ.

It is quite clear that, from the nature of this causation, the various diseases included in the last three groups are more or less preventable. Thus, sunstroke and heatstroke can be avoided by the exercise of reasonable care in safeguarding the head from the effects of the direct rays of a powerful sun and otherwise protecting the body from the effects of excessive heat. In the same way, venereal diseases can be avoided by the exercise of chastity and self-control, while, too, the effects of excessive eating and drinking are to be controlled by self-discipline, moderation, and common sense. The avoidance and prevention of the diseases in the remaining groups is not quite so simple, and involves a consideration of the nature and mode of action of the germs or the living things which are their cause.

37. Microbes or Germs.—The size and shape of the livings things which are sometimes called germs or microbes, and which are the cause of a number of diseases, vary ; their size may be anything from one five-thousandth to one ten-thousandth part of an inch, and their shape may be equally variable. Some are merely minute spherical granules, to which we give the name *micrococci* ; others, from their rod-like shape are known as *bacilli* whilst others, having a cork-screw or spiral form are known as *spirilla*. All these various forms are sometimes spoken of as *bacteria*, but no matter what is their shape or size, these various germs or microbes are living things and capable of producing others of their kind. The process of reproduction amongst the micro-organisms is generally a very simple one, and takes place under favourable conditions with enormous rapidity. The spherical micrococci and the majority of the bacilli and spirilla merely divide into two. In other cases, however, the bacilli multiply by the production within their substance of a round or oval, bead-like body. This is known as a *spore* or seed, and from it grows in due time another bacillus. These spores of bacteria are the hardiest forms of living matter of which we know, being able to resist extremes of heat, cold, and drying, conditions which would be immediately fatal to the parent bacilli from which they have sprung.

It must not be supposed that all bacteria or germs are hurtful and capable of producing disease; it is far otherwise. The majority of micro-organisms do good, and we could not carry on our lives without them; it is only a small number which are harmful to man and able to cause disease. Should, by chance, these disease-producing germs or bacteria gain access and a foothold, as it were, in man's body, they grow and increase in numbers. Sometimes they prefer to grow in the blood, at other times in the lungs, or spleen, or liver, or the bone marrow, while sometimes they prefer to grow inside the bowel, or perhaps outside the body on the skin or in the roots of the hair. The greater number of the disease-producing germs live and thrive in the blood and other juices of the body. While growing and multiplying there they make or excrete a poison or *toxin*, as it is called, and it is the circulation of this poison or toxin in the blood and body juices which makes a man ill and gives rise to the various symptoms of the particular disease which is being caused. Whether a person is going to recover or not from the effects of the growth of the disease germs in his body depends upon how well or how succesfully he can manufacture an antidote or corrective to the poison made and poured into his system by the germs. If sufficient of the antidote is made, then the germs are gradually killed and their poison neutralized, followed by the gradual recovery of the sick person. If, on the other hand, the germs make so much of the poison or the patient fails to make sufficient antidote to neutralize the germ poison, then he dies as the result of the disease caused.

This behaviour of these disease-producing germs in the human body is very similar to the action of yeast or other ferments when growing in sugar solutions, such as malt and water, or apple juice or grape juice. From these sugar solutions are made respectively beer, cider, wine, or brandy. Consider the case of wine for a moment. The vintner takes the ripe grapes and throws them into a vat or tub. By crushing them up he makes a sugary liquid into which pass various microbes, either from the air or by means of the skins of the grapes which are in the sugary mass. Certain of these germs or microbes from the air or attached to the grape-skins ferment the sugar, that is, split it up into carbonic acid gas and alcohol. This action of the ferment goes on until sufficient alcohol has been made so as to constitute 14 per cent. of the sugary juice.

When this amount of alcohol has been formed, fermentation ceases, owing to the excess of alcohol. This is very much the same as occurs in the human body when certain of the disease-producing germs gain access to it ; they go on growing and fermenting, as it were, in the blood and juices of the body until the body has manufactured a sufficiency of the antidote to stop their action. It is this curious resemblance between the two processes that has suggested the name of "fermentation-like" for many of these diseases, simply because their germs or causes behave in the human body like a ferment. Typical examples of diseases of this nature are smallpox, chicken-pox, measles, scarlet fever, enteric fever, plague, cholera, typhus, diphtheria, and many others. In all of them there is the introduction of a living germ or germs ; then a period of "incubation" or hatching, in which nothing can be observed ; then follows the active disturbance, and in the diseases, as well as in the fermentation of the sugary liquid, the process is stopped when the microbes have multiplied to a certain extent, a temporary or permanent protection being the result. Another name for diseases of this kind is "infective." A disease like smallpox or measles which can be passed from person to person without immediate contact between the two, is termed "infectious." In these cases the infection is conveyed by mucus expectorated by the first patient, or by dust blown about or carried in clothing, etc. Such diseases may also, of course, be communicated by direct contact. If direct contact between the sick and well is indispensable for the conveyance of a disease, it is called "contagious." In nature there is no such hard line drawn between contagion and infection, although some diseases can be more easily communicated than others. In this sense, then, the word "infectious" includes all the germ-caused diseases, however spread.

Throughout the progress of these diseases, except in the period of incubation, the patient is able to communicate his disease to persons about him who have not been rendered safe by a previous attack. The way in which he thus communicates his disease varies in different cases. In scarlet fever, the throat, nose, ears, and skin are the chief sources of contagion ; in diphtheria, influenza, measles, and whooping cough, the secretions from the throat and respiratory passages ; in enteric fever and cholera, the urine, stools and vomit. The protection afforded by one attack of an infective disease against its recurrence varies greatly ; speaking generally, they occur but once, but second attacks are not uncommon.

38. Means of Infection.—The modes by which infection is received vary greatly with different diseases ; the chief channels of infection are the skin and the mucous membranes, particularly of the digestive and respiratory tracts. This means, man can contract infection by means of cuts, scratches or wounds of the skin (inoculation), by means of the air, and by means of food and drink. Under the last head, milk and water are the two usual sources of infection, but uncooked food, especially oysters and mussels fed in sewage-polluted waters, may produce the same effect. Cholera, enteric fever and dysentery are the chief diseases from this source. Milk may be infected from having been handled by an infectious person, or it may convey infection of some disease from which the cow or other animal yielding the milk at the time is suffering, as, for instance, tuberculosis. Water may be contaminated with sewage, or the excreta of a single infectious person. When the air acts as a conveyor of infection, the infectious matter must generally be in the condition of dust. In this manner the contagion of small-pox can be carried considerable distances, that of tubercle possibly only a short space, and that of typhus but a few feet. Of diseases spread by inoculation or damage to the skin, notable examples are tetanus or lock-jaw following the fouling of wounds with earth, malaria and yellow fever resulting from bites of mosquitoes, plague from bites of fleas from rats, and sleeping sickness from the bites of a special fly found in various parts of Africa.

39. Susceptibility to Infection.—It may be asked, naturally, if, then, these disease-causing germs are so widely scattered and can reach man in such a variety of ways, why is it that man is not infected oftener than he is? The answer is that persons vary in suscep-tibility to attack by different infective diseases ; moreover, the possibility and intensity of an attack depend on the condition of the person, and on the number and virulence of the particular microbes infecting the person. The main protection against infection by germs exists in man's own body, more particularly in the blood, whose white corpuscles swallow up and destroy a certain number of bacteria after they have been damaged by means of a chemical substance dissolved in the watery part of the blood. This protective action varies in different persons, and in the same person at different times, the most important disturbing factors being age, fatigue, injury, exposure to climate, and errors in eating or drinking. As long as a person keeps fit and leads a wholesome life under wholesome surroundings, this protective action is at its best ; but when the vitality of the individual is lowered or the dose of infection is excessive, then the protection is proportionately over-come. The influence of age upon liability to infection by certain diseases is well known, notably in respect of enteric fever, which prevails more among young adults than among those of maturer age. So, again, fatigue or exhaustion plays a large part in rendering men susceptible to infection, especially that of enteric fever. This has been demonstrated experimentally, and there can be no doubt that much of the excessive incidence of this disease among young soldiers on field service can be explained by their greater suscepti-bility following exhaustion, fatigue, and the general stress of cam-paigning. The same can be said of both injury and exposure to variation or change of climate. We see this constantly in the greater prevalence of enteric fever among new arrivals in India. This is not the result of chance, but the outcome of their translation from a temperate to a more or less tropical climate, whereby their physiological equilibrium is profoundly disturbed, involving a corresponding loss of their natural ability to resist infection. Among the various dietetic errors and indiscretions which sensibly lower the vitality and healthy condition of the human body, the

foremost place must be given to alcoholic excess. The number of persons who contract infection by germs following the abuse of alcohol is much larger than many suppose, and in support of this view many interesting experiments have been made on animals. Thus, the disease-resisting power of the dog and pigeon against tetanus bacteria is so great that even large injections of these germs fail to affect them ; but both the dog and the pigeon are quickly killed by tetanus if twenty hours before injecting the bacteria the animal or bird be given a dose of whisky. In the same way, certain breeds of sheep are unaffected by anthrax germs, but this power to resist infection by this disease is taken away from the sheep by giving them alcohol.

CHAPTER VI.

THE PRINCIPLES OF DISEASE PREVENTION.

40. From what has been explained concerning the nature of disease, and the manner in which the causes act, it follows that the prevention of these diseases must include (1) measures to maintain or increase the resisting powers of the individual ; and (2) measures to prevent or lessen the possibilities of disease-germs entering the body. Among the former, a prominent place must be given to protective inoculations, while among the latter measures are such matters as personal cleanliness, clean air, clean barrack-rooms, clean food, clean water, and clean and wholesome camps. Further, there must be some system by which organized sanitary effort in the army is to be carried out to secure these details.

41. Protective Inoculation.—Mention has been made of the fact that in the case of the majority of the communicable or preventable diseases infection does not occur commonly a second time, notable examples in which this is the case being enteric fever and small-pox. This being so, the question suggests itself, why should not men be given or put in the way of acquiring a mild form of disease such as these, so that future infection of a severer nature may be rendered improbable if not impossible ? In the case of smallpox the inoculation of people with the disease was practised formerly, in the hope of giving them a mild form of the infection and so preventing the occurrence of severe cases. Owing to faulty methods of inoculation, severe cases did occur, and the disease got so much out of hand that the practice of inoculation with smallpox had to be forbidden. Its place is now taken by the modern procedure of vaccination. This is really nothing but the inoculation or infecting of human beings with the germ of smallpox after it has been through the cow or calf. In other words, the cow or calf is infected with human smallpox. This does not make the animal ill ; all that follows is the appearance of some blisters and sores on the animal, which yields a juice or lymph which, if inoculated (vaccination) into man, confers on him an ability to resist infection by the human smallpox. A very similar train of events occurs in the case of diphtheria in the horse. If inoculated with diphtheria germs, the animal does not get ill, but manufactures in its blood an antidote (antitoxin) to the diphtheria germs and their poison. If the animal be bled judiciously, its blood yields a watery fluid, rich in antitoxin, which, if injected into man, exercises both a preventive and curative influence on him against the human disease. The same idea is present in the attempts to ward off infection by enteric fever by injecting the killed germs into man, causing thereby the infected person to manufacture sufficient antitoxin to enable him to resist infection by natural means. The procedure is being constantly carried out in the Army, but, unfortunately, the protection against enteric infection which it gives is not as lasting or as complete as was hoped it would be. As a matter of fact, the protection lasts only some two years ; but even so, it is something worth having, especially if it covers or tides a young soldier over a critical or dangerous period, when his powers of resistance to the disease are likely to be at their lowest and the chances of infection are likely to be at their highest.

It may be asked what is the evidence in favour of the practice so far as relates to enteric fever in the Army ? All reports indicate that the admission rates for enteric fever are much less among the inoculated as compared with the uninoculated, while also the mortality rates from the disease compare favourably for the inoculated. Taking the experiences of the last three years, during which period the greatest care has been taken to secure accuracy of facts and figures, we find that 2,969 men were inoculated in various units, while 3,897 men in the same units were not inoculated. These represent 6,866 men belonging to different corps and all exposed to the same chances of infection. Among the 2,969 inoculated there have occurred 11 cases of enteric fever with 1 death, and among the uninoculated there have occurred 128 cases with 17 deaths. This means that for each 1,000 inoculated men there have been 3·7 cases of enteric fever, and for each 1,000 of the not-inoculated there have occurred 32·8 cases of the disease. It would be difficult to find a more striking series of figures, or one more suggestive of the efficacy of the procedure ; therefore, we are justified in believing that in protective inoculation we have a powerful aid in rendering the body more resistant to possible infection by the germs of enteric fever. Advantage of being so protected should be taken by every soldier, more especially when proceeding on foreign service.

It must be admitted that our ability to prevent or ward off infection from diseases of an infective nature by means of preventive inoculations is still limited to the three diseases, smallpox, diphtheria, and enteric fever ; still the principle is right and founded on scientific facts, and, as our knowledge becomes greater, will extend. Failing, then, a complete scheme of protection against all the infective diseases by means of preventive inoculations, on what must we depend ? Obviously, on a rational and wholesome mode of life, clean air, clean food, clean water, and cleanly surroundings as attainable by a proper removal of filth and waste materials, combined with the organized control and management of the infected, and the disinfection of their infected clothing, products, and surroundings.

42. Personal Cleanliness.—This is of the highest importance and involves not only attention to the skin, but to the hair, nails, mouth, and other parts of the body. The skin is a covering for protection, and for getting rid of water in the form of sweat. This latter function is increased by exercise as well as by other causes. If sweat be allowed continually to remain and dry on the surface of the skin, or soak into the clothing, it soon becomes irritating, unhealthy, and offensive. For these reasons we wash our bodies to remove, not only coarse dirt which we can see, but also the dried

sweat which we cannot see. The act of washing further improves the skin, opens and cleans its pores and keeps it sweet and healthy. Most persons wash their hands and faces, but often forget parts covered by clothes. Of these, the following should be washed every day when possible : (1) between the legs and buttocks ; (2) the arm-pits ; (3) the feet and toes. In addition to this daily washing, a bath once or twice a week is necessary, but a bath should not be taken within two hours of a meal. After bathing or washing, the skin should be well rubbed and dried, as this prevents a chill and improves the circulation of the blood. Hands should always be washed before eating, and when washing the hands care should be taken to trim and clean the nails. It is an important and simple matter to keep the nails clean and in good order ; the finger-nails should be cut round and the toe-nails straight across. Dirty nails and fingers are a common means of conveying infection.

The hair must be kept closely cut, be brushed and combed daily, and frequently washed. Pomades and grease are, as a rule, unnecessary. The mouth should be kept scrupulously clean, and the teeth cleaned at least once, if possible twice, a day by rubbing with a brush. The best time to use the tooth-brush is before going to bed, so as to remove particles of food adhering to the teeth after the evening meal. The mouth should be washed out with water both morning and evening. Decaying or painful teeth ought to be reported to the medical officer. Often the gums are soft and inclined to bleed ; because this is the case one must not cease to clean the teeth ; to those unaccustomed to use a tooth-brush regu-larly its employment may at first cause a little inconvenience, but continued use will harden the gums.

Closely connected with the care of the skin is clean clothing. Dirt from the clothes reaches the skin, and dirt and sweat from the skin soak into the clothing. For these reasons, it is important to change and wash underclothing at least once a week. The same clothes should not be worn by day and by night ; with a little management, every man should be able to keep a shirt and pair of drawers for night wear. Socks get dirty very quickly. Every man should try and have two pairs in use, one for the morning and one for evening wear ; there should be also two pairs for the wash. Unless care be taken in attention to details of this kind, it is impossible to keep the feet hard and clean. Underclothes as well as overclothes can be cleaned by brushing, shaking, and exposing to the air and sun. This is nearly always possible, even when washing cannot be managed, as, for instance, in camp and on the line of march. An article of kit which is often neglected is the hair-brush. It should be washed every three weeks or so. Soap or hot water should not be used, but the brush rinsed in a basin of cold water to which has been added a teaspoonful of washing soda ; this will remove all dirt and grease. Dry it by shaking or swinging it round, and place it to dry in the sun or wind.

48. Clean Air.—The importance of pure, clean, and fresh air cannot be over-estimated. Air is fouled by the breath we breathe from our lungs, by the effects of artificial lights, such as candles,

lamps, and gas, by the products given off by fires and other burning material, by the breath of animals, and by dust or other dirt lying about and collected in rooms and passage ways. To correct this constant fouling of the air in rooms and other inhabited places, provision has to be made to admit a constant stream of fresh air, and to pass out the foul or dirty air. For these purposes, windows and various ventilator openings are provided, and it is important to see that some are constantly open to allow the air to circulate in and out. There is no need to open these apertures to such an extent as to cause unpleasant draughts, because, by the exercise of a little common-sense, sufficient opening can be provided to let in sufficient fresh air without creating draughts. On the other hand, for fear of causing draughts, windows and ventilators must not be kept closed or blocked with paper and rags. A window is best kept open by lowering the upper sash some three inches; this will allow the incoming air to be directed well above the heads of the occupants of a room. Where an open fire is burning in a grate, this sets up a means of ventilation by drawing foul air up the chimney. Apart from securing clean air from the outside of a room or ward, much can be done to keep the air clean and sweet by keeping the person and clothing clean, as well as by taking care to prevent dust and dirt accumulating on floors, walls, shelves, cupboards, boxes, bedding, and benches. When possible, windows should be kept open all day, and the upper sashes open at least three inches at night, all the year round. The surest test of a room being properly ventilated and its air being clean and wholesome, is furnished by its being free from smell and stuffiness to anyone entering suddenly from the outside fresh air. It must be remembered that the constant breathing of foul air lowers the vitality of the body and so favours the possibility of infection by germs.

44. Clean Barracks.—All tables, chairs, and forms should be scrubbed weekly. Dry-scrubbing of floors should be a daily, and wet-scrubbing a weekly procedure. The sanding of floors is most objectionable, as tending to cause dust and untidiness. The custom of placing blankets on a recently washed floor to save it from getting dirtied is equally pernicious. By so doing the blanket gets full of dust and filth off boots, and, unless thoroughly well shaken in the outer air, affords a ready means of conveying all kinds of germs to the mouth and nostrils of the man who uses it as part of his bedding. All bedding should be systematically turned out of the room once a week, well aired and well shaken.

45. The desirability of keeping a room specially set apart for meals is now well recognized, and, when the accommodation permits, usually adhered to. The *fouling of food* in barracks is not uncommon. This is a matter largely connected with both personal cleanliness and the provision of clean air and cleanly surroundings. The following rules should be observed : (1) No food should be stored or kept in barrack rooms or wards. If it must be kept there, it should be placed in a covered jar or other receptacle. (2) The hands and clothes of all persons who handle food or cooking utensils should be scrupulously clean. (3) All bread and meat stores should be kept clean, tidy, ventilated, and not only free from, but rendered inaccessible to flies. (4) The kitchens and all fittings, such as tables, safes, shelves, as well as cooking utensils should be clean. Cooks and their assistants must be personally clean, and wear clean, washable over-clothing. As flies carry minute portions of filth and germs on their feet, contaminating all they touch, they should not be allowed to gain access to kitchens. Flies breed only in filth, and where there are many flies it is a certain sign that there is filth and dirt in the near neighbourhood. (5) Mess-orderly men should be personally clean, and not allowed to act as·such, or in any capacity connected with the serving of food, if recently recovering from any infective disease, but more especially from enteric fever. All cooks and their assistants must be supplied with a sufficiency of clean towels for washing up. All cans, dishes, plates, mugs, knives, forks, tubs, and other utensils used at meal times or for food storage should be scoured and cleaned on a table, and not placed on the floor or taken to outside taps. Utensils of this nature should be washed in a large tin or tub reserved and marked for this and no other purpose. All cloths used in the cook-houses or sculleries must be washed daily and dried. For scouring of tea-cans, meat-dishes, knives, and forks, clean bath-brick shaken from a tin kept for the purpose alone should be used. The use of casually collected sand must be forbidden for this scouring work.

46. Closely associated with the cleanliness of barracks and the health of the occupants is the proper *disposal of refuse*, and the use and care of urinals and latrines. Kitchen refuse must invariably be placed in the special receptacles provided. As far as possible liquid refuse should be kept distinct from the dry or solid material ; but in both cases the receptacle must be kept covered in order to avoid smells and to prevent the access of flies to the contents. Its removal from barracks must be performed daily. Paper and other rubbish must be placed in the receptacles provided, and whenever possible these should be kept closed. General untidiness quickly follows any failure to attend to this detail.

47. *Latrine* accommodation in barracks is on a sufficiently liberal scale. The proper use and care of these sanitary conveniences is a matter of the first importance, as, if neglected, these places rapidly become centres for infection. In most barracks at home, water carriage of sewage is available and the type of closet of a simple nature ; in these water-closets, the flushing is done either automatically or by hand. In the newer barracks, ordinary water-closets with individual flush-tanks are provided, and it is the duty of every user of these closets not only so to seat himself that he does not unnecessarily foul the seat, but also to see that the contents of the pan are properly washed away by pulling the chain of the flushing tank. Another detail requiring attention is that of using paper torn or cut to a size not larger than that of an ordinary hand. In all well-regulated barracks suitable toilet paper is provided, but in spite of this, it is not unusual to find large sheets of newspaper thrown into the closet-pans. The very bulkiness

of these masses of paper prevents the pan being properly cleaned and facilitates rapid clogging up of the discharge pipe. For the same reason pieces of cloth, rags, boot-laces, string, and other articles of the kind must never be thrown into a closet, the proper place for these waste products is the ash-bin.

In a few places at home and in most garrisons abroad, the dry-earth closet exists; the usual arrangement being the provision of a pail or portable midden placed under apertures in a well-fitted seat, with boxes of dry earth from which, by means of a scoop, the user covers over the excreta. The pail contents must be removed daily. As in the case of water-closets, the user must take care not to foul the seat, and take special care to throw a sufficiency of the dry earth available over the filth in the pail. The object of this is to remove the smell and to prevent flies gaining access to this objectionable material.

No matter whether it be a water-closet or a dry-earth closet, all woodwork and fittings must be kept scrupulously clean. The seats must be scrubbed daily with soap and water, the scrubbing to embrace both upper and under surfaces of the seat. The pans or pails must be kept clean, and every collection of filth must be covered with either water or earth. Where earth-closets are in use the proper employment of the earth must be enforced, and an adequate supply of finely powdered dry soil and a sufficiency of scoops must always be available. The pails must be of a size to fit closely under the seat. There should be no gap or space between the top of the pail and the seat; if there is, it means certain fouling of the floor with urine or other matter. The latrine floor must be suitably sloped, and made of some hard impermeable material. A sufficiency of pails must be available, so as to allow those which have been fouled to be cleaned and sweetened. This will be best secured by first washing out the contents with water, drying and airing by exposure for a few hours to the sun if possible, and then scrubbing over the inner surface with the heavy cresol oil supplied for the purpose by the barrack department. The coating of these utensils with tar is most objectionable, as it renders them unsightly and tends to conceal rather than remove dirt. The contents of each pail must be transferred without spilling to a suitably covered water and air-tight receptacle for daily removal.

48. *Urinals* need to be managed on similar lines. The slabs of slate or glazed earthenware must be adequately flushed with water either automatically or by hand, and twice a week scrubbed over with the heavy cresol oil supplied for the purpose. This does not need to be applied in excess; just sufficient to impart a greasy surface is ample. Well-managed latrines and urinals should be devoid of smell and free from flies, even in warm weather. The presence of flies in these places is a sure sign that something is wrong. For night convenience it is not unusual to find a urine-tub placed immediately outside each barrack-room. Gradually, this objectionable feature is being obviated by the provision of fixed urinals on the stairway landings; these urinals to be used only at night and kept locked during the day. Urine-tubs, if in use, must be treated in precisely the same way as closet-pails. Their contents need to be carefully emptied each morning, with special precautions taken to see that no splashing or spilling occurs on the landings or stairways. If such does occur it should be immediately dusted over with dry earth and the place swept clean. All men engaged in the handling of urine-tubs or in the care and cleaning of urinals, closets, or latrines must remember that they are handling dangerous material capable of giving infection to either themselves or others, often both. To reduce these risks to the lowest point, men engaged on these duties should carefully wash their hands immediately on completion of the work, and certainly before they handle food. No men employed in cook-houses or as mess-orderlies should ever be allowed to have anything to do with the removal of urine-tubs or with the care and cleansing of urinals or latrines ; further, it is advisable that no men who have ever suffered from enteric fever should be employed in either the preparing or serving of food.

49. The *water supply* of permanent barracks hardly comes within the personal sphere of duty of the individual soldier. It is almost invariably of good quality and obtained from some larger scheme of supply. The problem of securing and maintaining an adequate quantity of safe water concerns the individual soldier mainly in camps or in the circumstances of campaigning. As this is essentially a question presenting peculiar difficulties it is dealt with in a separate chapter.

CHAPTER VII.

THE CONTROL OF INFECTION.

50. The occurrence of a case of infectious disease calls for prompt measures to be taken (1) to find out how and why it has occurred; (2) to safeguard or prevent its extension to others. These are essentially matters of executive by the medical corps, and the greatest importance attaches to their faithful performance.

The first step to be taken is that of isolation, segregation, or the separation of the sufferer from others not similarly attacked. In the case of soldiers this means removal to the infectious disease hospital or such other place as may conveniently lend itself for the reception of an infective disease. In the case of children or other persons resident in married quarters, a similar procedure must be adopted, unless exceptional circumstances exist which either preclude the removal of the case with safety, or permit of adequate and complete isolation. It may be accepted that this latter contingency will rarely be possible. Concurrent with these procedures it may be necessary to isolate or arrange for the segregation of others who may have been exposed to infection. The term infectious disease, as applied to the preceding requirements, includes smallpox, measles, diphtheria, scarlet fever, typhus fever, enteric fever, cholera, yellow fever, plague, and erysipelas.

The second step must be the careful collection of all clothing, bedding, and other articles which have been used or presumably infected by the infected person. These should be carefully set aside and promptly despatched for disinfection by steam.

Having taken these initial precautions, the case should be at once notified on Army Form A 35, to the principal medical officer, who will pass it to the sanitary officer. Notification of infectious disease will include the occurrence not only of those enumerated above as requiring prompt isolation, but also the following, namely, cerebro-spinal fever, Malta fever, puerperal pyæmia, puerperal septicæmia, and tuberculosis of the lungs, larynx, or intestine. In some cases it may be desirable to carry out isolation in these diseases also, but this discretion rests with the officer in medical charge of or reporting the case, on whom primarily rests the responsibility of carrying out these initial steps for the control of infection.

In cases of infectious or contagious diseases, special care must be taken to prevent children of the family affected, or those on whom suspicion may rest as having possibly been exposed to infection, from attending school until the period of incubation has elapsed. The closing of schools should only be done in times of exceptional prevalence of infectious disease. It is far better to keep the children of one or more families away from school than to close it altogether.

The segregation of contacts or possible carriers of infection is one of great importance, more especially in diseases such as scarlet fever, diphtheria, measles, and enteric fever. Where there is reason to think that such exist, their detection and separation must be secured. The detection is a matter involving usually much labour, and is eminently a service in which the utility of the specialist sanitary officer manifests itself. It is more particularly feasible in the case of diphtheria and enteric fever, these being two diseases in which the least suspected carrier is often to be found by the careful bacteriological inspection of faucal mucus in the one case and of urine and fæces in the other. The occurrence of enteric fever among soldiers should invariably be followed by an examination of the medical history sheets of all immediate comrades, and the technical examination of all who have previously suffered from the disease. In foreign garrisons, in war-time, or such occasions when batches of men arrive from, or come through infected areas, it is desirable that these new arrivals should remain apart until sufficient time has elapsed to cover the incubation period. This policy is of especial value in the case of both enteric fever and cholera, care, of course, being taken to see that the suspects use only their own latrines and other domestic or sanitary conveniences.

Complementary to these precautions is the necessity for prompt inquiry, not only of the infected person but also of his associates, as to movements, habits, and possible sources of infection having arisen through water and food, more particularly shell-fish, water-cress, lettuces, milk, and other articles eaten in an uncooked state. The evidence forthcoming is often negative, but cannot be ignored, and wherever there is reason for doubt or suspicion, all those possible sources of infection should be looked into and personally verified by either the sanitary officer or the medical officer originally reporting the case. Action on these lines must be prompt and never deferred.

51. **Disinfection.**—There remains one other procedure to be considered in detail ; it has already been referred to. Disinfection means the application of some procedure to kill or destroy actual germs of disease. The mere removal of a smell or the delaying of the growth of bacteria is not disinfection. The actual practice of disinfection is essentially a matter for the medical corps, and any failure on its part to carry out this detail efficiently renders all other efforts to control infection valueless.

Disinfection may be effected in a variety of ways, but practically we employ disinfectants for one or other of the following purposes:— (1) to disinfect the clothing and bedding used or soiled by infected persons ; (2) to disinfect the rooms or places occupied by infected persons ; (3) to disinfect discharges from infected persons.

52. *Cotton and linen goods*, such as sheets, pillow-slips, and shirts, are readily disinfected by boiling. Before despatching them to the laundry for this purpose or in cases where boiling of these articles is not practicable, they should be soaked for half an hour in a 2½ per cent. cresol solution, made by taking 1½ fluid ounces of liquor cresoli saponatus fortis and diluting to one gallon.

53. *Blankets and woollen* articles, when suspected of serious infection, should be disinfected by steam in a proper disinfecting apparatus ; but if only dirty and not under suspicion of infection,

they may be soaked in cresol solution for half an hour and then sent to the laundry.

54. *Mattresses and pillows* are frequently seriously fouled and often awkward articles to disinfect and handle. They should be thoroughly well sprayed with a solution of formaldehyde, made by diluting eight fluid ounces of formalin solution to one gallon. The spraying should be done by means of a Mackenzie spray as officially issued. The articles should be efficiently sprayed on all surfaces, then rolled up and taken to the disinfecting apparatus for disinfection by steam. When no steam-disinfector is available, mattresses and pillows should be opened up, and the stuffing as well as the covers well wetted with the formaldehyde solution. In many cases, especially in married quarters, it is desirable thoroughly to saturate the bedstead and its fittings with the same solution.

55. *Cloth goods, uniform, and ordinary suits* should be disinfected by means of steam and removed to the disinfector for that purpose. Leather goods are not to be treated by steam, they are best disinfected by spraying with the formaldehyde solution, and should then be exposed to the air and dried. When steam-disinfection is not available, suits, overcoats, and cloth goods generally may be similarly treated. Toys and small articles much handled by infected children are better burnt ; if not so destroyed, they should be sprayed with formaldehyde solution, well aired and dried. All articles which do not admit of adequate disinfection should be destroyed by fire.

56. *Steam-disinfection* has now quite superseded treatment by hot air or dry heat, as the latter procedure is slow, unreliable in its effect, and often tends to scorch the articles. To disinfect by steam a special apparatus is required. There are a variety of these available. A form in general use in the Army, more particularly in camps, is that known as Thresh's portable or field disinfector. A

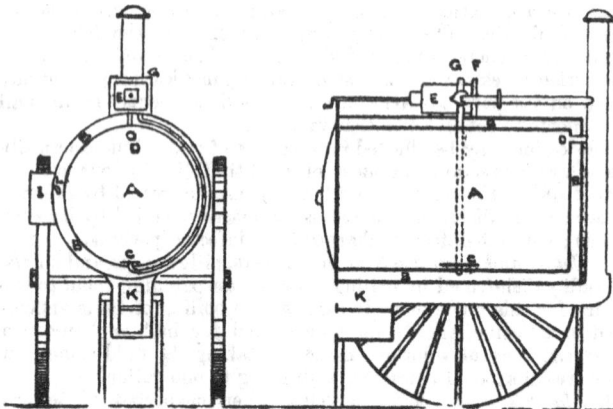

Fig. 1.—Portable Steam Disinfecting Apparatus (Thresh's).

diagram of this apparatus is shown in Fig. 1. It employs non-pressure steam derived from water, to which salt or other saline ingredients have been added in order to raise its boiling temperature to 220° or 225° F. The machine can be used equally well with ordinary water, in which case the boiling temperature will be 212° F. at sea level.

From the diagram it will be seen that the central chamber for infected articles, A, is surrounded by a jacket, B, containing the water which is heated by the furnace K. The steam given off is directed either to the chamber or to the chimney by a valve, G, and in the former case is distributed in the disinfecting chamber by a plate, C, before passing off into the chimney by a pipe D. As the water evaporates, an equivalent supply is introduced automatically from a cistern, I, with a ball-valve arrangement, and supplied by a pipe L. After the disinfecting process is over, and it should extend or cover at least half an hour, the steam is turned off from the chamber and allowed to escape into the furnace flue, and, by means of a coil of tubes, E, immersed in the water or saline solution, air, which enters at the valve, F, is heated and passing through the chamber dries the articles which have been wetted by contact with the steam. The proper drying of the articles by exposure to this heated and dry air in the chamber for a quarter of an hour constitutes a most important part of the act of disinfecting in this or any other kind of disinfecting apparatus, as, if the articles are taken out whilst still wet and damp from the steam, they will shrink and be damaged.

57. For use on field service a portable steam-disinfector has been designed at the School of Army Sanitation, Aldershot. It consists of a rectangular wooden box, 2 feet 9 inches by 2 feet 9 inches by 1 foot 6 inches. The box is zinc-lined, and between the zinc and wood is a layer of felt. A wire cage, 2 feet 6 inches by 2 feet 6 inches by 1 foot 3 inches, fits inside the box. Both the box and the cage have lift-off lids, that of the box being fixed by hinged wing-nuts, a layer of felt making the joint steam-tight. A steam inlet is provided near the bottom and is protected by a baffle on the inside. The outlet, protected by a sliding shutter, is on the opposite side. Steam is generated in a 10-gallon metal drum placed over a camp fire. An iron pipe with a push-in joint conducts the steam from the boiler and is joined on to a flexible metal pipe which carries the steam into the box. The boiler and tubing are carried inside the box during transport. The disinfector will hold four or five field service kits, and weighs 1 cwt. 60 lb.

58. In tropical countries where the sun is powerful, considerable surface disinfection of clothing and other articles can be secured by exposing them to the sun and wind.

59. *Rooms or quarters* which have been occupied by infected persons can only be disinfected after the people have left them. The aim or object is the disinfection of all exposed surfaces, as on them germs are liable to be lodged or resting. The disinfection of the air in infected rooms is effected sufficiently by opening windows and admitting fresh air and sunlight. Except in the case of places which have been occupied for some time by those suffering from smallpox,

scarlet fever, and tuberculosis of the lungs, or where three or more cases of an infectious disease have occurred in one room, it is rarely necessary to disinfect a room simply because a case of infectious disease has occurred among its occupants. The reason for this is the fact that the germs or causative agents of the majority of the infectious diseases attach themselves to the persons, bedding, clothing, and other personal articles of the infected, and not to the walls, ceilings, fittings, and floors of their rooms. In the majority of cases these latter can be rendered sanitarily safe by the exercise of free ventilation, admission of light, and scrubbing with soap and water. Where rooms are very dirty, ceilings need to be whitewashed and the walls either re-papered or colour-washed.

There are four chief means of disinfecting room surfaces : (a) Dry-rubbing the walls, etc., by means of bread or dough. This sterilizes them by mechanically removing microbes and germs of disease. The bread is cut into pieces suitable for grasping in the hand, the cut surface being applied to the ceiling, wall, etc. The crumbs must afterwards be carefully collected and burnt in the room itself. (b) Washing or scrubbing with soap and water or some ordinary disinfectant solution, as for instance the 2½ per cent. cresol solution already mentioned. This is an excellent way of dealing with floors, forms, tables, and other wooden pieces of furniture, or washable surfaces. For walls and ceilings it is somewhat laborious and best replaced by spraying. (c) Spraying the ceilings, walls, floors, and furniture with a disinfectant solution is a common and fairly convenient method of disinfecting surfaces. It is less laborious than dry-rubbing or even wet rubbing, and less likely to damage paint or wall-paper than brushing a disinfectant solution on them. But for all that, it is a slow procedure requiring much patience and time. A special spray apparatus is employed, the most effective disinfectant solution, for the purpose, being made by taking eight fluid ounces of formalin and making up to one gallon with water. This solution is effective if carefully applied ; one gallon will suffice to spray some 400 square feet of surface, and care must be taken to see that patches are not left uncovered with the solution. The spray must be applied from below upwards, this secures an even application of the disinfectant and prevents the marking of the wall by streaks. The operator will experience some discomfort from the formaldehyde vapour giving rise to smarting of the eyes, but in time this effect wears off. On completion of the spraying of all surfaces in a room, all drawers and cupboard doors should be left open and the apartment left closed for four hours, so as to allow the full effect of the vapour given off to be exercised on any germs which may be present. (d) Fumigation constitutes the remaining method of disinfecting a surface, and probably is the most easy and least troublesome mode. It can be carried out by a variety of chemical agents or gases, but that most commonly used in the army is sulphur dioxide.

When fumigation of a room has to be carried out, the measurements or size in cubic feet of the room must be taken. Next, all crevices, cracks, apertures, and holes, not forgetting the throat of the fire-place chimney must be carefully closed by pasting over with paper to prevent air or gas escaping. If this is not done the act of fumigation is more or less useless.

Sulphur dioxide can be generated by burning 3 lb. of sulphur in a metal dish or dishes for every thousand cubic feet of space in the room. The sulphur must be broken up and placed in a saucepan or other metal vessel, supported over a bucket of water, and its ignition aided by pouring some methylated spirit over the sulphur and then setting it alight. It is advisable to have a sufficiency of metal containers, so as to cause not more than one pound of the sulphur being burnt in any one dish. These vessels containing the sulphur should be evenly distributed over the room, and not all concentrated in the centre or any one part of the apartment. The same effect is secured by discharging the contents of specially prepared cylinders containing liquefied sulphurous acid gas : one 20-oz. cylinder of this compressed gas is sufficient for a space of a thousand cubic feet. The room must be left carefully closed and kept so for quite three hours. In using the cylinders of gas, the same care must be taken to distribute them equally through the room, as has been explained when using ordinary roll sulphur. Sulphur dioxide or sulphurous acid gas is not very reliable as a disinfectant ; it has a low penetrating power and is more or less non-effective in very dry weather.

The disinfection of a room by means of spraying the walls with diluted formalin, or by fumigation with sulphur dioxide will be carried out only when specially ordered. The usual procedure to be adopted when a case of infectious disease occurs in a barrack-room, after removal of the case to hospital, is to remove all the man's bedding and clothing and disinfect them by means of steam ; on this being done, the floor under the man's bed for a distance of six feet all round the bed, the bedstead, chair, locker, or other article of furniture used by the infected person will be scrubbed with a 2½ per cent. solution of cresol. In married quarters, the same procedure will be adopted after a case of infectious disease, but in addition, the whole floor and all wood-work and wooden furniture in the room will be scrubbed with cresol solution. Carpets, curtains, and other draperies will be sprayed with the formaldehyde solution, removed into the outer air, dried, dusted, and shaken before being taken back into the room. If these procedures be carefully and intelligently carried out, it will be rarely necessary to limewash or distemper walls or ceilings, or to strip and renew wall-papers of rooms after the occurrence of an infectious disease.

60. The *treatment of discharges from patients* is an important point in the control or management of infection. The stools or motions should be received into a bed-pan containing a 5 per cent. solution of carbolic acid, or a 2½ per cent. solution of cresol, or a 2 per cent. solution of either cyllin, izal, or kerol. The urine and vomit, if any, must be treated in exactly the same way, taking care that an amount of the disinfectant solution, equal in bulk to that of the material to be disinfected, be added. In the case of motions or stools, this may be taken to be quite eight fluid ounces, and this same volume of disinfectant solution must be added and mixed with the

excreta by means of a piece of stick. To urine and vomit, at least four ounces of the above solutions should be added each time, and well mixed. The urine from enteric fever patients should always be carefully disinfected. In circumstances when none of the disinfectant solutions are available, efficient disinfection of excreta or other discharges from the sick can be attained by pouring on to and well mixing with them plain boiling water. Hot water will not do, it must be boiling water.

61. *Discharges from the throat, nose, and mouth* of patients should be received into any one of the above-named disinfectant solutions. Pocket-handkerchiefs should be avoided if possible, using linen rags instead, which should be placed at once in one of the above solutions, or burnt.

62. The *skin* may scatter infection, especially in smallpox, chicken-pox, and scarlet fever. Frequent baths and smearing over with vaseline or oil are useful.

63. The *disinfection of hands* is most important for all attendants on the infectious sick. The simplest means of securing this is the free use of the nail-brush with soap and hot water. In special cases, the hands may be cleansed in any of the above-mentioned disinfectant solutions, or in a 1 in 1,000 solution of perchloride of mercury (corrosive sublimate). This is made by dissolving half an ounce of the perchloride in three gallons of water, adding one ounce of strong hydrochloric acid. It is best to colour this solution with either a little aniline blue or fuchsin ; the colouring is added to avoid accidental poisoning and to serve as a warning.

CHAPTER VIII.

WATER SUPPLIES.

64. In the army, this question presents certain special features, but, in respect of general principles, it differs little from the corresponding problem in civil life. In both communities the supply of wholesome water in sufficient quantity is a fundamental sanitary necessity. Without water, injury to health follows invariably either simply from deficiency of quantity, or more frequently from the presence of impurities.

65. Amount of water required.—In estimating the amount of water required daily for each person, it is necessary to allow a liberal quantity. There must be avoidance of waste, but still any error in supply had far better be on the side of excess. In civil communities the daily allowance per head of the population varies immensely, but includes water for municipal and trade purposes. The average daily allowance per head in civil life is 30 gallons ; in the Army, 20 gallons per day are allowed for each adult, and 10 gallons for every child. In addition, 20 gallons are allowed daily for each horse during peace. These figures make the official allowance of water approximate for all purposes to the corresponding issue in civil life. For soldiers living in camps, these figures need to be modified considerably. Under circumstances of stress, one gallon per head daily might suffice ; including animals, the lowest allowance may be put at three gallons per head each day. As a general statement, a daily allowance of five gallons per man may be taken as the usual water requirement in camp, with at least as much again for each horse or camel. Apart from the difficulties experienced in supplying more, it is desirable not to exceed this amount in camps, as any excess means waste, with corresponding difficulties in surface drainage.

66. Sources of water supply.—All our water supplies are derived in the first instance from rain, which, falling from the clouds, reaches the earth and there either lodges and lies on the surface or soaks and sinks into the ground according to the nature and arrangement of the soil. The water which lodges on the surface or top of the earth is familiar to us in the form of puddles, ponds, pools, lakes, ditches, and rivers. The water which soaks and sinks into the earth is the underground water, which we gain access to either by means of springs or wells. For these reasons, we may speak of the chief sources of water supply as being :—(1) rain ; (2) surface waters from hills, or high lands, and that lying on the top of the earth in ponds, pools, lakes, ditches, and rivers; (3) the underground waters cropping up to us as springs or that obtained by means of borings, shafts, or wells. Each of these supplies may yield either clean or unclean water, according to the nature of the circumstances.

67. *Rainwater* approaches nearer to absolute purity than any other kind of natural water. When collected in clean vessels it contains only such dissolved substances as it can take up from the air. As it falls through the air, it becomes highly aerated, but in inland districts the amount of impurities which rain washes out of the air is often considerable. It is, however, mainly from the surfaces on which rain falls that the chief impurities result. These consist generally of bird droppings, decayed leaves, soot, and such matters as collect on roofs, platforms, in gutters and receiving vessels. For these reasons, rain water, as ordinarily collected, is an impure and dirty water, and its use as a supply for drinking purposes is only justified in places where no better source is available. The chief merit of rain-water is its softness, owing to the absence of salts of lime and magnesia. On this account it is good for washing or cooking purposes, although this very attribute of softness renders it less palatable than other kinds of water for drinking. Owing to its richness in dissolved air, rain-water has frequently a considerable action on lead. This is a feature of some importance in connection with pipes, fittings, and cisterns or tanks to be used for its storage.

Apart from these drawbacks, rain as a general source of water supply is unsatisfactory, owing to the uncertainty of the rainfall, the length of the dry season in many countries, and the large size of the reservoirs which are then required.

The amount of water given by rain can be calculated easily if two facts are known; namely, the amount of rainfall and the area of the receiving surface. The rainfall can only be determined by a rain-gauge, the area of the receiving surface must be measured. A fall of one inch of rain delivers 4·6 gallons on every square yard or 22,617 gallons on each acre. All of this will not be available ; some will sink into the ground, and some will evaporate. The quantity lost in this way will vary with the soil and the season.

The utility of ice and snow water is very limited ; moreover, its use is not free from danger, especially in the case of ice derived from polluted water. The mere act of freezing has a feeble effect in destroying bacteria, and on this account because water has been frozen it cannot necessarily be deemed safe. In its general qualities, water derived from dew or melted snow may be regarded as similar to ordinary rain.

68. *Surface water* running off uplands or hills may be clean or dirty, according to the nature of the land or country over which it flows. Such water, running off hills over which neither man nor animal goes, will naturally be cleaner than similar water flowing over manured land or over country which men and animals frequent. The same must be said of other surface waters in pools, lakes, ditches, and streams or rivers. Sometimes this water will be clean sometimes not, according to the nature of the banks and neighbouring country, and according to what opportunities exist for the filth of man and animals to gain access to it. As a rule, it may be assumed that water obtained from these sources is unclean. There are, of course, exceptions, and each case must be judged on its merits, as disclosed by a scrutiny of local conditions. Many communities obtain safe water from upland surface supplies. But the gathering grounds are usually well safeguarded from casual

pollution by adequate patrolling. Rivers are fed from such a variety of sources that the quality of the water they yield is extremely variable. A stream running through a sparsely occupied district will obviously be cleaner than one passing through a more densely populated area. Equally, facts as to local methods of sewage disposal will materially affect the opinion to be formed as to the probable quality of water yielded by a pool, pond, stream, or river. The rule should be : *regard all surface waters with suspicion.*

69. *Underground water* is the vast volume of water which exists at varying depths below the earth's surface, representing the water which, having fallen as rain, has soaked through the soil layers. The amount of, and facility of access to, water underground varies with the configuration and density of the earth's crust. In some places this water may be abundant at a depth of only a few feet, while elsewhere it may be scanty or only obtainable at considerable depths. Man gains access to this ground water either by springs or wells.

70. *Springs* are natural out-crops or overflows of the underground water. The rain which falls on a permeable soil percolates downward until it is arrested by a bed of clay or other impermeable stratum, and there becomes stored underground until it rises to a point of level at which it can appear spontaneously at the surface. Springs are found commonly on the side or foot of a hill, in valleys, and near the beds of rivers. The water obtained from springs is usually good, though often hard and loaded with mineral salts such as lime, which have been dissolved out of the soil. Spring water is clear and bright, in consequence of the great degree of filtration which it naturally undergoes, in percolating through the soil layers, between the gathering ground and the point from which it issues again from the earth. Spring water is both pure and impure in different cases, and the mere fact of water being derived from a spring is not necessarily a guarantee of its goodness, though in the majority of cases it may be regarded as safe.

The yield of a spring is determined most readily by receiving the water into a vessel of known capacity and timing the rate of filling. The spring should have been opened up previously, and the receptacle employed should be of large size. In cases where a spring yields a steady but small volume of water, an increased supply may be frequently obtained by digging out the spring head. The chief risk attaching to springs is the facility of pollution of the issuing water by surface washing ; hence, when used for any length of time, a spring should be enclosed, its level raised, and the ground made to slope away from rather than towards it. If this is impracticable, the vicinity should be so ditched that all surface drainage from higher ground is intercepted and conducted to a point below the level of the spring.

71. *Wells* may be divided into two classes, shallow and deep ; in both cases they represent shafts or borings sunk by man to tap or gain access to the underground water. Shallow wells draw their water supply from the subsoil, while deep wells tap the water-bearing layer beneath some impervious soil stratum which separates it from

the subsoil above. By far the larger number of wells met with belong to the first class. Shallow wells may yield good water provided there is no risk of pollution from surface washings or from their proximity to cesspools or leaky drains. In or near towns, villages, or farmyards this pollution is very liable to occur, so much so that the water from shallow wells, say from ten to fifty feet deep, is always to be regarded with suspicion. The distance drained by wells is undetermined, the area varying with the nature and porosity of the soil, but in the majority of cases the radius of the area drained is equal to four times the depth, at least, and may even exceed this. A porous soil, with no impervious superficial stratum, will admit of impurities reaching a well from the surface which a clay soil would shut off. The movement and course of the ground-water being in the direction of the nearest watercourse or the sea, to protect the water-supply from any soakage from leaky drains or cesspools in the vicinity, a well should be placed above all such possible sources of contamination. A well which yields a moderate quantity of good water may, if the demand on it be increased, draw in water from the surrounding parts, and thus tap sources of impurity which a moderate demand left untouched. A sudden rise in the ground-water, as after heavy rain, may lead to direct communication between a cesspool and a well, by the water tapping the former in its flow.

In some cases a well at a lower level may receive the drainage of surrounding hills flowing down to it from great distances. Good coping stones, so as to protect from surface washings, and good masonry for several feet below the surface of wells in very loose soils, so as to prevent superficial soakage, are necessary in all shallow wells. In the majority of cases where shallow wells yield polluted water, this is due to defects in their construction. The growth of trees should not be encouraged in the vicinity of wells, as their roots are apt to cause facilities for the inlet of surface water. For similar reasons, moles and rats should be prevented from burrowing near wells.

Deep wells, artesian and tube wells, are generally of great depth, passing through an impermeable stratum, such as clay or rock, and penetrating a water-bearing soil which crops up elsewhere at some higher point, and below which again is another impermeable stratum. From the nature of these facts, it is easy to understand that the water from those deep wells or borings is nearly always good. Like the shallow wells, these must be adequately protected at the surface to avoid pollution at that point.

72. *Distilled water* needs a short reference, as distillation is one of the most effectual modes of freeing water from impurities. On board ships, distillation of sea water is resorted to in order to render salt water fit for drinking ; and although the water thus obtained is pure, yet, all the gases having been driven from it by the boiling, it is unpalatable, and by some supposed to be indigestible. Distilled water may be aerated by allowing it to trickle slowly down through a long column of wood-charcoal, or by filtration through some porous substance. In all distillation apparatus, care needs to be taken that the distilled water is not left in contact with lead, zinc, or copper fittings, as the water has a curious ability to dissolve and attack these metals.

73. Comparative qualities of water supplies.—This depends on many circumstances. Rain-water, if properly collected and stored, affords an excellent supply when other sources are not available, especially in country or sparsely populated areas. The uncertainty of the supply often necessitates a considerable storage capacity ; this is not very desirable. Rain-water should be clarified or filtered to remove suspended matters before being stored, and the tanks protected from surface or other workings, also from light and heat. Spring-water is usually good, but there are cases in which a spring may yield a bad water. Much depends upon the geological formation and how well the spring is protected from surface pollution. When springs arise from sand or gravel the immediate neighbourhood needs careful scrutiny ; as a rule, from two to five acres above and around a spring should be free from all manurial matter, and that portion of the area immediately affecting the spring should be enclosed to prevent access of men and animals. If heavy rainfall renders a spring-water turbid, it is highly suggestive that the source is unsatisfactory. Shallow well water is always to be viewed with suspicion ; the same must be said of most river water, as a river is the natural point to which the drainage of a good deal of surrounding land tends, and heavy rains will often wash many substances into it. Apart from this, few rivers are free from the discharge into them of much objectionable matter, if not actual sewage. Upland surface-waters are, as a rule, safe, but much depends upon the presence or absence of houses, flocks, or herds of animals, and adequate policing of the collecting area.

74. Storage and Delivery.—The methods of storing and delivering water will vary with its source. In upland surface schemes, storage reservoirs are a necessity to equalize the supply and demand ; in all cases these collections of water are best left uncovered, but suitably protected from the access of men and animals. They need periodical cleaning.

When water is obtained from a river, the intake should be placed where a good stream is constantly flowing ; stagnant and shallow parts should be avoided. The water is best taken some three feet below the surface. If storage is required, reservoirs will need to be constructed. River water undergoes notable improvement during storage in large reservoirs, and all experience shows that the larger the storage reservoirs and the longer the water can be retained in them, the greater is the self-purification obtained.

Occasionally, rain-water collected from the roofs of buildings is the only available source of supply. The storage of this water is of importance, but it needs care, as it has an erosive and solvent action on lead. For this reason rain-water storage tanks are best made of slate or galvanized iron. The tanks must be well protected by covers, ventilated, and periodically cleaned out.

In all water schemes, the water must, if possible, be conducted

D

in pipes from the reservoirs or other sources of supply to barracks. In camps, this is equally desirable, but not always possible. Distribution by hand or by open channels is crude and objectionable, for it is impossible to guard altogether from casual contamination. If hand-carriage is unavoidable it should be done only by means of tanks on wheels, provided with covers which should be kept closed down. These movable tanks need periodical cleaning just the same as fixed tanks. The best way of cleaning tanks is to fill them with water, add sufficient permanganate of potash crystals to make the water a blood-red colour, allow it to stand for six hours, and then empty. In barracks, cisterns are often provided; these must be kept covered, ventilated, and periodically cleaned. Each such cistern must have an overflow pipe, discharging into the open air and well away from all drain gullies. A cistern supplying a water-closet should not be used to supply cooking and drinking water, as the pipes leading to the closet often conduct closet air to the cistern. Hence a small cistern should be used for the flushing requirements of each closet.

75. Impurities in water.—The impurities which gain access to water and so render it unclean are various. Some reach the water at its source, some during its storage, and some during its distribution. No matter how or where these impurities reach water, they exist practically in two states or conditions; they are either dissolved in the water, that is they are in solution, or they are merely floating in the water, that is are in suspension. Experience has taught us that the various substances which are dissolved in ordinary waters are not, as a rule, hurtful; it is otherwise, however, with the suspended matter in waters. This suspended material is the true impurity in most waters, and may be in the form of fine sand, clay, grit, or mud, that is, suspended matter which we can see with our unaided eyes; or it may be germs and similar living substances which, although floating and suspended in the water, are so small that they are not to be seen by the naked eye. In other words, an absolutely clear and crystal-like water may be full of harmful germs and most hurtful to anyone drinking it. As a matter of fact, the visible and invisible suspended impurities in water are usually associated, and it is rare to find one without the other; but it is important to remember that it may be otherwise. It is, then, the suspended impurities in water which we have to fear as giving rise to disease. How the minute and invisible germs do so has been explained. The coarser suspended matter in the form of sand and grit is only a degree less harmful; if this matter be taken into the body, it acts as an irritant to the lining membrane of the bowel, irritates and renders it inflamed; of itself, perhaps, this will not cause actual disease, but as this material is usually associated with harmful germs, the damage done to the bowel surface favours their penetration and entry into the blood and consequent ability to give rise to infection. In this manner, coarse dirt and mud, though not itself causing infection, sets up conditions in the body favouring infection by germs in the water.

76. Effects of drinking impure water.—The diseases which are associated with the use of impure water are cholera, enteric fever, dysentery, diarrhœa, parasitic intestinal worms, and some obscure forms of metallic poisoning. The virulence of a water-borne disease has some definite relation to the original purity of the supply, for, once seeded with the specific germs, a dirty water appears to act more virulently than one that was originally clean. From our knowledge of the history of infective micro-organisms, it would appear doubtful whether they survive in good water for any lengthened period. Laboratory experiments show that from 14 to 40 days has been the maximum period of their vitality, and probably under less favourable conditions a much shorter period would complete their life.

The intimate association of both cholera and enteric fever with foul water is beyond dispute. In both diseases, the specific germs gain access to the water by the discharges of those suffering from these diseases being allowed to enter defective drains, etc., the contents of which infect the subsoil water or are carried direct into rivers or streams from which drinking water is taken. That dysentery is caused by the drinking of impure water there is ample evidence; in nearly every instance the water was polluted with fæcal or dysenteric discharges, and where the supply was discontinued the disease disappeared. It may also be said that diarrhœa among soldiers has frequently been caused by the fine or gross suspended mineral matters in water. These act as mechanical irritants to the bowel, and a bowel so damaged is consequently placed in an eminently receptive state for infection by various virulent germs, should they be swallowed subsequently. The ova or eggs of various parasitic intestinal worms are frequently found in water, particularly in the tropics ; their presence and ingestion by man constitutes one of the channels of this kind of infection. Metallic poisoning may result from the absorption by water of the metal used in the making of service pipes, cisterns, etc. The water may also be contaminated at its source by passing through a soil in which a metal is present, as in some mining districts. Copper, lead, zinc, and arsenic are the most probable poisonous metals which may gain access to water in this way. As affecting the daily life of the soldier this is not a practical question.

CHAPTER IX.

PURIFICATION OF WATER.

77. If it is realized what are the impurities likely to be met with in water, the principles on which and the practice by which they are to be removed will be readily understood. It may be accepted that we need not trouble about what is in solution, but aim simply to remove or render harmless that which is really suspended in water. This may be either coarse mineral grit, sand and mud, which is more or less obvious to the naked eye, or it may be germs and similar living bodies, which although floating and suspended in water, are so small that they are not to be seen by the unaided eye. A variety of procedures have been suggested and used for these purposes, and their applicability depends much upon whether it is intended to purify water in bulk or large volumes or whether the act of purification is to be applied to small quantities only. In civil life it is the exception rather than the rule for water to be purified in small quantities by the consumer, owing to the fact that water is nearly always submitted to some process of purification by the companies before distribution to the public. In military life, it is rare to find any organized attempt made to purify water in bulk, but if it is of indifferent quality the act of purification is applied to relatively small quantities only. As suitable for the various conditions of army life, there are four main methods by which we can purify water, namely clarification, filtration, sterilization by heat, and sterilization by chemicals. Each of these methods has its advantages and disadvantages, and may be employed separately or in combination.

78. Clarification.—This is the simplest and often the readiest method which can be applied for rendering a dirty water reasonably safe. Clarification or coarse straining of water removes only the mud and grosser impurities, and unless very specially conducted fails to remove the smaller suspended particles such as germs. In spite of this limitation, clarification is a procedure always worth doing; far better to do this much than do nothing at all, while as a preliminary procedure it has the greatest value.

The simplest way of accomplishing clarification is to pass the water through blanket or canvas sacking or canvas stretched on an improvised wooden frame, dusting over the fabric ordinary wood ashes from a camp fire. The strained water is received in any suitable receptacle placed beneath. If the water is not sufficiently cleaned it may be passed again through the strainer or through another one conveniently placed. The straining power of devices of this nature can be much increased if alum be added to the water before being poured on to the fabric. The alum forms gelatinous particles in the water and on the straining surface which entangle and hold back the suspended matter. An alternative device may well take the form of a canvas cone attached to a metal ring, having cords by which it can be hung from a tree branch. Such an improvised strainer can be used with or without wood-ashes or alum, and provided too much hurry is not exercised or the water not made to pass through too rapidly, it can and will remove not only coarse mud but a great portion of the associated germs ; by this means often an otherwise undrinkable water can be rendered reasonably safe. Many occasions on field service afford opportunities for the exercise of iniative on those lines, which can and should be turned to good account by the soldier.

79. Another simple way of securing quick clarification, especially of river water, consists in digging a pit near the proposed source of supply, so that the water may percolate through the soil before being used ; the arrangement will work better if time be allowed for the water to settle, and, when water is withdrawn, care must be taken not to stir up the mud.

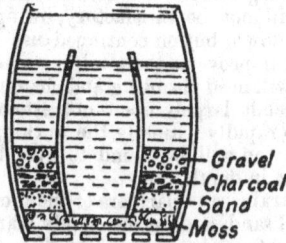

Fig. 2.   Improvised Barrel-filter.

80. If two barrels of unequal size be available, one may be placed inside the other and the interspace filled with clean sand or wood-ashes. The outer barrel bottom is pierced with small holes, and the inner barrel similarly pierced round its upper rim. If the whole be partially submerged in the water to be cleared, an excellent supply of clean water can be obtained by suction from the inner barrel (Fig. 2). When the supply is smaller, this method may be reversed, the space between the barrels being partially filled with clarifying material and the bottom of the inner barrel either removed or better

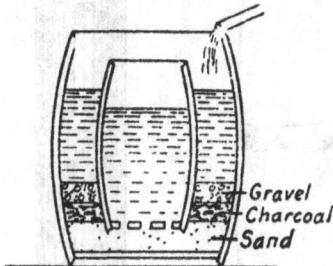

Fig. 3.   Improvised Barrel-filter.

still perforated with holes. If water be poured into the outer barrel on to the straining material it will percolate down through this and rise to its proper level in the inner barrel, whence it can be withdrawn (Fig. 3). Care must be taken to ram the straining material down, and to fix the inner barrel firmly in and hold it there till the weight of water within it is sufficient to keep it in position.

81. An effective strainer may be improvised by boring a small hole in the bottom of a barrel or other suitable receptacle, and partially filling the latter with layers of gravel, fine sand, and wood-ashes from below upwards. The gravel should be three inches in depth and the sand some twelve to fifteen inches deep, with some three inches of wood-ashes on the top. These thicknesses can be increased if the receptacle is large enough. The water to be clarified is poured in at the top, passes down through these layers, and is collected as it emerges from the hole in the bottom. On first using, the water will not be satisfactory, owing to the materials not having settled down, but on continued use the quality of the strained water will improve as the straining mass ripens. Periodically, the material will need cleansing and changing. The success of these methods depends largely upon not attempting to pass the water through too rapidly; usually the working head or layer of dirty water on the top will be found to give best results if not exceeding six inches in depth.

In improvising strainers or clarifiers of the above types, care must be taken to get real sand, and not use sandy marl in which there is much clay. This latter, when wetted, binds and forms so dense a mass that percolation of water is slow and often absent. It must further be remembered that all improvisations of the kind are mere makeshifts and, unless the material be periodically renewed and the water not allowed to rush through too quickly, may be a source of danger. The addition of a small amount of alum is an advantage, since it produces a jelly-like precipitate which helps in arresting and entangling the more minute particles held in suspension.

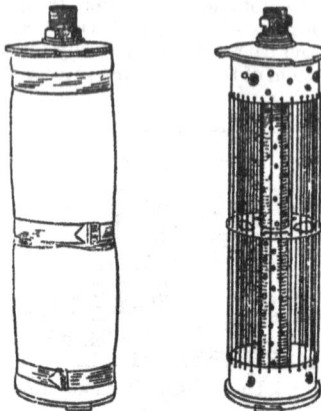

FIG. 4. CAGE AND FLANNELETTE STRAINER.

82. A more elaborate arrangement, and one well suited for fixed posts or camps, is that of making a stout wire cage (Fig. 4) and rolling round it the best and stoutest flannelette which can be obtained, and securing this firmly by means of broad tapes. The flannelette should be applied not less than four folds thick round the wire drum or cage. This strainer has a central axis or perforated tube closed at one end, but discharging through the other end-plate of the drum or cage-strainer. The whole needs to be enclosed in a properly fitting case or container. One end of this container has a central hole with piping attached, while the other end has a removable plate or lid capable of being securely clamped and rendered water-tight by means of hinged or detachable wing-nuts. In the centre of this detachable lid is a hole through which issues the outlet tube of the strainer when placed in position. This joint must be provided with a rubber washer and made water-tight by a proper screw union. The hosing or pipe from the other end of the casing is coupled up with a tap or other convenient exit in the lower part of a barrel or tank mounted on a wooden platform at a suitable height (Fig. 5).

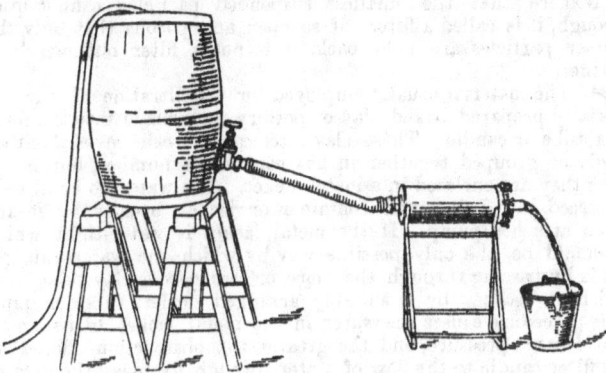

FIG. 5. BARREL AND STRAINER CONNECTED UP.

If this receptacle be filled with water, this flows by gravity along the pipe to the interior of the metal container from which it can escape only by passing through the flannelette strainer and thence out by the central outlet tube. The delivery of clear water by this arrangement varies naturally with its degree of muddiness and what head or drop is given to the water running from the barrel or tank to the strainer. For general efficiency the head or pressure should not exceed four feet. Excellent results have been obtained by this method, and if the water in the tank be dosed with alum or hydrogel, the quality of the strained water is very high. Practically, 99 per cent. of contained bacteria can be removed from dirty water by this method. When using a muddy water, the delivery falls off considerably, owing to the deposition of the suspended matter on the flannelette which gets clogged. Using a strainer of this kind, measuring 20 inches in length and 5 inches in diameter, and with a fall or head of three feet, the output varies from 200 to 300 gallons an hour, according to the original degree of muddiness of the water. When clogged up, as shown by the lessened outflow, the flannelette only needs washing and boiling, or to be replaced by fresh layers. The intelligent application of this system of water clarification affords a valuable means of purifying water when other and more elaborate procedures are not possible. It is specially suitable for camps or fixed posts. In place of flannelette, felt, blanketing, canvas, or other fabrics may be employed.

83. **Filtration** is really an exaggerated system of straining or clarifying, and aims at purifying water by catching or holding back the smallest particles of suspended matter, including germs, and allowing to pass whatever is in a state of solution or dissolved in the water. Ordinary clarification fails to remove the germs or very small suspended particles. The difference between filtration and clarification is merely a question of the size of the apertures in the straining material. When the material is so dense and close in texture that the smallest suspended particles cannot pass through, it is called a filter ; if so open and porous that only the coarser particles are held back, it is not a filter but merely a clarifier.

84. The material usually employed for the filtration of water is specially prepared baked clay or pottery ware made into the form of a tube or candle. These clay filter-candles can be used either singly or grouped together in any convenient number, but in all cases they are enclosed in a metal jacket. The water to be filtered is forced into this metal container or jacket, usually by means of an attached pump. If the metal jacket is water-tight, which it should be, the only possible way by which the water can get out is by passing through the more or less porous clay tube, from which it escapes by a suitably arranged outlet, tube, or pipe. This procedure causes the water in the metal jacket to be under considerable pressure, and the greater the obstruction offered by the filter-candle to the flow of water through its mass, the greater will be the pressure under which the water is forced through the filter. The average pressure developed in this attempt to force water through filters of this nature varies from 40 to 50 lb on the square inch. The result of this forced passage of the water through the tube is that all suspended matter is left on the surface of the filter-candle, and, if this candle be sound and free from flaws or cracks, the water which passes through is quite sterile and free from germs.

It will be obvious that the success of this method of filtration depends absolutely upon the freedom of the filter-candle from flaws or cracks. The weakest point in all these candles is the line of junction between the clay and the metal ends. Mere inspection will not detect any but large cracks or fissures. For the routine examination of filter-candles, it suffices first carefully to damp the surface of the clay with a little water, then carefully to close the open end of the candle by pressing the finger over the aperture and then gently hold the candle at a depth of an inch under clean water taking care all the time to keep the open end closed by pressure of the finger. Air will be imprisoned inside the filter-candle as the result of closing its aperture, and its only possible means of escape will be through the porous clay or by a hole or crack. While immersed under water, any escaping air will be manifest as air-bubbles arising to the surface. If the candle is quite sound, the escaping air will be apparent only as minute air bubbles issuing evenly from the whole surface of the candle. There will be no large bubbles. If there are large air-bubbles rising from any point, it indicates some flaw, crack, or weak point. If this be observed, the candle must be rejected as unsound ; if, on the other hand, the air issues evenly and only as very tiny bubbles then it may be presumed to be good and sound. The examination can be conducted in a similar way by connecting the aperture with an ordinary bicycle pump by means of some rubber tubing, and then, after laying the candle under water, forcing gently some air into its interior cavity. It is not a fair or reliable test to force the air in vigorously ; a gentle pressure or working of the pump suffices.

The action of the filters being merely to hold back the suspended matter in water which is collected on their surface, it follows that a gradual clogging of their pores, with a corresponding lessened flow of water through them, results. When the output becomes diminished the filter-candle needs cleaning by brushing the surface under water. This process in course of time weakens the filter by removing some of its substance, but with care the life of an individual tube can be made to extend over a couple of years. A more serious risk attaching to the routine use of filters of this kind lies in the fact that in the course of time germs, if present in the water under filtration, are capable of working their way into the pores of the medium, and even through its mass, so as to appear in the filtered water. In their passage through the actual filter they are helped by the pressure under which the water is forced through. The result of this is that filter-candles, if used for the filtration of dirty water, frequently become a seriously infected mass, and a possible means of polluting an uninfected water passing through them, consequently we must for safety's sake sterilize these candles every fourth day by boiling them in water for one minute. This is the regular practice in the army and must be rigidly carried out.

85. Excellent as these clay or pottery ware filters are for removing germs and other minute suspended matter, their employment is often difficult when very muddy water has to be filtered, owing to the mud, fine sand, or clay collecting on the filter surface and clogging up its pores so much that the water cannot get through. To avoid this and the consequent repeated brushings and cleanings, it is usual to submit the water to a preliminary clarification before it reaches the filter-candle.

Designed on these principles there is a filter-tank now in general use ; its weight when empty is 13 cwt., when full of water it weighs 23 cwt. It delivers 200 gallons of water per hour. It consists of an iron tank, holding 110 gallons mounted on two wheels. It is fitted with two pumps, two clarifying chambers and, for sterilizing purposes, eight filter-candles arranged in two batteries of four each. The filter-candles are of a standard size and make. Behind the main tank is a small seven-gallon tank which receives the sterilized water from the filters, and fitted to this are taps by which water can be drawn off and water-bottles filled. A locker is placed on the top of the fore-part of the main tank for carrying spare parts. A kettle is attached for boiling and sterilizing the filter-candles ; it can take four of the candles at once and when filled with water, the whole contents can be readily boiled over a camp fire. Two lengths of hose-pipe for connecting the pumps with the source of supply are carried coiled round hooks on the top of the large tank.

The main tank carries water which can be freed from coarse suspended matter by first passing it through the clarifying chambers. The clarifying chambers are placed horizontally on either side of the top of the hinder part of the large tank. Sponges have been placed in the clarifying chamber ; they are not very effective in removing suspended material, moreover they rapidly rot and wear away. It is preferable to employ flannelette wrapped on a cylindrical frame, which is fitted into the clarifying chamber. When the water is treated with a small quantity of alum, a very efficient filtering layer rapidly forms on the surface of the flannelette. The alum required is placed in a small box fitted in one end of the clarifying chamber, and is dissolved by the water in its passage to the flannelette cylinder. Water can be sterilized as required by pumping it through the filter candles. The eight filter-candles are in two sets of four, placed in separate chambers, fitted vertically inside the back part of the tank. Each filter-candle is covered with an asbestos cloth in order to lessen clogging of the tube. The clarified water from the main tank is pumped through the sterilizing candles. Each set or battery of candles with its associated clarifying chamber and pump is independent of the other, so that either half of the cart or tank can be worked regardless of the other. Each filter-candle has its own delivery tube or "swan-neck" as it is called, which discharges separately into the small storage tank behind. The multiplicity of these discharging tubes gives the appearance of complexity but it has the advantage of showing how each individual filter-candle is working. (Fig. 6.)

A store of sterilized water is not intended to be carried, and is limited to the capacity of the seven-gallon tank behind. The reason for this is that the water can be filtered as fast as it can be distributed, and the possibility of this safe water becoming contaminated during storage is reduced to a minimum. Both tanks should be kept closed by fastening their lids, and each is accessible for cleansing. The main tank can be filled with clarified water, using both pumps, in half an hour. It can be emptied through the filter-candles in about the same time. Each pump serves one clarifying chamber and one filtering chamber on its own side.

In working this filter-tank, the water may be pumped in one of three ways, namely, (a) through the clarifying chamber D, direct from the pond or stream into the main tank A, or (b) direct

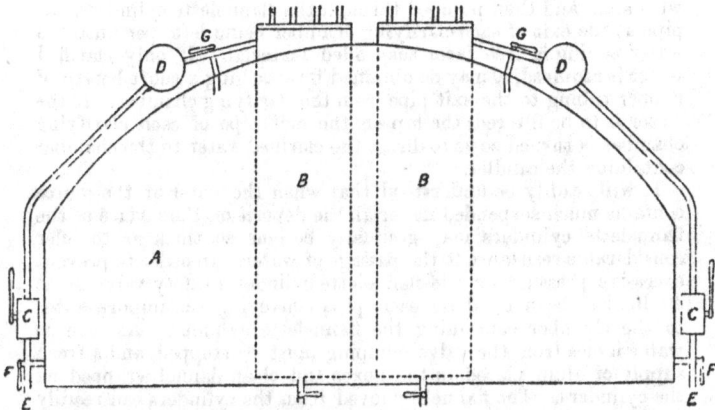

Fig. 6. Section of Filter-tank.

from the pond or stream through the clarifying chamber D and filter chamber B, or (c) from the main tank A through the clarifying chamber D and filter chamber B. In the two latter cases, the water is filtered and passes through into the small storage tank, while in the first case, the water is not filtered but merely clarified and passed into the main tank.

When a water containing much suspended material has to be dealt with, it is advisable to place the required amount of alum in the boxes contained in the clarifying chambers and then pump the water from the source through the boxes and flannelette cylinders. A tube at the exit from each clarifying chamber is left open until the water issuing is free from suspended material. A tap at the exit from each clarifying chamber is then turned so as to direct the clarified water into the body of the cart. Water for washing and cooking can be obtained by means of a pipe passing from the bottom of the tank to the rear of the cart. Water for drinking purposes requires to be filtered by passage through the filter-candles; accordingly the taps are turned so that by working the pump clarified water is taken from the tank and forced through the candles. Filtered water issues from the swan-necks and can be used at once or stored in the 7-gallon tank at the back of the cart.

When the cart is already full of clarified water it is possible to continue the delivery of filtered water by turning the taps on the cart so that the water passes from the source, through the alum box and clarifying chamber, straight to the candles.

The alum box is constructed in such a simple manner that rough usage on active service is unlikely to render inoperative the procedure just described.

Should, however, the box be damaged in any way, water can be pumped from the source into the tank where it can be treated with alum and then pumped through the flannelette cylinders, the pipe at the exit of each clarifying chamber being left open until the water issuing is free from suspended material. If only clarified water is required, it may be obtained by attaching a short length of rubber tubing to the exit pipe from the clarifying chamber. If the water is to be filtered, the tap on the exit pipe of each clarifying chamber is turned so as to direct the clarified water to the chamber containing the candles.

It will readily be understood that when the water at the source contains much suspended material, the deposit on the surface of the flannelette cylinders may gradually become so thick as to offer considerable resistance to the passage of water. In order to prevent excessive pressure on the flannelette cylinder a safety valve set at 40 lb. has been fixed on each pipe conveying the impure water to the chamber containing the flannelette cylinder. As soon as water issues from the valve pumping must be stopped, and a fresh supply of alum placed in the boxes and clean flannel wrapped on the cylinders. The flannel removed from the cylinders can readily be cleansed in some of the clarified water and kept ready for further use should occasion arise.

The main tank and the small storage tank behind should be flushed out every week. If possible, the small tank should be flushed out with boiling water. If there is reason to think the tanks are unusually dirty, it is advisable to fill them with as clean water as can be obtained, add a sufficiency of permanganate of potash to make the water a blood-red, and allow it to stand for a few hours. It may be then either simply drained out, or even pumped out through the clarifiers and filters. When a tank has been standing disused for some time, its various parts need to be cleaned out carefully before the apparatus is taken into use.

All filter-candles should be removed every three days, and, without removing the cloth in which they are wrapped, they should be placed in cold water in the kettle supplied, and the water raised to and maintained at boiling point for at least a minute. Once a week each filter-candle should be carefully inspected by removing its surrounding cloth. The cloth should be rinsed in boiling water but never brushed or scrubbed, and then replaced. If the filter-candle is dirty or working badly, remove the cloth and scrub the candle well with the brush supplied among the spare parts ; rinse the candle in clean water, replace the cloth, and boil cloth and candle. No difficulty is experienced in removing filter-candles ; the lid of the filter chamber is unclamped and then lifted bodily up, having attached to it the four candles and their associated swan-necks, if these have not been detached already. The whole set should be placed on the ground and the bottom or foot-plate which holds them together at the lower end unscrewed. Next the individual candles must be unscrewed from their swan-necks and the lid or plate to which they are attached. Once released, they are readily withdrawn, cleaned, and replaced, or others substituted for them. It only remains, then, to re-fix the foot-plate and re-adapt the top plate with swan-necks, and replace the whole in the filter chamber.

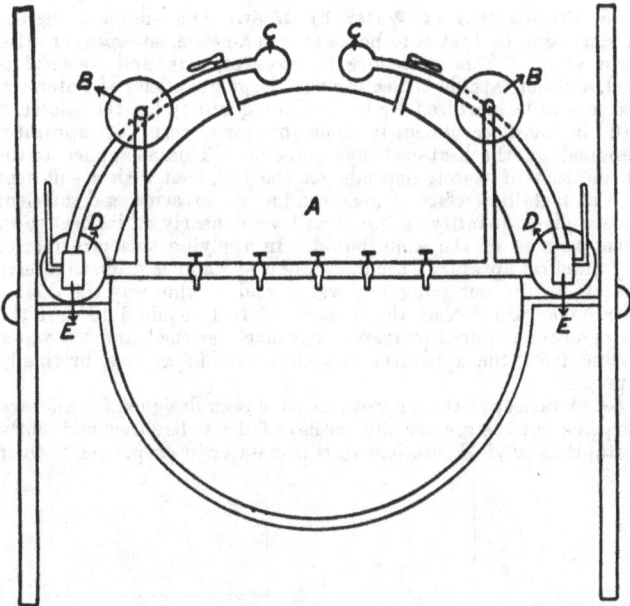

FIG. 7.   FILTER-TANK (CYLINDRICAL TYPE).

86. An alternate design of filter-tank may be met with. Its general arrangement and appearance is shown in Fig. 7. In principle it is the same as the more common rectangular filter-tank. The main tank is a cylindrical metal drum, A, capable of holding 110 gallons of water, this is mounted on a pair of wheels. Attached to the main tank are two filter chambers, B, two clarifying chambers, C, two cylindrical storage tanks, D, and two pumps, E. The pump, clarifier, filter, and storage tank on each side are independent. Apart from the shape of the main tank, the distinguishing feature of this filter-tank is that the filter chambers contain but one large filter tube instead of four, and the storage tanks are cylindrical and placed one on either side of the main tank. In the later pattern of this design the single candle is replaced by four candles of the standard type. The working and management of this type is precisely the same as that of the other; its advantage is that it is well-balanced. Its working is simple, and delivery of filtered water equal to about 200 gallons an hour. It is fitted with the usual spare-part box and a kettle or container in which to sterilize the filter tubes.

87. There is also under trial a filter consisting of a clarifying chamber containing an alum box and flannelette cylinder, and two standard candles. This filter is intended for pack saddle transport.

88. Sterilization of Water by Heat.—The simplest method of sterilizing by heat is to boil water in a kettle, saucepan, or other open vessel. This procedure is, however, slow and wasteful of fuel, and not capable of dealing with large quantities of water. If water is to be sterilized by heat in any quantity for the soldier, it will be most economically done by some form of apparatus designed on the heat-exchange principle. This, as applied to the purification of water, depends on the fact that with a sufficient area of metallic surface of good conducting capacity, and sufficient time, a given quantity of liquid will yield nearly all its heat to an equal volume of the same liquid. In applying this principle to any practical apparatus, the incoming cold water is made to receive heat from the out-going hot water, and in this way the double advantage gained that the amount of fuel required to raise the water to the required temperature is much lessened, and the water issuing from the apparatus is almost as cold as that originally supplied.

89. A variety of these apparatus have been designed for military purposes, but the greater number have failed to be either sufficiently portable as to yield sufficient sterilized water in proportion to their

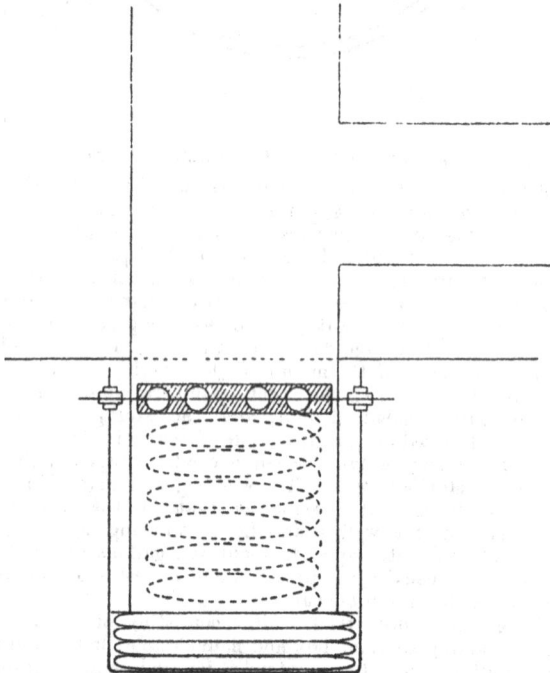

Fig. 8.

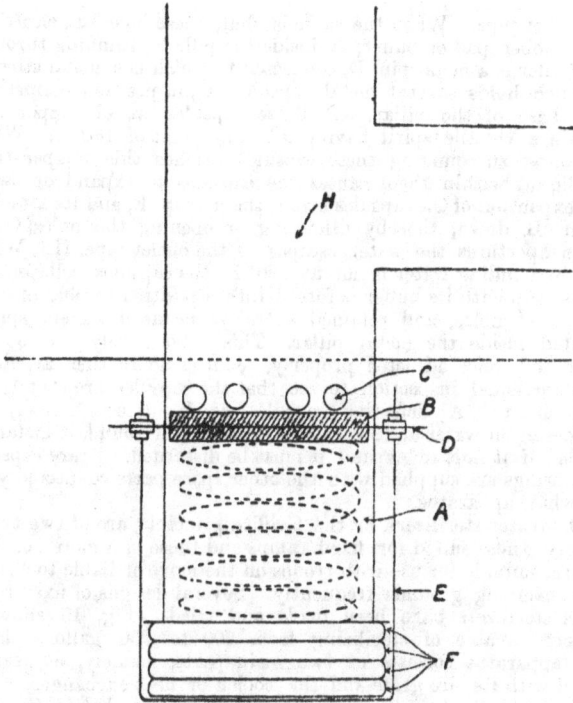

FIG. 9.

FIGS. 8 AND 9. VALVE IN WATER-STERILIZER.

size and weight. The particular sterilizer of this kind at present
under trial in the service is one known as the "Griffith." The
essential novelty in the Griffith water sterilizer is the recognition of
the fact that a momentary exposure of water to a temperature of
180° F., is sufficient to destroy all disease-producing germs that
are conveyed commonly by water.

The vital part of the apparatus is a valve which controls the
passage of the water from the sterilizing chamber to the cooler.
This valve is immersed in the water which is being heated, and is
so made that it opens only when the surrounding water attains
a temperature of 180° F., or 81° C., and closes automatically when
this temperature is not maintained. Fig. 8 gives a sectional
view of the valve when closed, and Fig. 9 when open. The
valve consists of a hollow metal pillar, A, placed inside the heating
chamber and connected to an outlet pipe, H, leading to an exchange
heater or cooler. The pillar has a solid base, but is perforated with
several outlet holes, C, at its upper end, near to its connection with

the outlet pipe. When the valve is shut, these holes are closed up by a rubber pad or buffer, B, inside the pillar. Running through this buffer is a metal pin, D, connected to which is a metal stirrup, E, which holds several metal capsules, F., in position against the solid base of the pillar, A. These capsules are of copper and contain a volatile spirit having a boiling point of 180° F. When the water surrounding these capsules reaches this temperature, the liquid within them causes the capsules to expand or swell. The expansion of the capsules brings the stirrup, E, and its attached buffer, B, down, thereby disclosing or opening the holes, C, by which apertures the water escapes to the outlet pipe, H. When the surrounding water is not at 180° F., the capsules collapse and the stirrup with its buffer is forced into a position to plug or close the outlet holes, and retained there by means of a metal spring situated inside the metal pillar. This valve rarely gets out of order and, once adjusted properly, requires no further attention than occasional inspection to see that the capsules are sound and in position. A defective capsule can be detected easily by immersing in water at 180° F., or over when, if sound, it instantly swells ; if it fails to expand it must be discarded. Spare capsules and springs are supplied with the other spare parts connected with the whole apparatus.

90. Water-sterilizers, on the Griffith principle, are of two types, namely, those suited for fixed camps and those of a more portable nature, suitable for use with troops on the move or liable to change their camping grounds frequently. Several designs of fixed camp water-sterilizers have been made and tried. Fig. 10 shows a pattern capable of sterilizing from 200 to 250 gallons daily. The apparatus consists of two main parts, namely, a heating vessel with its fire grate and the cooler or heat-exchanger. The heating vessel, A, is a cylindrical column expanded at its base into a barrel shape. The vertical part has a central air-way which allows of the smoke and gases from the fire to escape up to the chimney ; this airway is completely surrounded by the water-heating chamber. The horizontal portion of the water-heating chamber surrounds or forms a jacket to the fire grate which is thus placed in the most favourable position for heating the water. The cooler or heat-exchanger, B, is a vertical metal case having in its centre a number of copper tubes. On the top of the cooler is a small cistern, C, fitted with a gauge glass to show the varying level of the water. At the top of the heating vessel is the automatic valve, D, which controls the outflow of the water from the heater. From the back of the heating chamber runs a pipe, E, which can only be partly seen in the diagram. This pipe connects the heating vessel with the upper end of the cooler. Another pipe, F, is seen passing from the valve at top of heater to the top of the cooler in front. A third pipe, G, is to be seen issuing from the bottom of the cistern, it passes vertically down-wards and ends by discharging into the lower part of the cold water section of the cooler. A fourth pipe, H, is attached to the lower

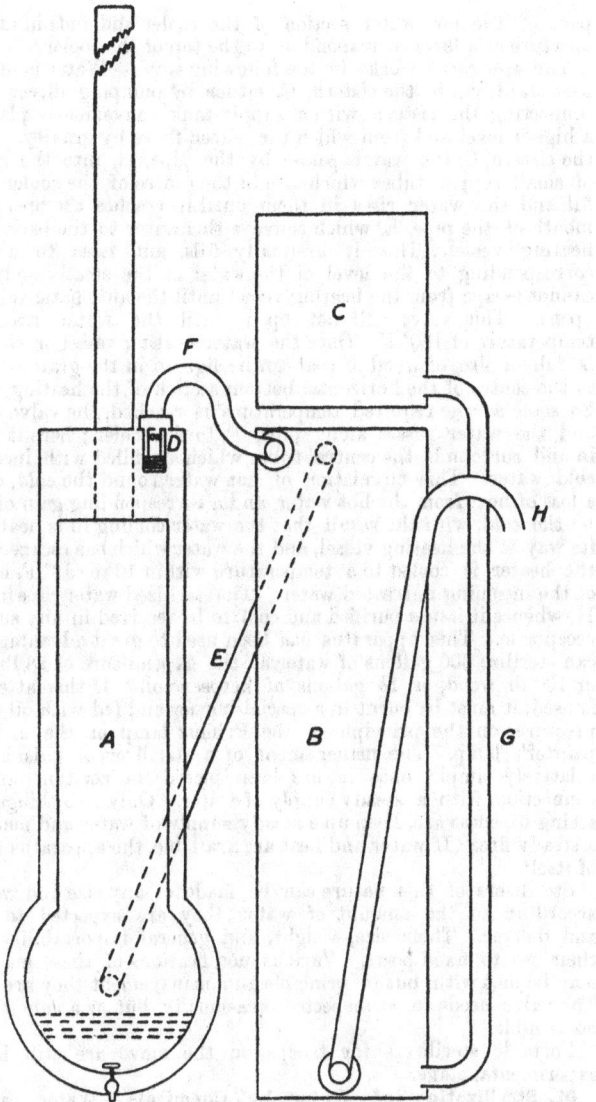

Fig. 10. Fixed Type of Water-sterilizer.

E

part of the hot water section of the cooler and ends in an open aperture at a level corresponding to the top of the cooler.

The apparatus works in the following way :—Water is made to pass steadily into the cistern, C, either by pumping direct or by connecting the cistern with a supply tank conveniently placed at a higher level and from which the water flows by gravity. From the cistern, C, the water passes by the pipe, G, into the system of small copper tubes which are in the centre of the cooler, these fill and the water rises in them until it reaches the opening or mouth of the pipe, E, which conveys this water to the back of the heating vessel. This it gradually fills, and rises to a point corresponding to the level of the water in the small cistern. It cannot escape from the heating vessel until the automatic valve, D, opens. This valve will not open until the water reaches a temperature of 180° F. Once the water-heating vessel or chamber is full, a fire of wood or coal can be lighted in the grate which is in the centre of the horizontal bottom section of the heating vessel. So soon as the required temperature is reached, the valve opens, and the water passes along pipe, F, to the cooler ; here it passes in and surrounds the central tubes which are filled with incoming cold water. This circulation of hot water round the cold, causes a loss of heat from the hot water and a corresponding gain of heat by the cold, with the result that the water coming in is heated on its way to the heating vessel, and the water which has escaped from the heater is cooled to a temperature within 10° or 12° F. of that of the incoming untreated water. The sterilized water rises in pipe, H, whence it issues purified and cool to be received in any suitable receptacle. This apparatus has been used to great advantage and can sterilize 600 gallons of water at the expenditure of 28 lb. coal, or 100 lb. wood, or 1½ gallons of kerosene oil. If this latter fuel is used, it must be burnt in a special burner and fed with oil under pressure, on the principle of the Primus lamp or the ordinary painter's lamp. The management of a sterilizer of this kind is relatively simple, once it has been placed in position and in connection with a steady supply of water. Only two things need seeing to, these are, keep up a steady supply of water and maintain a steady fire. If water and heat are available, the apparatus works of itself.

Sterilizers of this nature can be made of any size and weight, according to the amount of water they are expected to treat and deliver. Their size, weight, and general importability limit their use to fixed posts. Various modifications of these machines may be met with, but in principle and management they are alike. The valve needs to be inspected occasionally, but as a rule it gives no trouble.

Portable sterilizers for troops on the move are still in the experimental stage.

91. Sterilization of Water by Chemicals.—Water can be sterilized and purified undoubtedly by means of chemicals, but as a practical method for soldiers it presents many difficulties. The chief

are :—The necessity of portability, simplicity in working, rapidity
of action, and that the treated water be free from taste or smell.
A large number of chemicals have been suggested and tried for
water purification, of these the most useful for soldiers in camp or
in the field are alum, permanganate of potash, and the acid sulphate
of soda.

92. If *alum* be added to a muddy water in the proportion of a teaspoonful to a bucketful, and well stirred, a gelatinous cloud will form
and slowly fall to the bottom, carrying with it most of the mud and
other suspended matter, leaving a clear liquid which can then be
drawn off. This action of alum will not sterilize the water, but
merely clear it; it is, however, rather slow, taking an hour or more
to act properly, but when time is no object and a muddy water has
to be cleared when no filters or strainers are available, alum is a
useful stand-by. Alum does not act well with all waters, its best
effect being obtained in waters which contain lime; rain and other
soft waters do not readily clear by means of this chemical. It must
not be forgotten that alum will not kill the germs; it removes a
great number by throwing them to the bottom, but to make certain
the cleared water should be boiled or strained afterwards. The
use of alum in conjunction with straining and filtering has been
previously mentioned. As a useful help for the more rapid clarification of water by improvised methods, alum or some mixture
containing alum is a most valuable chemical.

93. *Permanganate of potash*, if added to water in sufficient
quantity to make it pink, is another useful means of purifying water.
It acts like alum in making a sediment and causing the water to clear
gradually if allowed to stand; it also has a mild action on germs,
killing them. This germ-killing power is, however, somewhat slow
and feeble; for this reason, reliance cannot be placed on permanganate to purify very foul waters. The germ which is most readily
killed by this chemical is the microbe which causes cholera. For
cleaning out barrels, tanks, cisterns, and other receptacles for storing
water, the addition of the permanganate is extremely useful. Sufficient should be added to make the water a good rose-pink colour.
The water should then be well stirred and allowed to stand for quite
three hours. Permanganate gives no taste to the water, and is quite
harmless to anyone drinking the pinked water.

94. The *acid sulphate of soda* is practically so much sulphuric acid
in a solid form. It is supplied conveniently in tablets, sweetened with
saxine and flavoured with oil of lemon; if one of these be dissolved
in 1¾ pints of water or the contents of a water-bottle, it yields enough
acid to that water to kill any disease-producing germs, which may
be in that water, in twenty minutes to half an hour. The water will
taste faintly acid and not unlike an inferior or flat lemonade; this
acid water is quite harmless and fit to drink. By the issue of these
tablets to soldiers, it is hoped that each man will be able to keep his
water-bottle sweet and clean and free from germs. Thus, say a man
fills his bottle full of water overnight, drops in one of the acid tablets

and allows it to dissolve and remain in that water till the morning, the contents of the bottle will be quite free from disease-producing germs. He can either use that same water for drinking purposes, or he can pour it away and refill the bottle with filtered or boiled water. By so doing, he will be certain, however, that his bottle is clean and free from germs. A more preferable way is not to allow the acid tablet to remain such a long time as ten or twelve hours in the bottle-full of water, but to add it to the water only about an hour before he is likely to want to drink some of the water. It must be remembered that the adding of these acids to a muddy water will not clear that water—that must be done by straining ; the acid tablet will only kill germs in water, not remove mud, and the germs are not killed until after at least twenty minutes. Used in this way these tablets should be of great value to soldiers and others who are unable to get their water properly filtered, or boiled, or otherwise sterilized by heat. The proper use of these tablets, if issued, is entirely a matter for the soldier himself ; he must understand what he is doing and why he is doing it.

95. *Chlorine,* derived from the electrical decomposition of a salt solution, presents some promise as a means of purifying water in bulk, but, as in the case of using *ozone* for a similar purpose, the procedure has not reached a practical form. If chlorine is used at all, for soldiers, it is best applied to water in the form of pellets or tablets of bleaching powder. Some success has attended this method, but the chief objection is that the water acquires an unpleasant taste. True, this unpleasantness can be removed by adding another tablet containing hyposulphite of soda, but this introduces the complication of having two chemicals instead of one. For this reason, the method is unsuitable for soldiers. The same objection applies to the use of *iodine* or *bromine* for the purification of water. Both these chemicals rapidly purify water, killing germs within five minutes, but the water is undrinkable until the iodine or bromide is removed by the hyposulphite of soda.

96. The utilization of chemicals for purifying water in camps and in the field is very promising theoretically, but its practical application in military life is full of difficulties. It is not implied by this that the matter is to be dismissed from further consideration ; on the contrary, every endeavour should be made to develop the idea, but until we can obtain a chemical at once more simple and efficient than any as yet suggested, it must be admitted that the use of chemical methods by individual soldiers offers but a slender prospect of being generally applied with success. It can be carried out successfully only for large quantities of water, say 100 gallons at a time. Used in this way for the contents of an ordinary water-cart, the iodine method is quite practicable. It is done in the following way :—Three sets of tablets are made up and packed together in a small box. One set of tablets is red, another is white, and the third is blue. The tablets are made up in sets of ten or a sufficiency for 100 gallons of water. The red and white tablets are broken up and dissolved in a little water in a metal cup; the water turns brown and smells strongly of iodine. This is now emptied into and well mixed with 100 gallons of water, say the contents of a water-cart. If allowed to act for ten minutes, the iodine kills all germs in the water. At the end of the ten minutes, but not before, in order to remove the iodine and so make it fit to drink, the blue tablets are added to a little water, broken up and then well stirred in the 100 gallons which have been treated with iodine. After a few minutes, the iodine will have been removed and the water found to be sterile, free from smell or taste and quite fit to drink. The only care needed is to use the red and white tablets together, allowing them to act for ten minutes; the blue tablets must not be added to the water until after the ten minutes.

CHAPTER X.

THE FOOD OF THE SOLDIER.

97. A food has been defined as "anything which, when taken into the body, is capable either of repairing its waste or of furnishing it with material from which to produce heat or nervous and muscular work." In other words, food has two main functions, *i.e.*, (1) to provide for the growth and repair of the tissues of the body, and (2) to act as a source of energy which can be converted into heat and work. Most articles of diet are made up of mixtures of various chemical substances, the nutritive constituents of which may be classified into:—(1) those that contain nitrogen, (2) those that do not contain nitrogen, (3) salts, (4) water. The nitrogen-containing foods or proteins are present in the flesh of various animals, also in eggs, cheese, the curd of milk, and in a few vegetables like peas, beans, and lentils. The non-nitrogenous foods consist of (1) carbohydrates such as sugar and starch, and (2) fats, animal or vegetable. The function of building up and repairing the tissues can be fulfilled by the nitrogenous foods, and by these alone.

The function of supplying energy is the property of both the nitrogenous and non-nitrogenous foods.

98. It is thus apparent that the nitrogenous foods alone are able to fulfil both the functions of a food ; without them life is impossible. With nitrogenous food, water, and salts, the body may be maintained in a healthy condition for a considerable time ; but for the best forms of diet, both fat and sugar, or starch, are required in addition to nitrogenous foods.

99. Salts, especially common salt, are essential to health ; the various salts of the body, such as those of calcium, iron, sodium, potassium, and phosphorus are all derived from the nitrogenous and non-nitrogenous foods.

100. Water serves for the solution and conveyance of food to the various parts of the body, and also for the excretion of useless products. It is not received into the body solely as a liquid, but forms a large proportion of the solids taken. Meat contains 72 per cent., and bread 38 per cent. of water.

101. Such being the uses of foods in the body, how is their relative value to be judged ? Chemical analyses will tell us how much of the nutritive substances a hundred parts of the food contain. In this way, an idea is obtained of the value of the food as a source of tissue building material and energy. At the present time, however, it is usual to estimate the energy value of a food by means of the amount of heat produced when it is completely burnt or oxidized. There is a definite relation between heat produced and work done.

102. The standard employed is the amount of heat which is required to raise 1 lb. of water 4° F. (or 1 kilogramme of water 1° C.). This amount of heat is called a Calorie (written with a capital letter). To apply this test, it is only necessary to ascertain how many pounds of water will be raised 4° F. (or kilogrammes of water 1° C.) in temperature, by completely burning 15·5 grains (or 1 gramme) of the food. The result gives the value of this amount of food in terms of Calories. Tested in this way it has been found that the complete combustion of 15·5 grains of fat ribs of fresh beef yield 3·6 Calories. Though the Calorie test is useful for comparing the value of foods, it must not be supposed that the food will necessarily give the amount of energy when taken into the body. In order that the energy may be obtained the food must be properly digested and more or less completely absorbed into the blood.

103. The quantity of food which a man should receive depends mainly on the amount of work which he is obliged to do. Food is required to furnish energy for the internal work of the body, i.e., the heart's work, etc., and to maintain the body temperature. This amount must be supplied whether at work or at rest in order to maintain life. But if a man does external work, such as marching, fighting, or any labouring work, he must have more food to supply energy for the work done. With regard to the external work and the amount of power required to be supplied by food to produce that work, it is estimated that in ordinary circumstances a man transforms about one-sixth of the total available energy of his food into work, the rest being lost in the form of heat. This loss is inevitable, but it compares favourably with that experienced in a steam engine, where the work done is about one-eighth of the total energy supplied by the fuel consumed. If a soldier were simply doing the usual parades and fatigues, the work would correspond to between 500 and 600 Calories and his food should then contain not less than from 3,000 to 3,500 Calories. If the muscular work be increased as on manœuvres and on active service, then there must be a corresponding increase in the amount of food consumed. On manœuvres at least 4,000 Calories should be supplied, and during active service a diet containing from 4,500 to 5,000 Calories should be given. Though work is the most important condition which influences the amount of food required, build, weight, age, and climate have also to be taken into consideration.

104. Build is more important than weight ; the larger the surface of the body in relation to its bulk, the greater is the loss of heat by radiation, and the greater the amount of food required to maintain the body temperature. A thin man requires more food than a fat man of the same cubic content, because the former has a greater amount of surface exposed. A child, relatively to its weight, requires more food, because it has a large surface in proportion to its bulk. A man whose weight is due mainly to muscle will require relatively more food, especially nitrogenous food, than one who owes his weight to bone or fat. Young men also require more food than those of maturer age.

105. As regards climate, the temperature of the body is mainly adjusted by regulating the amount of heat lost. As the external temperature rises, the body requires less heat, and the balance is usually adjusted, not by eating less food, but by increasing the loss of heat through wearing thinner clothes. When the external temperature falls, the loss of heat is diminished by wearing thicker clothes. In very cold climates, the demand for heat is so great that a greater consumption of food, particularly fatty food, is necessary.

In very hot climates, on the other hand, the demand for heat is much less, and a man instinctively avoids the nitrogen-containing foods and the fats, from which a large quantity of heat is produced in a short time, and resorts to vegetable food-stuffs.

106. Admitting that with an increased amount of work there should be a corresponding increase in the amount of food, arrangements must be made to increase all the nutritive constituents, proteins, fats, and carbohydrates. A mixed diet is essential ; no one article of food contains the different nutritive constituents in proper proportion, and the excess of a particular constituent in one article must be played off against its deficiency in another. Experience has shown this to be necessary, hence the usual combinations of bread and cheese, potatoes and beef, in which the excess of the carbohydrates in the bread and the potatoes is balanced by the proteins and fat in the cheese and beef. Variety is of paramount importance. An unvaried diet may be not only extremely distasteful, but may have serious consequences as regards general health and liability to disease. The causes of this are not quite clear, but there is no reason to doubt that the varying appetite for different kinds of food is an expression of bodily requirements of which we cannot give a strict scientific account. Also the constituents of a mixed diet are better absorbed than any one article of food when taken by itself.

107. In peace, the diet of the soldier consists of the government ration of 1 lb. of bread and ¾ lb. of meat, supplemented by articles purchased with the messing allowance of 3d. per diem. The average value of the food thus obtained has been calculated to be 3,369 Calories, which, as has already been stated, supplies sufficient energy for the work performed by a soldier doing ordinary parades and fatigues.

108. In addition to the above diet, the soldier constantly obtains, at his own expense, a supper which generally contains meat ; but there are no data from which the value of this meal can be calculated. The amount thus bought gives elasticity to the diet, as each man can select the quality and amount of food which suits him. In war, the amount of physical work done varies considerably, and there is no doubt that a man constantly engaged in marching and fighting will require a ration amounting to about 4,500 Calories. The Secretary of State fixes the special ration to be issued for active service in the field according to the climate and circumstances of the expedition.

109. The diet suggested in the Allowance Regulations consists of : 1¼ lb. fresh, or 1 lb. salt or preserved meat ; 1¼ lb. of bread or 1 lb. biscuit or 1 lb. of flour ; ⅝ oz. tea ; 2 oz. sugar ; ½ oz. salt ; ₁/₃₆ oz. pepper ; ½ lb. fresh vegetables or 2 oz. compressed vegetables or 4 oz. preserved fruit ; and 4 oz. jam. This ration is not sufficiently varied, and in South Africa it was supplemented by issues of cheese pickles, etc. Recent experimental marches have shown that a better diet is obtained by substituting oatmeal, peas, bacon, and cheese, for 4 oz. of biscuit and 4 oz. of meat. The total weight carried is thereby not increased, but variety is obtained and also more energy.

CHAPTER XI.

THE HYGIENE OF THE MARCH.

110. This is a matter which deserves the earnest consideration of every soldier, as apparently trivial mistakes made under these circumstances have often far-reaching effects. Further, these mistakes have reference mainly to a variety of details which are intimately concerned with the acts of the individual ; in other words, their remedy lies not so much in the issuing of orders as in the inculcation of knowledge and sense of responsibility in the mind of the soldier himself. Given the knowledge as to what is right and what is wrong, the soldier must stand or fall by his own actions.

111. Preparation for the March.—In preparing for a campaign or a series of marches, it is important that all cases of disability should be segregated and left behind, since such soldiers are certain, sooner or later, to become encumbrances to the marching column. Especially does this apply to the detection and elimination of concealed or partly cured venereal disease. Great care, therefore, must be taken that only fit men are permitted to join the columns. The next essential preliminary to every march is to see that the men do not start on empty stomachs. This does not mean the issue of a large meal, but rather the consumption of light refreshment, such as tea or coffee with bread or biscuit ; this is particularly desirable when the men break camp and move off in the early dawn, as at such times a little food and a warm drink does much to lessen fatigue and increase resistance to disease.

112. Time, Length and Speed of the March.—The hour of starting and the length of the march are matters upon which any precise rules are impossible, since any movement of troops is influenced by weather, roads, and military necessity. The custom in our service is to march in the early morning ; the men are fresh, the air is cool, and the main effort can be completed before the heat of the day comes on. Night marches are to be deprecated ; except under the stress of military necessity, the loss of sleep and general discomfort occasioned by night marches may be considered far to outweigh the ordinary advantages to be gained thereby.

As to the length of the march, a fair day's effort for infantry under usual conditions may be said to be from twelve to fifteen miles. Of course much more than this can be done, but a greater average than fifteen miles daily is rarely achieved, except by small bodies of men and for short periods. The severity of a march is not to be measured so much by its mere length in miles, but rather by other factors, such as pace or time in which done, load carried, and formation or position in the column.

The rate of speed and individual ease with which a march can be done depends largely on the size of the command. An infantry battalion will cover a fifteen-mile march in something under six hours, but an infantry brigade will need nearer seven hours for the same distance, and a division will require eight or nine hours. The question of individual ease when on the march is complicated by the fact that the movements of the soldier are to a certain degree unnatural or constrained. It is true these disabilities are much less manifest now than formerly, but even so the weak man has to keep up with the strong, the man of short stride with the one of long, and the very regularity of the step tends to make military marching wearisome. As far as possible the movements of the individual soldier should not be impeded by restrictions of an unnecessary nature, and every endeavour made to turn what is a compulsory military movement into a salutary and stimulant exercise. Thus in hot weather, men should be made to unbutton their coats, turn them well back and present as few obstacles to free expansion of the chest and personal comfort as possible. Where weights or loads are carried, the length of the step must be shortened. This question of the load or equipment obviously has an important bearing upon the facility with which men will be able to complete a march. At the present time, it is doubtful whether the British soldier suffers any serious disability under this heading. The question of formation and position in the column are details of great moment to the individual. On dusty roads, close order becomes particularly trying to the foot soldier, and for this reason it is a good rule that, if the military situation permits, infantry on the march should preserve a wide front and as open a formation as possible, in order to avoid the effects of crowding. Without ventilation through the ranks the air soon becomes very foul.

113. **Mental Occupation.**—Few things harass troops on the line of march more than straggling. It is an evil which demoralizes the men and needs to be firmly controlled. Its prevention depends upon a careful elimination of the sick, the encouragement and assistance of the tired, and the application of suitable measures to the undisciplined and lazy. To occupy the minds of the men on the march is probably the surest way of preventing fatigue ; to this end a band or singing does much to lessen the tedium of a journey.

114. **Foot-soreness.**—The proper care of the feet, while rightly within the purview of all officers, is mainly a matter for the individual soldier. Ill-fitting boots and socks, combined with uncleanliness of the feet, are the real causes of this disablement of the marching soldier. The ablution of the feet at least once daily should be compulsory for troops in the field. If facilities for complete washing of the feet are not available, the thorough wiping with a wet cloth, particularly of the toes, answers an excellent purpose in the removal of dirt and grease. Excessive sweating of the feet may be relieved by bathing in a solution made by diluting one ounce of formalin with two pints of water. For the same purpose, soaking the feet in water coloured red with permanganate of potash is useful, so also a 2 per cent. ointment of salicylic acid made up with tallow or vaseline is recommended, or a powder made up of salicylic acid 3 parts, starch 10 parts, and powdered talc 87 parts. These remedies are at best but palliatives ; the real remedy lies in the provision of a well-fitting boot and a soft, smooth sock to

cover the foot. Much of the soldier's difficulty turns on the fact that his sock tends to shrink quickly and so causes creases. To reduce this trouble, men should be taught to stretch their socks when they take them off, also at the end of a march to shake out and stretch the sock, then putting the sock which has been worn on the right foot on to the left and vice versa. The inside of the sock, too, should be greased with soap where it fits over tender parts of the feet. In cases where the sock is much shrunken and obviously ill-fitting, and where no spare pair is available, it is better for the man not to wear socks at all, but simply cover the foot over with ordinary newspaper. If the foot be placed in the centre of a page of any newspaper, the paper can be quickly wrapped round and so moulded to the shape of the foot as to make an excellent substitute for a sock. This covering will protect the foot for a day and be readily replaced by more paper. When blisters or chafes arise, they must be appropriately treated; the blisters must be pricked with a clean needle, and all tender parts covered with soap or some simple and clean grease. This question is not generally well understood by the soldier, few of whom realise that, for the prevention of injury to the feet by marching, three factors must ever receive consideration; these are, the elimination of men with badly-formed feet, the issue of well-fitting boots and socks, and the maintenance of clean feet. The ensurement of attention to these details is only to be secured by daily personal inspection by the company or unit commanders.

115. Smoking on the March.—The habit of smoking has an important bearing upon the ability of men to march. It is one of those questions as to which it is unwise to enforce prohibitive orders. It is easy to sympathize with a man, accustomed to smoke, who finds that he cannot have his pipe or cigarette; still the practice of smoking undoubtedly has a deleterious effect on a man engaged in a serious physical effort. This arises mainly from the poisonous or disturbing effect of tobacco upon the nervous control of the heart, combined with a tendency to make men dry-mouthed and consequently thirsty. For these reasons, men should be discouraged from smoking when marching. This discouragement should not take the form of prohibition, but rather by some simple explanation to the men of the reasons why the smoking of tobacco, when engaged in physical exercise, is likely to diminish their power of work. Further, it should be explained that, if smoking is such an acquired habit as to be a necessity, the least hurtful mode of smoking is the pipe and the most hurtful the cigarette; also that the best time for a smoke is when the work is done, that is after arrival in camp. To many, when tired, a smoke is eminently soothing, therefore its arbitrary prohibition should be exercised with care and discrimination.

116. Beer and Spirit Drinking.—Although, on the line of march, soldiers have not many opportunities to consume these beverages, still the due appreciation of the true value of these drinks is of great importance, more especially in regard to their influence on the body in respect of work to be done. In both beer and spirits, the essential dietetic element is alcohol which is present to the extent of about

4 per cent. in beer and from 40 to 50 per cent. in ordinary spirits, such as brandy, whisky, gin, or rum. Beer is the chief drink of a large number of soldiers; on some it acts as a depressant and, if taken in excess, is an intoxicant and stupor-producer. Beer tends to fatten and engender gout and rheumatism. When drunk to any excess it has a retarding influence on digestion, and produces the same injuries to health as over-indulgence in the stronger alcoholic liquors; taken in moderation, however, beer is not only an invigorating and refreshing beverage, but also a food.

As bearing on the true relation of beer or spirit drinking, when on the march or in circumstances when work has to be done, it is important to bear in mind that there is a distinction between the effects of alcohol taken in dietetic doses and when taken in excess. Moreover, it must not be forgotten that what is a dietetic dose for one man is an excess for another. Experiments indicate that alcohol in small doses may be regarded as capable of utilization in the body as a food; but when larger doses are taken more than half is excreted unused; in these latter circumstances it is clearly not a food. The experimental facts compel us to say that one and a half fluid ounces of pure alcohol in twenty-four hours is the maximum amount which a man should take. This is contained in about three ounces of ordinary brandy, whisky, gin, or rum; in three-fourths of a pint of the light wines; and in three pints of the ordinary ales or beers. Any consumption over these amounts, daily, means the dosing of the body with a quantity of alcohol with which it is incapable of dealing. If so, it can do no possible good, but much real harm.

Many people have an idea that beer and spirits make them feel warmer. This is very doubtful; certainly, if taken in any excess, these drinks really lower the body temperature and, on this account, are unsuited for those exposed to great cold. If taken too often, even in small doses, or taken in large quantity at one time, beer and spirits depress and paralyse the nervous system, delay digestion, and gradually set up disease in the stomach, liver, and kidneys which ultimately results in fatal illness.

How far alcohol is beneficial or not, when taken in small or dietetic doses, is still a matter of controversy between the teetotallers and those who advocate moderation. Of this, however, we are sure, that only in exceptional circumstances can alcoholic drinks be regarded as a food; also that they do not conduce to the doing of hard work. We can fully sympathize with a man, accustomed to an occasional glass of beer, finding himself quite deprived of this drink. We are bound to recognize that beer or spirits are often useful in disease and sometimes desirable in health, but in health neither beer nor spirits are a necessity, and the majority of persons are better without them. To men, tired and fagged out after a long march, a moderate issue of beer or spirits is not only an advantage, but almost a necessity. These considerations should influence our attitude in regard to these issues in the service. Where men are known habitually to abuse the consumption of these liquors they should be encouraged and helped to become total abstainers, but where such is not the case it is unwise to forbid the consumption of alcoholic drinks altogether, or to coerce men towards total abstinence. The only rules which should be laid down in regard to this matter are (1) beer or spirits should not be drunk during working hours ; (2) beer or spirits should only be drunk after the day's work is over, that is on the completion of the march and after arrival in camp or bivouac ; (3) the issue of beer or spirits at this time should be strictly limited to either two pints of beer or one and a half fluid ounces of one of the ordinary spirits ; (4) the alcoholic drink issued must not be taken fasting, but with the evening meal. If issued on these lines, there is much to suggest that, for those accustomed to drink one or other of these beverages, an allowance daily of either beer or spirits may be productive of more good than harm. In all cases, the circumstances must be taken into consideration, but, above all things, we must remember that the only hope of a rational use of alcoholic drinks by soldiers lies in the inculcation of sound knowledge as to their limited dietetic value.

117. **Water Discipline.**—A common fault, even among experienced soldiers, is a too free recourse to the contents of their water-bottles, and the tendency to drink each time they approach usable water. While arbitrary control over the use of the water-bottle on the march is as unwise as it is impracticable,still it is well to explain to the men the advantages of husbanding their resources and of developing a proper sense of water self-discipline. Much can be done to prevent the sensation of thirst by carrying a pebble in the mouth to excite the flow of saliva. To the same end, breathing through the nose rather than through the mouth should be encouraged, while tobacco chewing, and to a less degree smoking and spitting is inadvisable on the march as tending to increase thirst. The water-bottle should invariably be filled with approved water before starting on the march, or it may be filled with unsweetened tea or coffee ; never with beer or spirits. At all halts near water the quality should be determined by the medical officer, and on his verdict or advice should depend whether the men's bottles are refilled or not at that source. The various modes suggested for purifying water have been discussed. Mention may, however, be made here of the paramount importance of all officers exercising a supervision as to the general cleanliness of the men's water-bottles and the regimental water-tanks. The successful carrying out of this detail is merely a matter of initiative and a little trouble. Washing out with boiling or very hot water is the most rational method of cleansing the bottles, but on field service this is impracticable owing to the lack of sufficient hot water. For similar reasons the use of permanganate of potash or other chemical is not always a practical procedure. Probably the best thing to do is to fill the bottles with very hot tea, and cause this hot liquid to be retained in the bottle for at least an hour. Hot tea is available in most camps or bivouacs, and if used in this way once a week as a mere means of washing out the water-bottles would do much good ; but to be of any use, the tea must be poured into the bottles in as

near a condition of boiling as possible. The practice of attempting to scour out the inside of a bottle by placing stones, sand, or gravel in it and then shaking, followed by washing out with water, should be discouraged. The sand or stones are usually dirty, and the last state of the water-bottle will be worse than the first. In circumstances where there is an ample supply of clean water the ordinary washing out with three or four fillings with this safe water is a reliable procedure, but to be of any use this and all similar methods must be carried out under the intelligent supervision of an officer. Water should never be kept in the bottles when the water-bottle is not in daily use.

118. The Halt.—Periodical halts must be made during all marches. These are generally for five minutes in each hour, while on long marches a halt for half an hour is made usually half-way. Some care needs to be exercised to prevent men getting chilled on these occasions ; shade should be taken advantage of in hot weather, but when the men have been perspiring freely, it is open to risk if any breeze be blowing. The most important sanitary question connected with all halts is the need of sanitary police to control and prevent the reckless fouling of the vicinity of the halting places by men who retire to ease themselves. Too much stress cannot be laid on this point ; the essential need is for the officer in command to allocate at once areas to which the men may resort, and to place piquets or sanitary police over these places to see that the men, using the same, cover up all excretal matter deposited there. The covering of this material with earth need be no elaborate effort, nor involve more than the preliminary scratching of a shallow hole with the point of the boot, sword, bayonet, or a stick, and the depositing of the excreta in this shallow depression, taking care on completion of the act to cover the ordure over with the displaced earth. Failure to comply with this practice, should be made the subject of disciplinary measures.

A more preferable routine is for the sanitary duty men to proceed with their companies or units, each carrying a pick and spade. As soon as the halting place is reached, these men should proceed at once to the easement areas and prepare urine pits or trenches and shallow latrine trenches. These sanitary detachment men should remain and see that those resorting to these trenches use them properly. Immediately the " fall in " sounds, they should fill in the trenches and pits, replace turf, and leave the spot clean, tidy, and wholesome. There can be no doubt that the strictest discipline is needed at all halting places, if only to check or prevent the wholesale fouling of wayside areas where marching columns halt. The remedy is comparatively simple, involves little personal effort, and is limited to the exercise of a small amount of administrative capacity and an attention to details as explained. This question is entirely one of discipline ; its fulfilment can only follow the awakening of a. sense of sanitary responsibility in the officer, coupled with intelligent obedience and co-operation on the part of the man.

On halting for the day, or arriving in camp, one of the first duties of the officer in command of the unit or party is to send out piquets to protect and safeguard the water supply from indiscriminate use and consequent probable pollution : this detail will embrace the allocation, when possible, of separate sources of supply for men and animals. Concurrent with this primary duty, will be the sending forward of the sanitary duty men to prepare latrines, urine pits, and other places for easement of men when they arrive in camp. These may be of a temporary nature only, but some must be provided without delay, if only to preclude casual easement and consequent rapid fouling of what otherwise must be maintained as a clean and wholesome area.

The duties of the sanitary duty men in this connection may be detailed as follows :—(1) Make a sufficiency of latrines for one day for (a) officers, (b) non-commissioned officers, and (c) men. (2) Make a urinal for (a) officers, (b) non-commissioned officers, and (c) men. (3) Dig a urine-pit to receive the contents of the night urine tubs if they are used, or dig a series of urine pits at end of lines for night use. (4) Make the necessary drains and pits for the disposal of waste water. (5) Make straining pits or traps for greasy water, namely, one for each cooking place, one for serjeants' mess and one for officers' mess. (6) Build such incinerators or refuse pits as may be needed. (7) Prepare drains for carrying off excess water from stand-pipes and around ablution or washing places.

As for the men who compose the main party, after settling down in camp or bivouac and getting food, every man should examine his feet. Blisters should be pricked, the feet cleaned, and the socks shaken out. After the feet have been attended to, the general body should be washed, or as much of it as is possible in the circumstances.

CHAPTER XII.

SANITATION OF CAMPS.

119. The same principles and ideas which animate our efforts to prevent disease in barracks must be applied to camps, and with doubled energy. The need of this will be at once apparent if we remember that the moment men go into camp or bivouac they revert to a simpler mode of life, and find themselves removed from all the more or less elaborate appliances of barracks.

120. Camp Sites.—The selection of a camp site is dominated largely by the facilities which exist for obtaining water, this is particularly so in regard to temporary camps ; but where camps are likely to be occupied any length of time the feasibility of bringing the water to the camp must be as much considered as taking the camp to the water. The proper location of a camp, as a matter having a definite influence on the health and efficiency of soldiers, demands intelligent consideration. It is a good rule to select a site as if for continued occupancy, since the mere bivouac may, through necessity, become a camp of a more or less permanent character.

When possible, camps should be placed on high ground, since not only is the surface drainage better, but exposure to air currents facilitates evaporation. Situations at the base of hills are usually damp, such a site may be acceptable if a transverse ravine intercepts the drainage from the higher ground. No camp should be placed in ravines or the dry beds of water courses. Low plains surrounded by high land, valleys, and hollows are often hot and damp. The vicinity of marshes or irrigated lands, as well as areas periodically under water, are always unhealthy and favourable to mosquitoes. Similarly, situations at the mouths of rivers or places to which surface or subsoil water gravitates are always undesirable, for obvious reasons. An abandoned camp site should never be utilized, except in circumstances of great necessity. Old camping grounds must be considered as more or less permeated with the organic soakage incidental to human occupation. As regards actual soil, it may be said the more porous the better, but if a camp must be pitched upon an impermeable soil, like clay or rock, the locality affording the best surface drainage should be chosen. Ploughed land should be avoided, so, too, should very dusty areas ; in all cases grass covered soil is preferable. In the selection of camp sites apart from the question of water supply, the golden rule to follow is :—Choose areas which are not only dry but clean, that is, have not been occupied recently for encampments, and are not fouled or in any way encumbered with the recent filth of man and animals.

121. Camp Space.—Although certain regulations exist as to the manner and place of laying out various camps, it will readily be understood that these are subject to constant variations, owing to physical difficulties connected with the locality. The minimum camp and bivouac spaces allowed for certain units are as follows :—

A Cavalry Regiment	Length 161 yds.,	depth 150 yds.
A Battery or Ammunition Column	„ 75 „	„ 150 „
An Infantry Battalion	„ 65 „	„ 150 „
A Field Ambulance	„ 120 „	„ 200 „
A Cavalry Field Ambulance ...	„ 80 „	„ 180 „
A General Hospital	„ 550 „	„ 400 „
A Brigade of Infantry	„ 280 „	„ 150 „
A Brigade of Cavalry	„ 515 „	„ 150 „

Each horse requires 6 feet by 18 feet, and each mule 4 feet by 15 feet.

If the ground is not very good, the above areas are insufficient ; further, some extra depth is needed to allow for suitable latrines to be constructed. This extra depth can be estimated in yards by taking two-thirds of the number of days of probable occupation. Thus, a fifteen-day occupation would mean 10 yards extra depth ; therefore, a general hospital, likely to remain a month on a given site, would need a minimum space of 550 by 420 yards.

The figures given in the table, expressed in terms of so many men per acre, do not show any excessive density of population on the gross area ; but it is only when we come to note the extent of crowding together of men in individual houses or tents that we come to realize what life in camps really means. In the most favourable circumstances, the average soldier does not get a greater floor space in tents than 17 square feet, while in many cases it is as little as 10 square feet. This means crowding, and it is not difficult to understand the excessive incidents of some diseases among troops and others living in tents. The recognition of this sanitary danger suggests the disuse, as much as possible, of tents for troops in the field and allowing the men to bivouac in the open. In many foreign climates and in our own summer this is sound practice and may be followed with the best results. Experience goes to show that the risks attaching to exposure and vicissitudes of weather among well-fed and well-clad persons are comparatively small. On this question it can be affirmed that a field force without tents may be uncomfortable, but it will be healthy ; on the other hand, a similar force with tents may be comfortable, but it will be less healthy. Whatever may be the rule, tents or no tents, it is incumbent upon all to realize the risks attending the crowding of men together in tents, and to do their best to minimize the facilities for direct infection from man to man which tent-life does so much to foster.

All tent-walls should be looped up during fine weather, so that the tent area may be dried and disinfected by fresh air and sunlight. Even in cold and doubtful weather, the sides of the tents should be tied up during the absence of the occupants. If removal to a new camp site or fresh tent area be not practicable, all tents should be struck and their enclosed ground area sunned or aired for a few hours every four days. In a properly arranged camp, the intervals should be always sufficient to render the shifting of a tent to a new site possible. Where huts are used, the doors and windows must be opened to permit of aeration and the entrance of sunlight, and the roof, if of canvas, should be turned back. The digging up or excavation of the soil within a tent area should be discouraged, as tending to impede ventilation and due cleanliness; if floor-boards are not available, then the ground may be covered with either straw or a tarpaulin, but whatever is employed it must be turned out and well-aired and cleaned daily, so long as weather permits. Blankets and bedding must be sunned and aired each day, either by hanging on supports erected especially for the purpose, or by spreading on the sunny side of the tent roof; the former plan is preferable, as it allows access of light and air to both sides of the article.

122. Another important practice is to discourage the men, as far as possible, from eating their food in the tents, and also to forbid the storage or retention of food in them. This is admittedly a very difficult question on field service, when the renewal of supplies is often precarious and the need of economy of what is available an urgent necessity. Still, every effort should be made to reduce the amount of stored food, particularly cooked food, to a minimum. If food must be retained, every endeavour must be made to keep it in closed tins or boxes so that flies may not gain access to it. Food material attracts flies, is very difficult to keep sweet or clean, and in warm climates rapidly deteriorates. All remains of food, par-ticularly if not likely to be utilized in a few hours, should be either burnt or buried.

123. Official regulations do not refer to it, but an important point to be borne in mind when planning or laying out camp areas is the need to allow a sufficiency of ground for what may be termed the conservancy area, as distinguished from the inhabited area. No hard and fast rules can be laid down, but for general guidance it may be said that a depth of 20 yards should be allowed to intervene between the canteens, cook-houses, and washing places and the latrines, urinals, and incinerators. On a subsequent page a diagram is submitted as a type of how a suitably arranged encampment may be planned in regard to these details.

124. Water Supply.—The general principles affecting this question have been considered and need no detailed discussion in this place, except it be to emphasize the fact that it is the duty of the commanding officer on forming or occupying a camp or bivouac, to secure and protect the water supply. The question of the quality of the water available will be determined by the medical officer, and in accordance with his advice action must be taken as to treatment and general distribution. The protection of the supply from pollu-tion permits of no delay'; action must be prompt and thorough, in-volving the placing of piquets to warn off unauthorized access, and where only one source of supply is available, to prevent pollution by animals drinking before the men's supply has been drawn. Where the circumstances permit water for animals should be taken at a

point distinct from that supplying men ; in the case of running water the animals' drinking place must be below that whence the water for troops is taken.

In all circumstances, every endeavour should be made to prevent waste, pollution, and the turbidity which results from trampling the margin of a surface supply into mud. If the camp is of any permanency and the water be derived from a stream, the approach should be paved and so located that the water may be drawn from the main current, and not from the sides or from a foul eddy. If the supply be at all limited, the water will be best given to animals by receiving it first in troughs, as by so doing, less disturbance of the stream results. In cases where wells are the source of supply, the essential precaution to take is the safeguarding them from surface pollution. If they are covered this is comparatively simple, but if uncovered, special piquets may be needed to prevent access of unauthorized persons and the utilization of such places for ablution purposes. In commands consisting of both European and Oriental or native races it is advisable, if circumstances permit, to allocate certain wells exclusively to whites, and others to natives.

In camps, water is carried usually from its source to the lines in water-tanks on wheels ; but other vessels, such as pails, canvas troughs, barrels, chatties, and skins are used. In all cases the very greatest care is required to keep these receptacles clean. This is by no means easy to do, and whether it is done must depend largely on circumstances. There is no simple procedure, and the only all-round method is the washing or flushing out with ordinary water made a deep red colour by means of permanganate of potash, repeating the process so long as the water fails to remain of a pink colour after three hours. This will not sterilize these receptacles, but it will destroy the greater number of contained bacteria and render the vessels reasonably safe and clean. If water is kept stored in camp, the vessels must be protected by suitable covers. Men should not be allowed to drink direct from the taps of water tanks, or from the rim or spouts of other receptacles used for carrying or distributing water.

125. **Kitchens and Ablution Places.**—These are a fruitful source of untidiness in camps, and consequently need to be managed and so arranged that remains of food and all greasy water is rapidly and efficiently removed from the immediate vicinity. The most important details which need attention are :—(1) That the kitchens and washing places be located so as to be handy for water, but remote from latrines, urine-pits, or other receptacles for refuse and garbage ; (2) all greasy water must be made to pass readily away ; this will usually be effected by a passage into soakage-pits, and, if this does not suffice, then by drainage away along suitably-dug trenches. This waste-water is greasy, and if allowed to pass direct on to soil soon makes a felt-like scum, which not only impedes the soaking-in of the water, but also attracts flies. A useful plan is to fill the reception pits or the upper ends of the drainage channels with coarse brushwood ; if the greasy water be poured on to this mass of brushwood, the grease and other organic solids are entangled,

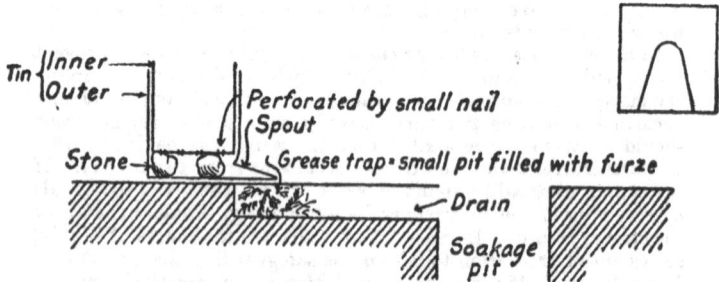

FIG. 11.—GREASE TRAP FOR CAMPS.

allowing the clearer liquid to run freely away. The brushwood, loaded with fatty matter, is conveniently burnt daily and replaced by fresh cuttings.

An alternative plan, which has been found to be effective and easily improvised, is the following :—Take two large biscuit tins, the upper acting as a coarse strainer, and the lower serving to direct the water over and into a small pit, which, filled with grass, heather, or brushwood, acts as a grease trap. From this small pit cut a shallow trench leading to a large soakage-pit (Fig. 11). The inner tin should rest on two or more stones, so as to allow an interspace. The lower tin can be given a spout, conveniently made by cutting an inverted U or V-shaped flap from one of the sides, turning down and rounding off. Modifications of the foregoing can be made by turning a box upside down over the pit or grease trap, the bottom of the box being perforated with a hole into which is fitted a

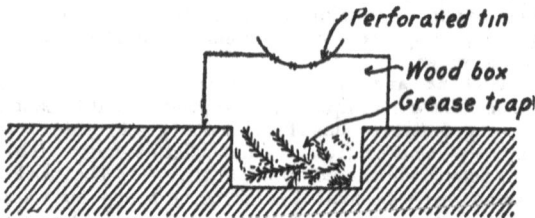

FIG. 12.—GREASE TRAP FOR CAMPS.

colander or piece of perforated tin (Fig. 12). An even simpler arrangement is that shown in Fig. 13, which consists merely of a grease trap filled with bracken or gorse, a drain from it and a final soakage-pit, the earth at the bottom of which has been loosened by a pick. In all cases the furze, grass, or brushwood used to entangle or trap the grease must be burnt and renewed daily.

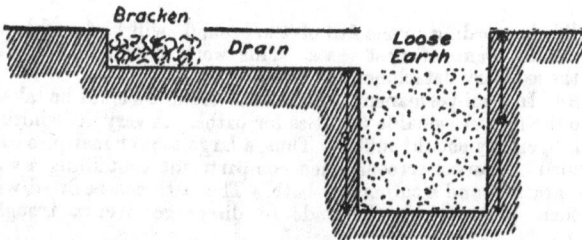

FIG. 13.—GREASE TRAP FOR CAMPS.

126. In connection with the kitchens and food supplies in camp, it is desirable that the arrangements for washing cooking utensils receive attention. At each kitchen or mess there should be an appointed place devoted solely to the cleaning up of utensils. This should have a table, or boxes to serve as a table, a suitable straining pit handy, a sufficiency of clean cloths, and a plentiful supply of hot water. If sand is used for cleaning vessels, this should be previously baked over a fire, collected and kept in a tin or box near the cleaning bench. Ashes from the wood fire may be used in place of sand. The whole process of washing up, collecting and baking of sand should be under the supervision of one of the men of the sanitary detachment or sanitary squad.

127. The ablution places need to be located conveniently near the men's tents, and the soiled or soapy water therefrom drained away on similar principles to those indicated for kitchen sullage-water. Where ordinary ablution-benches with foot-gratings are available, care needs to be taken to prevent the adjacent ground becoming sloppy. Whether benches are available or not, the water must be run away quickly and tidily ; the arrangement shown in Fig. 14,

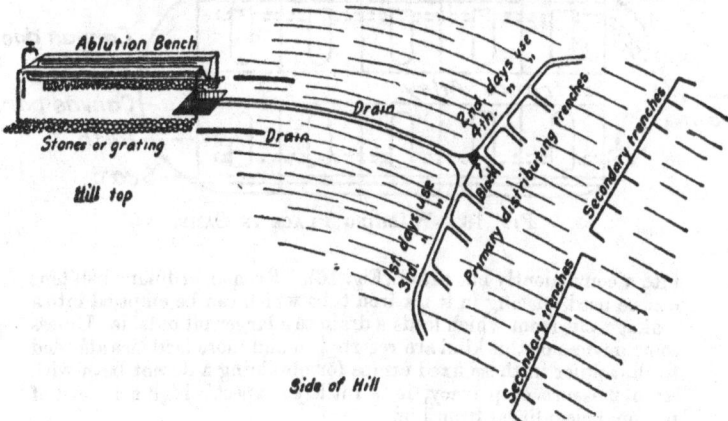

FIG. 14.—ABLUTION PLACE AND DRAINAGE IN CAMP.

modified according to the fall of the ground, will be found to meet the requirements of most cases. This work should be carried out by the sanitary detachment or sanitary squad.

128. In semi-permanent camps, some trouble should be taken to give the men reasonable facilities for baths. A very little initiative and ingenuity should suffice. Thus, a large tent or marquee can be divided by canvas screens, each compartment containing a seat, a foot-grating, and a tub or tin bath. The bath can be fitted with a wooden plug, which is made to discharge over a trough of

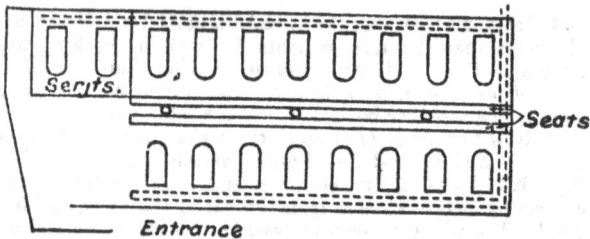

FIG. 15.—WASHING PLACE IN CAMP.

galvanized iron (Fig. 15). Or, a temporary hut can be made of canvas stretched over rough wood supports. A long seat should be arranged down each side, with a suitable number of foot-gratings and metal baths ; these latter can be emptied by tipping

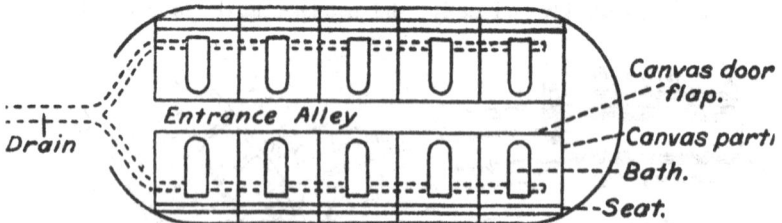

FIG. 16.—WASHING PLACE IN CAMP.

into a conveniently cut drain (Fig. 16). Even an ordinary bell tent can be used, placing in it six iron tubs which can be emptied into a soakage-pit, from which leads a drain to a larger pit outside. Unless some devices of this kind are resorted to and more facilities afforded to the soldier in these fixed camps for obtaining a decent bath with some measure of privacy, it is futile to expect a high standard of personal cleanliness from him.

129. In standing camps, unless the physical condition of the soil and the gradients are distinctly favourable for a rapid absorption and soakage away of all sullage and ablution water, it will be advisable either to shift the location of the kitchens and washing places every few days or to collect this liquid in watertight receptacles. Such receptacles should be placed on raised platforms for the better protection of themselves and the ground beneath them, and should be emptied daily and the contents disposed of outside the camp area. Before being returned to use, they should be cleaned and smeared over with a cloth soaked in crude creosote oil.

130. Drying of Clothes.—Closely associated with the personal hygiene and comfort of the soldier, both in camps and in bivouacs, is the question of drying clothing which has been wetted by rain. It is true the wearing of wet clothes conduces to much less ill-health than many suppose; still, a great deal of personal discomfort could be avoided if some simple means of drying clothes, at times when neither the sun nor wind can be utilized, could be devised. The following method is deserving of note:—Pitch as large a tent as is available, dig one or more holes, some two feet deep, within the tent, sufficiently far from the poles and canvas to minimize the risk of fire. Line the holes with stones, and carry the stones up so as to make a rim or parapet round the hole, some feet high. The stones must be fairly large, and the diameter of the hole quite three feet. If a fire be lighted in the hole and carefully tended, the stones soon get quite hot and radiate a good heat. The wet clothing should be hung round the hole as well as the appliances on the spot will allow, and the tent shut up. With a little care and initiative considerable numbers of wet garments can be dried in this way in a few hours. In place of a tent a rough shelter can be built, or use made of some outhouse on a farm. An alternative procedure is to rig up a simple

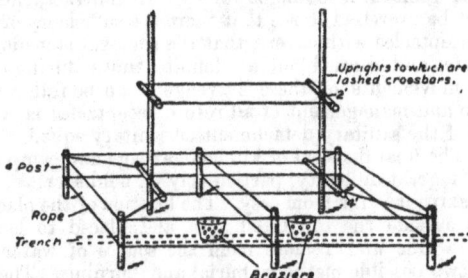

FIG. 17.—FRAME FOR DRYING CLOTHES IN CAMP.

framework, as shown in Fig. 17, by means of ropes, cords, or wire. This should be erected either within a large tent or under some rough shelter, and one or more braziers, improvised from buckets or tins, full of wood-ashes, placed at suitable intervals near to the wet clothing. These suggested methods are crude, but better than doing nothing to obviate the discomforts resulting from wet garments.

131. Disposal of Refuse.—The refuse of a camp consists of general rubbish strewn about tents, kitchen-garbage, bits of crockery, tins, paper, and rags. This material must never be thrown casually on the ground, but needs to be dealt with strictly on a definite system. It must be thrown invariably into special receptacles conveniently placed for the purpose. In camps which are of a temporary nature these receptacles best take the form of pits or holes, but where these are employed the contents must be covered over with at least six inches of earth three or four times a day, the constant endeavour being to protect the material from flies. Pits of this nature should be located near kitchens and one at the end of each line of tents, suitably marked with a notice, "rubbish to be thrown here." In more permanent camps, all this garbage and refuse should be placed in closed metal receptacles, the contents of which are removed and disposed of daily, as explained for sullage-water. In the absence of metal receptacles, the general refuse may be collected in sacks which are hung on posts placed at the end of the lines of tents. Kitchen-garbage can be collected in tubs, barrels, or boxes, which need to be raised on stands close to the cooking places; these stands may be made by four short posts supporting a rough wood frame-work. On no account, unless necessity compels, should the solid and liquid refuse be mixed. Carts or other vehicles used for the removal of this material to the place of disposal should be designed so as to prevent any escape of their contents. The casual and too frequent mode of disposal of this waste material from camps to civilians, who collect and cart it through lines and encampments without regard to elementary sanitary rules, should be strenuously opposed. The soldier should be made to dispose of this refuse himself. If removal is arranged for by civil contract, close super-vision must be exercised to see that there is a sufficiency of suitable tubs or receptacles with covers, that the removal is made daily in proper carts, and carried out at definite times during daylight, when the movements of these scavengers can be followed. The supervision and management of all refuse receptacles is a part of the duties of the sanitary detachment or sanitary squad.

132. (i) The final disposal of kitchen-garbage and camp-refuse is a matter of great difficulty, particularly on field service; even in standing camps it is far from easy. The location of the place should always be outside the inhabited area, and placed to leeward of prevailing winds and remote from the source of water supply. There are two possible methods, burial and burning. The former is suitable for cases where the amount of material to be disposed of is not excessive, but when much refuse is present the labour necessary to dig sufficiently large pits is almost prohibitive. In these cases, as much as possible should be destroyed by fire, and what is not so burnt, must be buried; in fact, it may be said that burning is the ideal mode of disposal in all cases. Theoretically this is so, but practically it is difficult to carry out, mainly on account of the natural dampness of the material. In wet weather the difficulties from this cause are much increased. In the field, the methods for the cremation of refuse vary from the use of the company kitchen fire to the employment of specially constructed crematories. Various portable destructors have been proposed and used in camps ; for the general requirements of field service, none can be said to be satisfactory. Failing any special apparatus being available for the burning of camp-garbage and refuse, ingenuity and common sense must be used as to the best method of effecting their combustion without offence.

(ii) Where crude mineral oil is available, its incorporation with the more combustible material constitutes an effective aid for the destruction of garbage by fire. In other cases, where iron rods or lengths of railway rails can be obtained, the construction of a simple grate or grid by placing these iron rods or rails on lateral supports made of turf or earth is eminently successful in maintaining a brisk fire, when fed with camp refuse. In any devices of this kind the great essential is to secure a draught of air under and through the material to be burnt ; and the damper the mass the greater the need of air. Once a draught is secured, the fire will burn, provided, of course, common sense is exercised in not being in too great a hurry and not feeding the fire too quickly with cold, damp refuse. The failure to appreciate the necessity of slow feeding or stoking is the great fault of all attempts to burn camp refuse in field incinerators. These have to be made by the men of the sanitary detachment or sanitary squad, and they must be taught and practised in their construction and use.

(iii) An improvised refuse-destructor of a simple nature can be made by digging two shallow trenches intersecting each other at right angles ; each trench should be 9 inches deep and 9 inches wide where they cross, and getting shallower and shallower to their ends. The length of each trench need not exceed five feet and may be advantageously made with an expanded or a trumpet-shaped mouth or end. Over the angles of intersection a chimney or shaft, some 3 feet high and 3 feet in diameter must be built up of turf-sods or bricks. Some ingenuity is needed to support the walls of the shaft or chimney where they cross the trenches. This can usually be overcome by utilizing bits of iron bands off bales or barrels, or even by knocking the bottom out of food tins and placing these metal

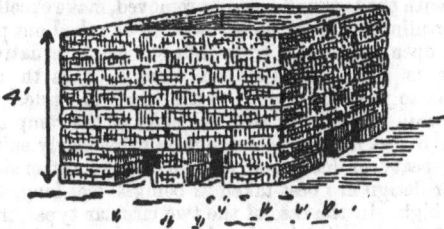

FIG. 18.—CAMP INCINERATOR—RECTANGULAR.

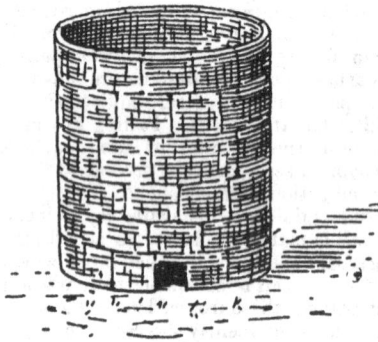

FIG. 19.—CAMP INCINERATOR—ROUND.

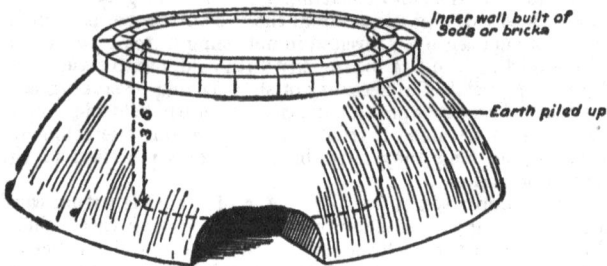

Inner wall built of Sods or bricks

Earth piled up

FIG. 20.—CAMP INCINERATOR—BEEHIVE.

tubes in the trenches, so as to support the walls of the shaft. A fire can be quickly lighted with any dry material at the bottom of the shaft, and fed steadily by throwing rubbish and refuse down the top. Modifications of this type of incinerator are shown in Figs. 18, 19 and 20 ; these can be built quite easily of turf-sods or bricks. The essential detail is to provide sufficient air inlets at the base. Disused meat-tins, with the tops and bottoms removed, make excellent frames for these openings. The air-inlets need to be raked out periodically and kept open and free from ashes. An alternative type of incinerator is a horseshoe-shaped mound of earth or sods, so arranged as to place the mouth to the windward side. The refuse is burnt within the ramped area, the sides of the ramp need not be more than 3 feet high. This design is particularly suitable when the soil is peaty or loose and crumbly. The dimensions of the rectangular design are best taken as being 4 feet long, 4 feet wide, and 3 feet high. In the case of the two circular types, the diameter should be 5 feet, and the height of wall or ramp 3 feet 6 inches.

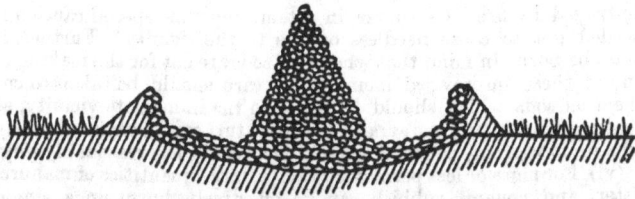

FIG. 21.—CAMP INCINERATOR (STONES).

(iv) Another effective camp incinerator is one suggested by the Americans. It consists of a circular, shallow, saucer-like depression dug out from the ground, measuring 10 feet in diameter, and not more than 2 feet deep in the centre, from which point it should gradually shelve up to the level of the ground at its edge. The whole of this saucer-like hollow must be lined with large stones or broken bricks, and with the same materials a low wall built up all round it, the excavated earth being packed against it to prevent surface water gaining access to the depression, and also to provide a sloping approach for tilting refuse into it. Next, a cairn or pyramid of large stones must be built up in the centre of the saucer-like basin; this pyramid should rise so as to have its top some two feet or more above the level of the rim or encircling wall (Fig. 21). The object of the central cairn is to provide a steady draught through the centre of the burning material. Ordinary dry wood or brushwood must be used to start the fire, and after it is well burning it can be maintained by steadily adding refuse. The stones soon become intensely hot, and serve to dispose of liquid and damp stuff with rapidity. This incinerator is eminently adapted for stony or rocky country. In places where boulders or large stones or broken bricks are not procurable, a similar crematory can be devised by using empty tins of all kinds and sizes. If not utilized in exactly the same way as suggested for the stone-made design, the tins may be stacked in heaps about 4 feet high; upon and around these heaps should be piled the miscellaneous combustible rubbish, and the whole then set alight. The tins serve to keep an air-space and generate an under draught causing the whole heap to burn fiercely. The burnt tins can be used over and over again. Ultimately all tins and broken hardware should be buried and on no account be left lying about to mark the site of an abandoned camping ground.

(v) No difficulty should be experienced by sanitary squad men or others in constructing and using camp incinerators of any of these designs, but it must be understood that initiative, ingenuity, and common sense must be shown. Assuming the refuse to be burnt be added with ordinary care and the potency of the draught-trenches or holes maintained by judicious raking out, an enormous amount of material can be disposed of in a few hours. Once a fire is burning fiercely in any of these incinerators, a considerable amount of even fæcal material from the latrine buckets can be disposed of and destroyed by fire. Of course, in attempting this, special caution is needed not to cause needless offence to the vicinity. Further, it must be borne in mind that when turf sods are cut for the making of any of these improvised incinerators, care should be taken to cut them as sods which should be stored in the immediate vicinity, so that on dismantling the arrangement the turf can be replaced neatly whence it was cut, patted down and the locality left reasonably tidy.

(vi) For more or less permanent camps, large quantities of manure, litter, and general rubbish can be effectively burnt in a single apparatus which may be described as a large trough made of iron-work raised two feet from the ground. Bands from forage bundles or any wire or pieces of iron can be utilized to make an arrange-

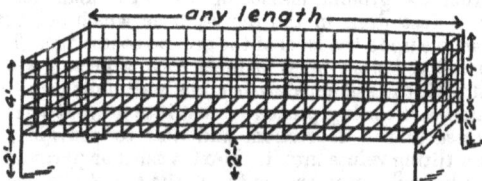

FIG. 22.—CAMP INCINERATOR (WIRE FRAME).

ment as shown in Fig. 22. Such a trough may be of any length, but should be 4 feet wide and deep. It must be placed broadside to the wind, and the bars forming the bottom made to run from side to side, not lengthwise. The mesh is best made five inches square. In this wire trough rubbish burns freely. If ordinary railway rails are available in any quantity an excellent grate or grid can be made by arranging a dozen rails each 10 feet long as a circular cone, with the upper ends securely lashed together by stout wire and the lower ends placed on the ground so as to form a circular base some 5 feet in diameter. Around the central pyramid of rails, grates are

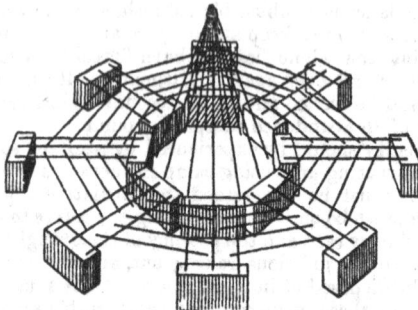

FIG. 23.—CAMP INCINERATOR (RAILWAY LINES OR GRID-TYPE).

arranged radially. These grids or grates are made of other lengths of rail resting on low turf or brick walls raised about one foot high. The radiating grids are joined together by lengths of rail. Seen from above the whole would have the appearance as shown in Fig. 23. On this large circular grid enormous masses of litter, refuse, manure, and even fæculant material can be made to burn freely, as the arrangement lends itself to free draughts of air through the mass. The only serious difficulty is to get a sufficiency of rails or iron rods so as to lay the horizontal grids close enough together to prevent litter falling through. This arrangement is obviously only feasible in a permanent camp, but once constructed is capable of coping with enormous quantities of combustible material.

133. Disposal of Dead Animals.—Closely associated with the question of disposing of camp-refuse is that of how to get rid of the carcasses of dead animals. This problem does not occur during ordinary peace manœuvres, but in time of actual war assumes serious proportions. Here again two methods of disposal are possible, namely, burial and burning. Unless special furnaces are available, the burning of the carcasses of large animals is impracticable ; it is difficult enough to burn the dead body of a single animal, but when it comes to having to cope with the carcasses of a dozen or more beasts, such as oxen, horses, and camels, the task is quite impossible. The only alternative is to bury, and even then this is far from easy. The time and labour needed to dig a pit to receive the body of a dead ox is appreciable, and when it comes to do the same for some dozen or more similar animals it will be readily understood that few units or commands can do it. What then, is to be done ? To leave the carcass to rot and decompose in the open is to establish a nuisance and general menace to the health of all around, and consequently not permissible. In ordinary circumstances of warfare the only course open is to disembowel the animals, bury the viscera as deeply as possible, and to leave the skeletal remains to be disposed of by nature. It is a crude proposal, but the only alternative. The defects of this procedure can to a certain extent be minimized by stuffing the eviscerated remains with straw or other combustible material and setting light to it. This will not consume the carcass, but it will do something towards drying it up and lessening the evils consequent on its subsequent gradual disintegration. This proposal is not put forward as the ideal or a desirable procedure ; it is merely the best that can be done in circumstances of great difficulty. In many cases, improvised crematories can be built up on which the bodies of animals can be burnt, and every endeavour to do so should be made in all camps. Experience has shown that the incinerator made of rails, or rather the collection of grids arranged round a central cone of rails or iron rods, offers the best means of burning dead animals, but, even then, a plentiful supply of dry material is needed to hasten combustion.

The final disposal of *all* refuse matter in camps should be under the direct control and direction of the sanitary officer of the command. His powers in this direction must be of the fullest and moreover, exercised with tact, firmness, and regard only for the sanitary interests of the individuals in his charge.

134. Disposal of Excreta.—The proper disposal of this material is vital to the sanitary interests of all, but provided ordinary intelligence be exercised it presents fewer difficulties than might be expected. The moment a camp or bivouac is about to be formed or occupied the first duty of the commanding officer is to secure and protect his water supply, and at the same time to send forward his sanitary duty men for the location and preparation of latrines and urinals. The construction of these necessaries must not be delayed until the tents are pitched and other camp duties have been performed ; no matter how temporary the halt may be, the location and completion of these places is an urgent necessity demanding prompt action, and to be supplemented by the detailing of sanitary police to prevent surface contamination of the camp area by casual easement. Certain military circumstances are conceivable when the construction of latrines may be delayed ; under these conditions, to avoid surface pollution, some carefully selected spot must be marked off for the reception of excreta, and sanitary discipline enforced to see that the men resort to this spot only. At the earliest opportunity all excrement so deposited must be buried or covered with earth by the sanitary duty men.

135. (i) The general location of latrines will depend upon the direction of the prevailing wind and the position of the water supply, the rule being to place them to leeward of the camp and in such a position that no possible fouling of the water supply can result. The exact position of these places should never be left to the discretion of any officer other than the sanitary officer or such other officer of the medical corps as may be exercising sanitary supervision of the command. Latrines and urinals should be as far removed from the tents as is compatible with convenience ; under ordinary conditions this may be put at 100 yards. The latrines must be placed as far as possible away from the kitchens and other places where food is prepared or stored. The extent of latrine accommodation in camps will vary according to whether the area is for temporary or permanent occupation ; in bivouacs it should be 3 per cent., for ordinary camps occupied for a few days it should be 5 per cent., and in those intended for longer occupation at least 8 per cent. These figures may be taken to represent either yards or actual seats, according to circumstances. The multiplication of latrines is undesirable, as one or two fairly large ones are easier of control than several smaller ones, and soil pollution is also more localized.

(ii) In permanent camps, latrine accommodation will best take the form of pail-middens with dry earth, fitted with rough wooden seats, and arranged as shown in Fig. 24. This design of fixed latrine provides urine-troughs for urination which may either drain into tubs or other receptacles or into soakage-pits conveniently placed. This latter arrangement is undesirable unless the ground is very porous and absorbent, but even then the liquid needs frequent covering over with fresh earth. In the majority of cases,

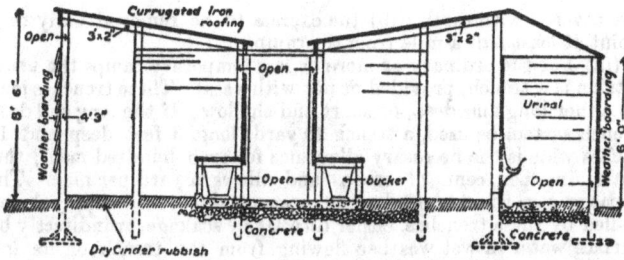

Fig. 24.—Diagram showing Latrines for Fixed Camp.

for the reception of urine iron tubs are usually provided, these being placed adjacent to the ordinary latrines for day use, and during the night at selected points convenient for the tents. The contents of the various receptacles should be removed daily and buried well away from the camp site. The ideal latrine is one provided with pails, each of which has a water-tight cover fixed by a bayonet catch. When the receptacles are full the covers are applied, and the covered receptacles are then placed in a cart for removal to the area chosen for disposal. Here the pails are emptied, thoroughly cleansed, and then brushed over with paraffin oil. This procedure is more sanitary than emptying the pails into a supposed water-tight cart, which has to be again emptied and cleaned on reaching the disposal area. In practice these carts are rarely water-tight, and the contents are often spilled during transit. The carts are also difficult to empty without fouling the ground adjacent to the pit or trench which receives the dejecta. If portable middens, such as pails, are not provided, then the seats must be placed over pits or trenches specially dug. Whatever form the latrine takes, its successful management depends absolutely upon rigid adherence to the rule that the excreta must be quickly and completely covered over with earth, and this depends again upon the enforcement of individual sanitary discipline, adequate personnel, and competent administrative control and supervision. To secure this, the following conditions must be observed : (1) the number of pails provided to be double the number of latrine seats ; (2) removal of the pails and their contents to be carried out in daylight, say between 5 and 7 a.m. ; (3) when the pails in use are removed, clean ones containing a little dry earth to be placed in position ; (4) the dry earth to be dry, not wet, and sufficiently broken up to pass through a half-inch mesh ; (5) the supply of earth to be kept under cover, this is conveniently divided into two compartments, namely, one for a supply of earth to get properly dry before the contents of the other are used ; (6) boxes or receptacles at each latrine seat to hold dry earth ; (7) a scoop to be provided for each of these small receptacles ; (8) the constant attendance from "reveillé" to "last post" of a man at the latrine to remove pails which are full, and to replace in lieu thereof clean ones, and to maintain constant supervision that the contents are covered with earth ; (9) the excreta to be removed daily to a point at least half a mile from the camp.

(iii) For the ordinary or more or less temporary camps the usual latrine is a trench, provided or not with a seat. These trenches may be either long and deep, or short and shallow. If the long and deep trench system be used, a trench 20 yards long, 3 feet deep, and 16 inches wide is the necessary allowance for each hundred men ; this seats five per cent. of troops and allows a yard per man. The greatest care should be taken to prevent the water supply being fouled by these trenches, either directly by soakage, or indirectly by surface water in wet weather flowing from the trench or its immediate neighbourhood. The great difficulty about all latrines of this kind, no matter whether they have seats or not, is the fact that the front edge of the trench soon gets wetted with urine, and the front of the latrine rapidly becomes a urine-sodden quagmire, the mud from which gets carried back into the lines and tents on the men's boots. In the not remote chance of there being one or more undetected cases of enteric fever among the command, the possibilities of infection from this source are not difficult to imagine. To remedy this, the later practice has been to dig not one long trench but a series of short trenches in parallel, across which the user straddles and readily directs both solid and liquid excreta clear into the cavity, without soiling the sides. The trench on the short and shallow system should be 3 feet long, 2 feet deep, and 1 foot wide, and the interspace between each trench not more than three feet—preferably two and a half feet if the nature of the soil permits, so as to preclude the men using the trench otherwise than in the straddling attitude. These short trenches are far cleaner than the long type, they entail less labour to dig, and are more efficiently filled up and renewed. If available, a seat in the form of a stout pole can be laid at right angles to the trenches, supported on forked uprights. A back-rest may be formed by a similar pole, but is often omitted.

(iv) It is usual to allow five short and shallow trenches for every 100 men, but when the numbers of men are 500 or upwards, three per cent. of trenches suffice, that is 500 men can do very well with 15 trenches. As a rule, a trench lasts only one day. A trench can be made to last longer if the contents, which tend to get heaped up in the centre, are levelled off and if the earth used for covering the excreta be finely broken up. If the space available is limited and the trenches are not filled in one day, a fewer number may be provided. The interspace of 2½ feet is convenient and usually ample when the soil is firm, not sandy or crumbly. It allows plenty of room for another trench to be dug in it and the men using the second trench have nine inches of firm ground for each foot and there is an economy of space. A 3-foot interspace has the advantage of allowing more room between trenches, but it entails a longer frontage, more than is available with a minimum camping ground, and it also requires a greater length of screen.

The method of making and laying out these short and shallow trenches will be gathered from Figs. 25 and 26. Suppose B is the

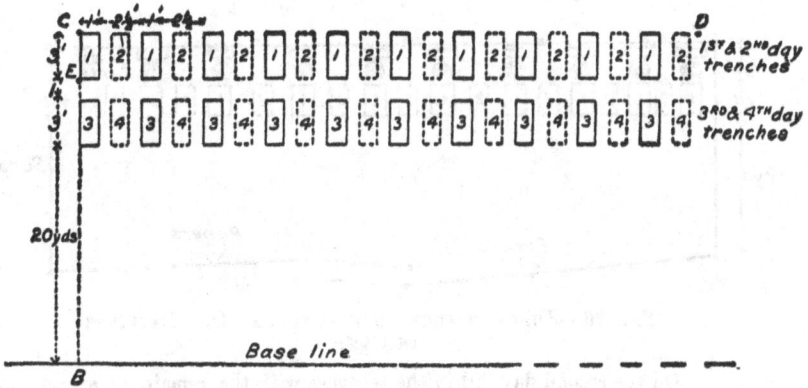

FIG. 25.—DIAGRAM SHOWING HOW TO LAY OUT LATRINES IN CAMP.

base line of the camp and that latrine trenches are to be dug to the rear; that the number of men is 200, and the probable length of occupation is thirty days. For this small number we must allow 5 per cent., or ten trenches daily, if over 500 men were present we could allow only 3 per cent. The frontage in yards required may be calculated as being six times the number of hundreds of men present, that is 200 men will need 12 yards of latrine frontage. The depth for latrine area is two-thirds the number of days' stay. In this case, the occupation being probably thirty days the required depth will be two-thirds of 30, or 20 yards.

From B, and at right angles, measure off twenty yards, or BC, and drive in a peg at C. From C, take the line CD parallel to the base of camp and measure 12 yards. This line CD equals the line of first row of trenches. From C, along CD, measure off 1-foot and 2½-feet spaces alternately, marking the spots with a spade till there are ten 1-foot spaces. To do this, it is convenient to use a stick which is 3 feet long and marked at 1 foot and 2½ feet, or a cord looped at one end and marked by pieces of coloured rag. From C measure three feet, CE. From E and parallel to CD mark off alternate spaces as before and join up. This outlines the first row of trenches. Next, remove the upper sod of each trench in one piece as far as possible, and put it about 3 feet behind the trench. Excavate the trenches till they are a clear foot deep, keeping the sides vertical, and placing the excavated earth immediately behind the trenches between it and the sod. This earth must be finely broken up. Surround the trenches with a canvas screen, the back being three feet behind and the fore-part at least six feet in front of the trenches. The entrance should be in the centre of the front and have a six-foot overlap. The length of screening necessary for 1,000 men on a 5 per cent. basis will be 130 yards; if twenty-five trenches are used, they will require 70 yards.

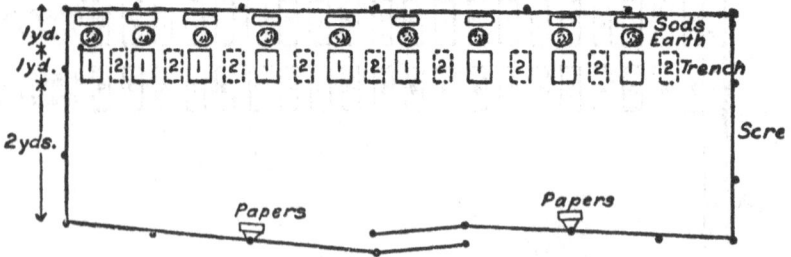

FIG. 26.—DIAGRAM SHOWING HOW TO LAY OUT LATRINES
IN CAMP.

On the second day, fill in the trenches with the remaining excavated earth, replace the sod, tread and beat down firmly. The advantage of the large upper sod is now obvious. Dig the second day's trenches in the interspaces of the first row. On the third day, dig a row of trenches similar to and parallel with the first row and one foot in front of them. Move the screening forward so as to surround them properly. Repeat the construction of trenches on the subsequent days in a precisely similar manner. After the latrine has been prepared, examine the slope of the ground and, if necessary, dig a shallow drain to divert surface water from the trenches, taking care that it does not flow on to the ground in front of the trenches, which will have to be used later on. This precaution applies also to urinals.

For covering the deposited excreta with earth, some kind of implement such as one or more spades, scoops, empty tins, or tin-lids must be provided near each trench for replacing earth and covering the filth over. Kicking the earth in by the foot is certain to be a failure and should be discouraged, as conducive to imperfect covering of the excreta, and consequent slackness. Men must be told the necessity for covering their dejecta; this precept cannot be impressed upon them too often. Failure on their part to cover their excreta properly should be made a matter of discipline, and systematically punished.

(v) Considerable supervision is required over all latrines, and their proper administration is a most important factor in the preservation of the health of men living in camps or bivouacs. One rule only must dominate the successful working of these places and that is all excreta must be covered up as soon as possible with earth, not only for mere purposes of deodorization, but to preclude the access to it of flies. These insects are one of the great means by which this filth and the associated germs are carried to man and his food. The practical problem is, how is this systematic and instant covering of excreta with earth to be secured and who is to do it? Is each individual man to cover his own filth or are special men to be detailed for this particular purpose? Where ordinary earth-closets or pail-middens are fixed in camps there should be no difficulty in providing a number of boxes of dry earth with the necessary scoops, and so enabling, with the least trouble, each individual to cover his own fæcal deposit. This is the proper way for it to be done. In other camps, where the ordinary trench-latrine only exists the situation is not so simple. In the first place the available soil is less conveniently placed, the provision of a sufficiency of spades or scoops is not always practicable, and the whole surroundings of the place conduce to a hurried rather than a leisured resort on the part of the individual. The remedy lies in strict enforcement of discipline and compulsion of the men to cover up their own excreta with earth at the latrines, moreover, a sanitary patrol or policeman must be placed over the latrine to see that each man fulfils his duty to himself and his neighbour. The only alternative to this is to place a man within the screen, provided with a spade, and direct him to cover each deposit with earth as each depositor moves off. In either case, the tour of this latrine duty should not exceed two hours, and in the early part of the day might well be limited to one hour. So long as the sanitary foresight of men remains at the present low level, the latrine sentry, however great the sentimental objections may appear, is a necessity. The question arises, where are the latrine sentries to come from ? Are they to be drawn only from the sanitary detachment or from the unit as a whole ? Clearly, the latrine sentry must come from the whole unit as being the best means of imbuing the minds of all concerned with their own personal responsibilities in protecting the health of their own unit and the army at large. The tour of duty should be short, say one to two hours, and the interval long. Consistent practice on these lines will soon lead to a great change for the better in the care and management of these places. When this is so, the incidence of filth originated or dust and fly-borne disease in camps will be sensibly lessened.

The condition of all latrines should be verified personally by the orderly officer of the day at least once during each twenty-four hours. So soon as the latrine trenches have been filled in to within six inches of the ground level their use should be discontinued, earth thrown in and the turf or sods replaced. On the abandonment of a camp or a bivouac, all the latrine trenches must be filled in and the site marked as foul ground.

(vi) From time to time a variety of excreta-incinerators have been suggested. Experience has shown them to be unsuccessful except when dealing with small quantities of fæcal material ; they certainly are not suited for general use by troops constantly on the move. In fixed camps, much more could be done than is usually attempted in this direction by burning the latrine-pail contents with ordinary refuse and litter in one or other of the refuse-incinerators which have been described. In so doing, care must be taken not to create an offensive smell or nuisance, but in the light of practical experience the objections from this cause are not so great as many suppose. The essentials for success are: (1) Start with and maintain a fierce fire ; (2) add the excreta slowly ; and (3) only attempt to burn the solid material ; the liquid must not and cannot be disposed of by fire.

186. In all camps, where ordinary receptacles are not provided, pits or trenches must be dug for the purposes of urination. For day use, these *urinals* are best placed within the screen and adjacent to the latrine trenches. Given a reasonably absorbent soil, the urine soon disappears, but it may be that such will not occur; in this case, care must be taken to make supplementary pits, while at all times the exposed urine-sodden soil must be covered at least three times a day with clean dry earth to protect it from flies. For night use, when special urine-tubs cannot be provided, or when the day urine-pits are any distance from the tents, it may be necessary to dig shallow urine-pits near the men's lines into which they can micturate at night. This is a practice which should be resorted to as rarely as possible ; at all times such pits must be carefully filled in at dawn. Urine-tubs can be extemporized easily from empty oil-tins, which may with advantage be partly filled with grass, chopped straw, sawdust, earth, or any other absorbent material. These tins should be mounted on boxes or on rough wooden trestles, to reduce to a minimum all chance of splashing or spilling.

A variety of improvised urinals can be planned for camp use. These will best take the form of shallow trenches, at least 2 feet wide leading into a pit filled with large stones, the trench being for urinating into, and the pit to take the excess which fails to soak into the soil. Roughly, two trenches, each 8 feet long, will suffice for a battalion of full strength. The gradient should be a fall of one inch to the foot. The catch-pit will vary in depth and size according to soil and number of men using the trenches; one 3 feet deep and 3 feet in diameter in a moderately porous soil should

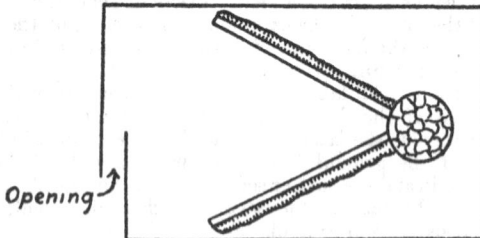

FIG. 27.—PLAN OF CAMP URINAL.

suffice for 800 to 1,000 men. Fig. 27 shows a typical example of one of these rough urinals. The trenches will last about two days and the pit some eight days; when foul, new trenches can be dug as radii from the pit and the old ones filled in and all grass sods replaced. In some cases it may be feasible to screen off the pit to prevent men actually micturating into it, shifting the screen with the trenches, or, better still, cover the pit with sods supported on stakes, and leave apertures by which the contributing trenches may drain into it. The ground around a urinal should be burnt when another has to be dug or the camp evacuated.

137. Much of the success or failure in regard to efficient sanitary control of an encampment depends upon the planning or arrangement of the area. To a large extent this again depends upon the extent of land available. Assuming that the space is equivalent to that officially laid down, the various sanitary arrangements, such as cooking places, washing places, incinerators, latrines, and urinals should be located in the rear of the tents in what can conveniently

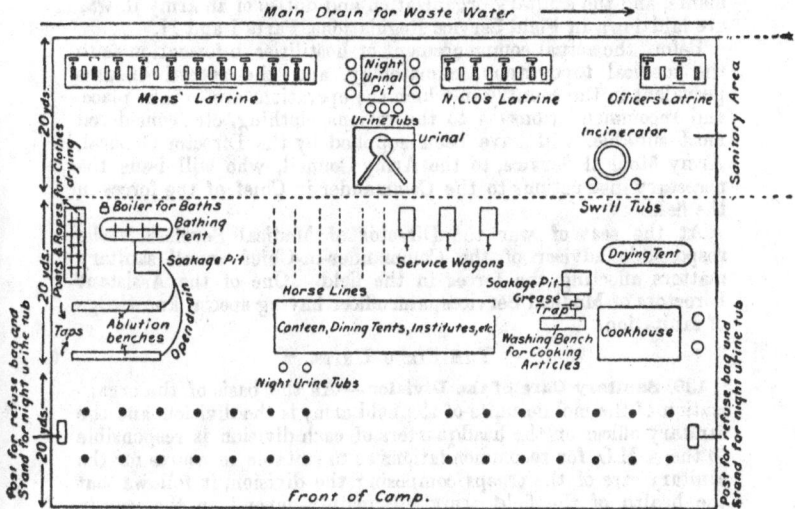

FIG. 28.—PLAN OF CAMP.

be termed the "sanitary area." As a general guide as to how these arrangements can be located, Fig. 28 may well serve as a type. Conditions vary so much that no official plan is recognized, but each case must be judged on its merits.

In closing this subject of the sanitary control of the camp, it is desirable to emphasize the fact that much of its successful practice depends upon the exercise of care and personal initiative. This is required not only of the men, but of the officer; there can be little doubt that the men in all these matters will and must take their cue from the officer. The essential principle of sanitation in the camp, as elsewhere, is *cleanliness*. This state of cleanness must not only be maintained while the camp is occupied, but on evacuation the camp area must be left sweet and tidy, so that those coming after may not suffer from a heritage of filth. The surest index of the cleanliness of men and places is the absence of flies, for if there is no dirt or filth to feed upon the fly will not be present

CHAPTER XIII.

SANITARY ORGANIZATION IN WAR.

188. In war the importance of an efficient sanitary organization whereby health is maintained cannot be over-estimated. Details of the number of officers and soldiers specially allotted for this purpose to the forces in the field are contained in War Establishments, and the sanitary organization and duties of an army in war are laid down in Field Service Regulations, Parts I and II.

Before the actual commencement of hostilities, information as to the medical topography, climatology, and the special diseases prevalent in the country in which the operations are to take place, and recommendations as to the rations, clothing, etc., considered most suitable, will have been supplied by the Director-General, Army Medical Service, to the Army Council, who will issue the necessary instructions to the Commander-in-Chief of the forces in the field.

At the seat of war the Director of Medical Services is the responsible adviser of the Commander-in-Chief on all sanitary matters affecting the forces in the field. One of the Assistant Directors of Medical Services is an officer having special knowledge of sanitation.

THE FIELD UNITS.

139. Sanitary Care of the Division.—As the basis of the organization of the mobile units of the field army is the division, and the sanitary officer on the headquarters of each division is responsible to the A.M.O. for recommendations as to suitable measures for the sanitary care of the troops composing the division, it follows that the health of the field army will mainly depend on the way in which the sanitary officer realizes his responsibilities and performs his duties.

140. Duties of the Sanitary Officer on the Headquarters of a Division.—(i) Subject to such other instructions as he may receive from the A.M.O., the sanitary officer will exercise general supervision over the sanitary condition of all places occupied by the troops of the division.

(ii) On the march he should accompany the staff officer charged with the selection of camps, billets, or bivouacs, and advise as to the selection from a sanitary point of view of sites for camps and bivouacs, and on questions relating to the sanitary condition of towns, villages, or buildings about to be occupied.

(iii) He will carefully inspect the water supplies available and will request the staff officer to take steps to ensure that sources obviously unsuitable may be policed before the arrival of the troops. He will also make careful inquiries from the local authorities of towns and villages as to the prevalence of infectious disease, and take all the necessary precautions. He will advise as to special methods required for the distribution and purification of water.

(iv) When the division is encamped on the banks of a river he should select and point out to the staff the place or places most suitable for the supply of drinking water, and also places for watering horses and bathing so situated as not to be likely to cause pollution of the drinking water. The individual units of the division should not be allowed to select these places, as watering and bathing parties might pollute the drinking water of units encamped lower down the stream. On the bank of a river there should be one place for obtaining drinking water, one place for watering animals, and one place for bathing ; and if possible, water for these purposes should be supplied direct to the units, so that in case of the division moving again over the same route, and still having to use the same stream as a source of supply, the water supply may be polluted as little as possible. These conditions, although the best, can only be obtained when there is time to erect stages into the river and pump water into troughs from which water-carts may be filled and animals "watered."

When springs and wells are the only source of supply, arrangements must be made for the distribution of water ; and after a rapid survey the sanitary officer should indicate the best general methods for this purpose.

(v) When advising as to sites for the various units of the division, the sanitary officer will have to indicate the best position for the sanitary area of each unit. The latrines, urinals, and destructor of one unit must on no account be placed in proximity to cookhouses of adjacent units. It is also of first importance to secure that during heavy rain the surface water from the sanitary area will not invade the drinking-water area.

When in touch with the enemy and the component parts of the division are advancing along different roads and on a wide front, much must be left to the initiative of the units themselves.

(vi) After an action the burial of the dead and destruction of the carcasses of slaughtered animals must be performed under the best sanitary conditions possible in the circumstances, and the sanitary officer will be required to advise as to the system which should be adopted.

(vii) The sanitary officer must at once investigate the cause of any unusual prevalence of disease among the troops or inhabitants of towns and villages occupied by, or in proximity to, the troops.

(viii) The detection of the earliest cases of enteric fever is of prime importance especially when the troops are under canvas or quartered in buildings. Under conditions of field service, infection by contact is one of the most common means of spreading the disease. It is essential to remove infected cases at once ; and, while it is also essential for the prevention of the spread of disease to isolate contacts as far as possible, care must be taken not to deplete the fighting ranks unnecessarily.

It should be possible in the majority of cases to isolate in all essential particulars a party of contacts without detaching them from their unit. By separate arrangements for messing, billeting, and sanitation, by disinfection of clothing, where possible, and by strictly enforced orders prohibiting unauthorized communication, it should be possible to prevent contacts being a source of danger to others. This is the problem the sanitary officer will have to face, and upon the timeliness of his advice and its practicability will largely depend the fighting value of the division.

(ix) He must impress upon all M.Os. of units the vital importance of detecting early cases of enteric fever. He must advise as to arrangements to be made for the isolation of all contacts with suspected cases of enteric fever, and for the disinfection of the clothing and blankets of contacts. This is admittedly difficult when the force is in actual touch with the enemy, but in the intermediate phases of operations it is quite possible to carry out these preventive measures.

(x) The A.M.O. may require the sanitary officer to prepare for his consideration drafts for insertion in divisional orders, or for publication to those concerned in other convenient form, embodying instructions for the sanitary measures which are to be adopted on the orders of the divisional commander.

141. Sanitary care of the Brigade.—There is no special sanitary organization for the brigade as a whole ; but, should it be acting independently, or should the division have such a wide front that the sanitary officer of the division cannot supervise the whole, the senior medical officer of the brigade will act as the sanitary adviser of the brigade commander and should carry out, as far as possible, the duties already outlined as pertaining to the sanitary officer of the division.

142. Sanitary care of the Unit.—The commander of every unit is responsible to superior authority for the sanitary condition of any area which it may occupy, and it is his duty to see that all ranks render loyal and intelligent assistance to the medical officer who is responsible to the C.O. for the efficient performance of the work of the regimental sanitary detachment.

143. The medical officer in charge of a unit, under the direction of the A.M.O. and with the advice of the sanitary officer of the division will be mainly responsible for the detection and prompt removal of all cases likely to prejudice the health of the unit. He must be alive to the protean types which enteric fever so often displays on field service. At the *commencement* of a campaign, when men have not become accustomed to field service conditions, atypical cases of enteric fever are very likely to occur. It is of vital importance, in these circumstances, to make frequent medical inspections of the unit and to send all febrile cases so detected to the medical unit detailed to receive them. When the men are housed in tents or permanent buildings there is a great probability of infection by contact, and when febrile cases develop in these circumstances, the men associated with them (contacts) should be regarded as possible sources of infection and should be medically examined as frequently as possible and especially from the 10th to 14th day after association with a febrile case.

The duties of a medical officer in charge of a unit are particularly onerous and responsible, because he is the first link in the chain of protective measures which safeguard the health of the division. While he must use every effort to prevent undue depletion of the fighting force, he must also remember that his paramount duty is to prevent an outbreak of infective disease, which, originating in his unit, may spread to the whole division. By careful attention to sanitary detail, he should be able to prevent the introduction of disease from *without*, but his chief difficulty will be to prevent the spread of infection originating *within* the unit. No matter how carefully men are inspected before being found "fit" for field service, it is certain that "enteric carriers" will be found amongst the men composing the field force. But if the medical officers in charge of units realize their responsibilities and take prompt action on the lines indicated, they should be able to prevent the "mass" infection which has hitherto attended all field operations.

144. The duties of the regimental sanitary detachment, which forms part of the regimental medical establishment, are as follows:—

(i) *Water duties:*—N.C.Os. and men are detailed for the daily supervision of the water supply and its purification for drinking purposes by heat, filtration, or the addition of chemicals, as may be directed. The men on water duty also take charge of all apparatus and stores connected with the water supply of the unit. They may also be required to carry out the disinfection of tents, quarters, and clothing as may be necessary, and to supervise contact cases, isolated by order of the C.O. on the advice of the M.O., and all cases of infectious disease segregated before removal from the unit. But whenever possible, men while actually employed on water duties should on no account handle infected clothing, or be brought in actual contact with the sick.

(ii) *Sanitary duties:*— N.C.Os. and men are also detailed to act as sanitary police, and to carry out, with such assistance as may be necessary, the preparation and care of latrines and urinals, including the filling in of the same and marking of old sites; the collection and disposal of refuse; the construction of ablution places and disposal of waste water; and the sanitation of cooking places, horse and mule lines, and slaughtering places in the area occupied by the unit. The men detailed as sanitary police may be provided regimentally with the badge (arm) lettered "R.P." worn by other regimental policemen.

The M.O. of the unit will allocate the various duties amongst the men composing the sanitary detachment, remembering, as has been indicated in the previous paragraph, that men employed on water-duties should on no account handle infected clothing or be brought in contact with the sick.

The Lines of Communication.

145. The sanitary service on the L. of C. is organized on a more permanent basis than that of the field units. A Deputy Director of Medical Services on the headquarters of the I.G.C. is his adviser on all sanitary measures affecting the whole L. of C., such as the selection of sites for hospitals, convalescent camps, methods of housing the troops, etc. One of the Assistant Deputy Directors of Medical Services is an officer having special knowledge of sanitation.

For purposes of sanitary administration the L. of C. is divided into sanitary districts and sanitary posts.

146. Sanitary Districts.—As a rule the base, advanced base, and any especially important part of the L. of C. will form a separate sanitary district. Towns and villages occupied by civil inhabitants may be included in a sanitary district. A sanitary officer is appointed to each district and a sanitary section is also allotted thereto to form the nucleus of a sanitary establishment, which is supplemented by such hired civilian labour as can be procured.

147. Duties of the Sanitary Officer of a District.—(i) The sanitary officer is the adviser of the administrative commandant, who is responsible to the I.G.C. for the sanitation of the district.

(ii) The duties of a sanitary officer of a district are analogous to those of a medical officer of health, and include, generally, the supervision of food and water supplies, the disposal of sewage and refuse, disinfection, and all measures necessary to prevent the introduction and spread of infectious disease. The sanitary officer must inform himself, as far as practicable, respecting all influences affecting or threatening to affect injuriously the public health within the district. Systematic inspection of towns and villages occupied by civil inhabitants will form an important part of his duties. He must inquire into the causes, origin and distribution of diseases within the district, and ascertain to what extent the same have depended on conditions capable of removal or mitigation. On receiving information of the outbreak of any infectious disease he must at once visit the spot where the cases have occurred, and inquire into the causes and circumstances of such outbreak, and take such measures as appear necessary to prevent the extension of the disease. He must keep records of his inspections and of recommendations made to the administrative commandant. When the lines of communication pass through a friendly country and there is a medical officer of health appointed by the civil administration, the sanitary officer should ascertain from him the sanitary circumstances of the town or village under his charge—and especially as to the existence and location of infectious disease likely to affect the health of the troops.

(iii) Fully equipped laboratories will be formed in the districts containing the base and advanced base, and the sanitary officers will supervise the chemical and bacteriological work performed therein. The chemical work will mainly consist in the analysis of water, foods, and sewage effluents. The bacteriological investigations will be chiefly directed towards the diagnosis of enteric fever, dysentery,

malaria, and, possibly, cholera. The examination of convalescent
enteric cases and the detection of "carrier" cases will form an
important part of the work performed at the railhead laboratory,
and an officer specially qualified in bacteriology will probably be
required to assist the sanitary officer in these examinations.

(iv) In the sanitary district formed at the base the sanitary officer
will be the adviser of the senior medical officer and through him of
the base commandant. If this sanitary district includes a seaport,
the sanitary officer will also perform the duties of port sanitary
officer, and may be assisted by one or more assistant sanitary
officers.

(v) A port sanitary officer must inform himself as far as practicable
of all conditions affecting the health of crews and other persons on
ship-board within the district. He must inquire into the causes,
origin, and distribution of diseases in the ships, and ascertain to what
extent the same have depended on conditions capable of removal or
mitigation. By inspection of all shipping he must keep himself
informed of the conditions injurious to health existing therein. On
receiving information of the arrival within the district of any ship
having infectious disease on board he must visit the vessel
without delay, and inquire into the causes and circumstances of
such outbreak and take such precautions as appear necessary to
prevent the introduction of the disease into the district. He must
make arrangements for the isolation of actual and suspected cases
of infectious disease, and for the control of "contacts." Specific
instructions regarding smallpox, plague, malarial and yellow fevers
are contained in the Regulations for the Army Medical Service.

148. Sanitary Sections.—(i) A section is allotted to each
district, and constitutes the sanitary personnel at the disposal
of the sanitary officer in charge. The duties of the personnel
will be allocated by the sanitary officer. They comprise
inspection work such as is performed by sanitary inspectors in civil
life; special duties in connection with the supply of water at, and the
conservancy of, railway stations; chemical and bacteriological work
in the laboratories at railhead and the base; and supervision of disinfecting stations.

(ii) The N.C.Os. and men composing a sanitary section must all
have been trained in sanitary or laboratory duties, and, in addition, a
proportion must be experienced soldiers suitable for employment as
sanitary police. When necessary, privates may be appointed acting
lance-corporals without additional pay, under the rules laid down in
the King's Regulations.

(iii) If the district contains a town or villages and there is no
regular civil staff of sanitary inspectors, the sanitary officer must
arrange for the inspection of these places by N.C.Os. and men of
the section. The actual personnel employed will depend on the
number of inhabitants, the proximity of the town or villages to the
troops, and the general sanitary condition of the places at the time.
If buildings are made use of for the location of troops, and for the
formation of rest and convalescent camps, a strict sanitary super-

vision of the civil inhabitants will be required, and special arrangements also will have to be made for the provision of sanitary appliances to be used by troops and convalescents; fatigue parties employed in this conservancy work must also be supervised by one or more men of the sanitary section. For this purpose the N.C.Os. and men are invested with the authority of military police and wear a police badge, lettered " M.P." as for other military policemen.

(iv) Sanitary supervision of railway stations will form an important duty of the section. Pure water must be supplied to the troops passing through, and the conservancy arrangements generally will require constant attention.

149. Sanitary Posts.—Sanitary posts are formed at the various road or railway posts along the L. of C. The administrative commandant is responsible to the I.G.C. for the sanitation of the post and receives technical advice from the senior medical officer of the post.

To each post a sanitary squad is allotted, and others may from time to time be added or the squad strengthened from military or civil sources as local circumstances demand.

150. Sanitary Squads.—The duties of a sanitary squad are as follows :—

(i) To execute skilled work in connection with disinfection ; the provision of pure water, including its collection, distribution, and storage ; construction of incinerators, etc.

(ii) One or more of the men will be specially detailed to supervise the work of permanent fatigue parties, employed for conservancy or other work in connection with sanitation.

(iii) To act as sanitary police. For this purpose the N.C.Os. and men of the squad are invested with the authority of military police and wear a police badge, lettered " M.P.," as for other military policemen.

(iv) If a post has a railway station under military control, the squad exercises sanitary supervision over the water supply to the troops passing through, and over the conservancy arrangements generally.

The N.C.Os. and men of a sanitary squad must all have been trained in sanitary duties, and, in addition, a proportion must be experienced soldiers suitable for employment as sanitary police.

Privates may be appointed acting lance-corporals as in the case of a sanitary section.

151. Convalescent Depots.—It is probable that at selected places on the L. of C., large convalescent camps or depots will be arranged for the reception of men discharged from hospital, but not yet fit for duty in the field. The convalescent depots, having no sanitary personnel of their own, will be supervised by men of the sanitary squads or sanitary section of the posts, under the direction of the commandant, who is a medical officer. The method of housing the convalescent soldiers whether in tents, huts, or in available buildings, the water supply and the necessary sanitary appliances for the depot, will be arranged for by the D.D.M.S. with the advice of the sanitary officer of the district in which the depots are formed. (See also paras. 285–287, Chap. XVII.)

152. Rest Camps.—The sanitation of rest camps for troops moving up to join the field army will also be in charge of the sanitary sections and squads. But as the units occupying such camps will usually have their own sanitary personnel, who should be responsible for the proper sanitary state of the camp during occupation by the unit, the sanitary squads will be mainly responsible for the care of permanent installations for the supply of water, and for the supervision of civilian labour employed in the removal of excreta, etc.

THE SANITARY INSPECTION COMMITTEE.

153. On mobilization being ordered, a sanitary inspection committee is formed consisting of a combatant officer as president, a field officer R.E., and a field officer R.A.M.C., as members. The committee receive the instructions of the C. in C. through the D.M.S. The duties of the committee are :—

(i) To assist commanders and the medical service in their efforts to maintain the health of the army, not only by co-ordinating the work of the different military branches, but also by co-ordinating the military with the civil sanitary organization of the country or area occupied.

(ii) To initiate important schemes of general sanitation, and to serve as a board of reference for the solution of sanitary problems.

(iii) To visit and inspect stations occupied by troops, to advise local authorities regarding necessary sanitary measures, and to further in every way the maintenance of satisfactory sanitary conditions, reporting to the D.M.S. any measures they consider necessary.

(iv) To ascertain what sanitary appliances and materials of all kinds are required for the army, and that an adequate reserve is maintained.

PART III.—TRAINING IN TECHNICAL DUTIES IN THE FIELD.

THE CARE OF THE SICK AND WOUNDED.

(*See Definitions on p.* viii.)

CHAPTER XIV.

GENERAL REMARKS.

154. The earlier a wounded man comes under medical care, and the better the arrangements made for his reception, the more will he be benefited by professional skill. In the performance of its duties in relation to the care of the sick and wounded, with the object of relieving the troops from the charge of their non-effectives, the medical service is also required to deal with the discipline, pay, clothing, and disposal of all sick and wounded from the time they come under its care until they are discharged to duty. In order that its duties may be carried out effectively and suitable medical arrangements formulated for the various strategical and tactical operations in which an army may be engaged, a general knowledge of the principles upon which these operations are conducted is necessary to officers of the Corps, and reference should be made for this purpose to Field Service Regulations, Parts I and II.

155. The medical organization designed to deal with these duties may be divided into three zones,* namely :—(i) The collecting zone, corresponding with the area occupied by the field units and containing the regimental medical establishments, field ambulances, and cavalry field ambulances. In this zone the points of medical assistance to the wounded are, first, the regimental aid posts of the regimental medical establishments, and second, the advanced dressing stations, dressing stations, and divisional collecting station or stations of field ambulances. Cavalry field ambulances form collecting posts or dressing stations according to the nature of the operations. (ii) The evacuating zone, corresponding with the Lines of Communication and containing the clearing hospitals, ambulance trains, advanced depots of medical stores, and, in certain circumstances,

---

* This division of the theatre of warfare into three zones of medical service was first described by the late Surgeon-General Sir Thomas Longmore, C.B., etc. ("Gunshot Injuries," 1877.)

general and stationary hospitals. (iii) The distributing zone, which includes a portion of the L. of C., the Base, and, in an oversea war, territory outside the theatre of operations. It contains stationary and general hospitals, convalescent depots, ambulance trains, base depots of medical stores, hospital ships, and the military hospitals in the United Kingdom.

Although distinct in theory, in practice the three zones form a single service like the links in a chain. A certain amount of overlapping must naturally occur, just as a link fits into the next ; but, as in one chain, unless each link supports its neighbour, the whole is useless.

156. The establishments of the medical service in these zones are regulated by War Establishments. Their organization is laid down in Field Service Regulations, Part II, and details of their medical and ordnance equipment are contained in the Field Service Manual, Army Medical Service.

157. The duties of the Director of Medical Services and his relationship towards the Commander-in-Chief and the staff are laid down in Field Service Regulations, Part II.

The representative of the D.M.S. on the headquarters of the Inspector-General of Communications is a D.D.M.S., who is responsible to the I.G.C. and D.M.S. for the medical service of the L. of C., which includes the evacuating zone and the distributing zone, less, in an expedition over seas, such part of the distributing zone as may be outside the theatre of operations. His duties are similar to those of the D.M.S., but are restricted to the region under the administration of the I.G.C. Whether the D.D.M.S. would perform similar duties towards the Commander of L. of C. defence troops and the troops under his orders, would be a matter for determination with reference to the special circumstances of a campaign.

The senior officer of the medical service in a unit or command represents the D.M.S. when no officer has been specially appointed to do so. The Principal Matron, Queen Alexandra's Imperial Military Nursing Service, is attached to the headquarters of the I.G.C.

158. It is necessary that officers and men should be trained in the details of their duties in order that they may be carried out with despatch and precision.

Exercises and preparations carried out for instructional purposes during peace should be performed as thoroughly as in the theatre of actual war ; otherwise the omission of some detail, thought to be unnecessary when real casualties are not to be dealt with, may be repeated at some critical period in a campaign. The conditions of actual warfare, such as the disposition and movements of other troops, the long range of modern weapons, and the limitations which these factors impose, must always be kept clearly in mind.

159. The units which differ most markedly in their organization and duties from a military hospital in peace are cavalry field ambulances, field ambulances, and clearing hospitals, and consequently one or all of these units should form the basis of training.

CHAPTER XV.

THE COLLECTING ZONE.

THE MEDICAL SERVICE WITH A DIVISION.

160. The medical service with a division comprises: (i) the A.M.O. of the division and his headquarters; (ii) the regimental medical establishments with units; (iii) field ambulances.

THE ADMINISTRATIVE MEDICAL OFFICER OF A DIVISION.

161. The A.M.O., as the representative of the D.M.S. on divisional headquarters, is the responsible adviser of the commander and staff on all technical matters connected with the medical service concerning the division. He commands the group of units of the R.A.M.C., and administers and is responsible for the distribution of the whole of the personnel of the corps in the division. As a commander (administrative commander), commanding the group of medical units, he receives and transmits to them the orders of the divisional commander, together with his own orders.

His relationship towards the personnel of the R.A.M.C. attached to units of other arms is that of administrator and superior officer in technical matters. The personnel of the corps so attached is under the orders of the officers commanding the units with which it is serving, and, while the A.M.O. is empowered to issue to all the R.A.M.C. in the division instructions in technical matters, and orders regarding medical stores and equipment, the ordinary channel for the communication of orders affecting the regimental medical establishments is by orders or instructions prepared by the A.M.O., but issued through the branch of the staff concerned to officers commanding brigades or units.

162. Under the orders of the divisional commander, and in consultation with the staff and officers of other administrative services concerned, the A.M.O. suggests, or drafts, as required, paragraphs for orders issued in the name of the divisional commander, notifying medical and sanitary matters which require to be known by the troops of the division.

As the O.C., R.A.M.C., he issues operation, routine, or other orders for the R.A.M.C., based on divisional orders. These should include orders for the medical units and medical arrangements approved by the divisional commander, as well as any divisional orders necessary. In routine orders he includes details affecting the services of the personnel of the corps, and sends extracts to the O.C. concerned if affecting the personnel of the corps attached to units of other arms or services.

General instructions on the subject of the preparation of orders are contained in Field Service Regulations, Part I, and by these the A.M.O. is guided in the preparation of drafts for divisional orders, and the issue of R.A.M.C. orders.

The Regimental Medical Establishments with Units.

163. Large units in the field, such as an infantry battalion, have a regimental medical establishment consisting of an officer in medical charge, orderlies for the M.O., stretcher bearers, N.C.Os. and men for sanitary duties, and N.C.Os. and men for water duties. Certain units, such as batteries, while they include men trained in first aid and the duties of stretcher bearers, have no stretcher bearers specially detailed for that purpose. The M.O's. orderlies and the stretcher bearers form the regimental medical detachment; the men for sanitary duties and men for water duties the regimental sanitary detachment. In addition to the medical and surgical equipment authorized for each unit, every officer and soldier carries a first field dressing. Medical and surgical equipment is replenished as necessary by the field ambulances.

164. Duties in the Field.—The regimental medical establishments of units carry out their duties under the orders of the officers commanding the units of which they form part, subject, however, to the administrative control of the A.M.O. in technical matters. The regimental stretcher bearers of a battalion remain with their companies until an action is imminent, when they are placed under the orders of the M.O. For their duties in action see paragraph 181.

The M.O's. orderlies are trained in first aid; the lance-corporal takes charge of the medical and surgical equipment, and attends the M.O. when seeing the sick. The second orderly, a private, drives the cart for medical equipment and is otherwise at the disposal of the M.O. For their duties in action see paragraph 180.

The duties of the regimental sanitary detachment are described in Chapter XIII.

The Field Ambulances.

165. Field ambulances are designed for the immediate medical assistance of the infantry and other troops in a division in war.

They are divisional troops, under the command of the A.M.O.; three field ambulances being included in each division. A field ambulance consists of a bearer division for the early medical assistance and collection of wounded, and a tent division for their reception, temporary treatment, and care; and is divisible into three sections, A, B, and C, each capable of acting independently, or even of being mobilized separately. Each section is organized as a bearer sub-division and a tent sub-division. The transport consists of ambulance wagons for the carriage of sick and wounded, and transport wagons and carts for the carriage of medical and surgical stores, equipment, and water. An ambulance being an administrative unit, its transport marches with it as a whole.

A field ambulance like other British medical establishments in the field is distinguished during the day by a flag bearing the Geneva Cross on a white ground and a Union Jack flying side by side on a cross-bar, and during the night by two white lamps placed horizontally.

166. General duties in the Field.—The general military duties of all arms in the field are laid down in Field Service Regulations, Parts I and II.

167. The disposition of a field ambulance in action varies with the nature of the operations, *e.g.*, according as it forms part of a force carrying out a deliberate attack, holding a defensive position, engaged in an encounter battle requiring the arrangements to be carried out unexpectedly from the line of march, or during a retirement. Operations of a different nature and each requiring appropriate medical arrangements may be in progress at the same time.

As a general rule the disposition of a field ambulance in action is :—(i) the whole bearer division or one or two sub-divisions in advance ; (ii) the ambulance wagons working between the bearer division and the dressing station or advanced dressing station ; (iii) the last-named posts, formed by one or more tent sub-divisions with the medical store carts and water-carts of the section or sections ; and (iv) the remainder of the unit, *i.e.*, the sections, sub-divisions, or transport held in reserve.

168. On the line of march, field ambulances, each of which occupies 380 yards of road space, follow their own divisions unless otherwise ordered, and usually march in rear of the brigade ammunition columns. The military situation may require medical units or sections to be placed nearer the head of a main body, *e.g.*, owing to the length of the column, or the possibility of an engagement necessitating a rapid deployment ; but should it be considered that wheeled ambulance-transport is required with the fighting troops on the line of march, the commander's orders will be taken on the subject ; however, the possibility of placing personnel, without transport, nearer the head of the column should be considered.

The ambulance wagons of one or more of the field ambulances may be distributed to battalions or other formations for the purpose of carrying casualties ; but whether ambulance transport may be detached from medical units in this manner will depend upon the circumstances and must be subservient to the purpose of the march, and the likelihood of immediate battle.

169. On the line of march, and on arrival in camp, the sick of units will be received by a field medical unit detailed by the A.M.O., and notified to the troops, and will thereafter be disposed of under his orders in accordance with arrangements made by the D.M.S. and notified from general headquarters.

170. In a concentration area, and during periods of inactivity, the medical units should be placed on the natural line of evacuation from the area, and sick from outlying posts should be brought in by ambulance wagons detailed for the purpose, at fixed hours daily.

171. Strong outposts in isolated positions may require medical personnel and transport to be temporarily allotted to them from the medical units.

THE DISPOSITION OF THE MEDICAL SERVICE WITH A DIVISION CARRYING OUT AN ATTACK.

ADMINISTRATIVE ARRANGEMENTS.

172. The A.M.O. should be present when the staff are preparing divisional operation orders for an engagement. On receiving information as to the military situation and on being made acquainted with the intentions of the commander and the orders to be issued to the fighting troops, he will propose medical arrangements suitable for the fight, having regard to the object in view.

173. He will state the number of field ambulances or sections of field ambulances he intends to employ, and the areas he proposes to allot to them, specifying as far as possible the actual limits of the frontages, the positions at which the units should be at a given hour, and, if he is able to select them beforehand, the number and sites of dressing stations and the hour at which they should be formed.

He will also suggest a position for the divisional collecting station for slightly wounded men, if the probable nature of the fight renders it desirable to establish one.

He then drafts, as occasion requires, paragraphs for insertion in divisional operation orders notifying such of the foregoing arrangements, as finally determined, that it is necessary for the troops generally to know.

He should also arrange with the staff regarding the routes to be followed by the medical units, and the time and order of march.

174. All men unfit to remain with their units, and who cannot be utilized to assist the medical service, will be sent to the ambulance detailed in divisional routine orders to receive them, and they with other sick in the field medical units will usually be evacuated by means of the supply vehicles which serve the division, when returning empty. Should it be impossible to evacuate all, on account of their condition or because transport is not available at the time, a sufficient detachment, with equipment, will be left in charge of them, general headquarters being informed so that the detachment may be relieved by a medical unit from the L. of C. and sent to rejoin the division as early as possible.

175. Regard must be had to the subsequent evacuation of wounded from the battle. Normally, this will be arranged under the orders of the I.G.C., the means employed being the empty supply column vehicles referred to above, supplemented by local transport when necessary. The arrangements made in this respect and the clearing hospitals or other medical units to receive sick and wounded are notified from time to time from general headquarters to commanders of divisions. The divisional authorities will require to arrange for the conveyance of wounded to the supply vehicles, or to a clearing hospital should one have been brought up close to the division. For this purpose the ambulance wagons of the divisional medical units may be supplemented by transport obtained locally by divisional headquarters.

Further details regarding this subject are contained in paras. 262 to 274, Chapter XVI. The A.M.O. will state his proposals in this matter when divisional operation orders or instructions consequent on them are being prepared, in order that the scheme decided on may be included in the general administrative arrangements for the division.

176. The possibility of a large number of wounded having to be fed by the medical service should not be lost sight of.

177. The general scheme of the medical arrangements having been agreed upon by divisional headquarters, and the necessary drafts of orders prepared, the A.M.O. will next issue R.A.M.C. operation orders for the units under his command. He will include information regarding the general situation, but only so much, if any, of the divisional commander's intention as may be necessary for the proper performance of the duties allotted to the medical units. If it will assist Os.C. ambulances, he will intimate the general plan of the medical arrangements, *e.g.*, the position of a clearing hospital, or the arrangements made for evacuation.

He will embody the divisional operation orders for the medical units, amplifying them where necessary, and giving particulars of the route to be followed ; the time and order of march ; the areas allotted, their limits, and the troops to be engaged in them ; the positions to be reached and the hour.

If, as is generally the case, the nature of the fight has not permitted the selection of dressing stations beforehand, the A.M.O. may direct the Os.C. ambulances to select sites on arrival at the position assigned to their units, after reconnaissance of the ground and observation of the action ; or he may order them to await his decision. When the A.M.O. reconnoitres the ground he should be accompanied by the Os.C. ambulances or their representatives.

R.A.M.C. orders will also state the position and the personnel and equipment detailed for the divisional collecting station, if one is to be opened; the arrangements made for evacuation, and the duties of the ambulances in this respect ; the units or sections which are to be held in reserve, specifying the locality ; and the place, usually divisional headquarters, to which reports to the A.M.O. will be sent.

The reserves are kept for use when the action develops and it becomes known where the greatest number of casualties is taking place.

178. Officers detailed for reconnaissance with a view to selecting sites for dressing stations should bear in mind the requirements mentioned in para. 202, and the provisions of para. 204, and should supplement their reports with simple field sketches, if such would facilitate the choice of a position.

179. In the case of a night attack, sites for regimental aid posts and dressing stations should be selected, and if possible pointed out to the troops during daylight with proper safeguards to prevent disclosure of the intention to the enemy. In certain circumstances, it may be expedient to direct the personnel for duty at these posts to proceed there independently of the troops to which they are attached.

THE REGIMENTAL MEDICAL ESTABLISHMENTS.

180. The medical arrangements notified in divisional or brigade operation orders are communicated to the M.Os. by officers commanding units. The regimental medical establishments accompany their units and remain with them throughout the action. Before the action commences, the stretcher bearers (without arms, which will be in the medical equipment cart) will be placed under the orders of the M.O. They will be provided with stretchers from the medical equipment cart of the unit, and will wear the stretcher bearers' armlet (S.B.) on the left arm. One of the bearers may be provided with a surgical haversack and water-bottle.

The M.O's. orderly lance corporal will carry the field medical companion and water-bottle and accompany the M.O.

The medical equipment cart, after the above material has been taken out, will remain, under the charge of the second orderly, in some suitable position which can be used as a regimental aid post or with the first line transport of the unit until required.

In units which have no stretcher bearers, such as artillery, the M.O. and his orderlies render what assistance they can to the wounded who may be unable to walk, obtaining assistance from the unit if it can be afforded to carry them to a place under shelter. Otherwise their duties in action are as herein described.

181. During the engagement, the regimental medical detachments will render first aid to the wounded and will remove them, if possible, from the firing line and place them under cover. If they cannot be brought to the regimental aid post, it will facilitate their subsequent removal if they are collected in groups. The movement of stretcher squads in an exposed position is apt to draw fire, but, individuals taking every advantage of cover may frequently render valuable immediate assistance. Serious cases should be attended to first, if practicable. The immediate treatment should be confined to the arrest of hæmorrhage, the application of the first field or other dressing, the relief of pain,* and the application of support to a broken limb.

A guiding principle, after immediate treatment has been rendered, is to leave a seriously wounded man where he lies, giving him as much cover as possible, until there is a pause in the fighting or until the progress of the action permits the systematic removal of the wounded to take place. Specification-tallies should be attached to each wounded man. (See para. 197.)

182. Regimental Aid Posts.—Each medical officer with a unit, under the orders of the C.O., will endeavour to select suitable places which may be used as regimental aid posts, to which the regimental stretcher bearers will bring the wounded, and where they can be attended to and left until taken over by the field ambulances.

---

* For the relief of pain, a hypodermic tabloid of morphia placed under the tongue is rapidly absorbed and the difficulty of using syringes and solutions is avoided. Opiates should only be used under the orders of a medical officer.

A regimental aid post should be under cover or out of the line of fire, but sufficiently near the firing line as to be readily accessible. One or more will be selected for each battalion or other unit.

183. Information regarding wounded left under cover or in villages, should be communicated to the inhabitants so that they may be easily found by the field ambulances; a message should also be sent back, if possible, to the field ambulances indicating where they will be found. The occasions on which field ambulances cannot keep touch with the regimental medical establishments are rare.

THE FIELD AMBULANCES.

184. R.A.M.C. orders having been received, the manner in which the task allotted to each unit is carried out will rest with the O.C., who will in turn issue orders to his unit. Guided by the information and orders given him, he must rely upon his own initiative in unforeseen contingencies. He will inform his superior officer of important developments which it is necessary for that officer to know, especially as regards the accumulation of wounded. Whether the selection of dressing stations has been made by the A.M.O., or left to the discretion of unit commanders, the principle will always be observed of not employing more sections of ambulances at first than are absolutely necessary, in order that some may be kept in hand to meet any development of the action.

185. The Divisional Collecting Station is the place where slightly wounded men, able to walk, are collected, treated, fed, and rested before further evacuation or return to their units. If large numbers of wounded have to be dealt with, it should be a village or prominent feature in the landscape which can be easily seen and reached, but should be well to the rear and not on the main line of evacuation. It may be in the locality of, or attached to, a selected dressing station when the number of casualties is not large. Other places are where the units or sections are being held in reserve, or where transport is collected for the subsequent evacuation of the wounded, in which case the detachment preparing the wagons for sick transport (see para. 268, Chapter XVI) could give such attention as is required to the slightly wounded men arriving there. A unit may be ordered to detail a tent sub-division or other detachment for duty at the collecting station.

Preparation for feeding the wounded may be necessary, and if possible some shelter should be available.

In the event of there being large numbers of slightly wounded, any of the officers or N.C.Os. not incapacitated from assisting in maintaining discipline among them should be ordered to do so, and in practice the slightly wounded may be formed into squads, under N.C.Os. of their own regiments if possible, in order that proper control may be maintained.

186. A unit to be employed in an area of the field, or as many sections as are ordered to proceed, will move off to the position assigned. There the bearer division or sub-divisions will be disengaged from the remainder of the unit, and the stretcher squads formed up, ready to advance when ordered, accompanied, if the military situation permits and the ground is suitable, by the ambulance wagons of the sections employed.

187. If a dressing station is to be opened at this point, it will be prepared by a dressing station party consisting of one or more of the tent sub-divisions. One tent sub-division with medical store cart and water-cart will be held in readiness to advance with the bearer division for the purpose of forming an advanced dressing station where the stretcher squads transfer to the ambulance wagons.

If only one tent sub-division forms a dressing station at first, additional personnel from the remaining tent sub-divisions may be added subsequently as required.

188. Any portions of the tent division not brought into action at once will stand fast in reserve, with the wagons drawn up on the side of the road, or parked in its immediate vicinity so as to avoid interference with movements. They will be ready to open where halted, and receive wounded brought in by the ambulance wagons ; or to move forward to any position where a dressing station is to be established ; or to go further forward and augment the advanced dressing station, the ambulance wagons then working between that point and a clearing hospital (if available and within reach), or to a tent sub-division forming a link between the dressing station and the clearing hospital. Communication should be maintained between the several portions of the unit.

As a rule dressing stations will be opened as soon as the troops in the area become engaged ; but this should not be done when the enemy is falling back, as a dressing station opened too early would, in that case, soon become out of touch with the troops.

189. During the progress of the attack, if the troops move so far forward that a further advanced dressing station is required, another tent sub-division with the necessary equipment will advance and open ; or, if the troops are more or less stationary and casualties accumulate, more tent sub-divisions may be ordered up to assist at the dressing station.

The whole field ambulance may encamp at one or other of the dressing stations ; but the principle of getting the wounded, by continuous removal, as far back at the earliest possible moment and in the smallest number of moves should never be lost sight of. This may involve keeping one or more sub-divisions open, 3, 4, or 5 miles back, as a link between the fighting line and the clearing hospital.

It is a bad plan to open far in advance unless victory is assured and a retreat of the enemy has commenced. It is only for the severe cases unfit for removal that tent divisions should be immobilized in advanced positions.

190. The C.O., while exercising supervision over the whole of the unit, should, as a rule, select a position which will be sufficiently central to facilitate the receipt of reports and the issue of orders. The sectional organization will be maintained as far as possible especially when two or more tent sub-divisions form a dressing station at the same place. If the C.O. detaches a section to work independently he will give to the section commander such special instructions as may be necessary.

191. The Bearer Division.—The first duty of the bearer division in advancing over an area where casualties are lying, is to establish communication with the regimental medical establishments of the troops engaged, with a view to ascertaining where the wounded are and taking them over.

The transmission of information regarding the sick and wounded and its speedy communication to the proper quarter, with a view to their early succour and disposal, is a duty in which all arms can assist the medical service.

The advance of the bearer division must necessarily depend upon circumstances, such as the area being no longer subjected to the enemy's fire, or the possibility of advancing under cover when rifle and shell fire render it unsafe to carry on the work of removing wounded without this protection. By taking advantage of cover, single bearers may often be able to reach wounded and give valuable help where it would be impossible for a squad to advance and carry off a wounded man. But a bearer division with an advanced dressing station party is justified in advancing over rather exposed ground if thereby it can reach "dead ground" nearer the front, where it can more effectively set up a dressing station. Whether any vehicles can accompany it must depend upon circumstances ; if necessary a few light articles and some material must be carried by hand.

192. It will seldom be possible to commence the collection of wounded until the firing line has advanced, or the successful delivery of the assault has left the ground clear for the stretcher squads and ambulance wagons to come up. The main work of collecting wounded takes place after a battle. Each sub-division, and each squad within it should work over a definite area. Careful search, especially of places affording concealment and cover, is necessary, particularly after nightfall, when the squads will require lanterns to aid them if their use is permissible. But even with lanterns the collection of wounded after nightfall takes longer than by day ; small obstacles are not seen, hence the bearers are more liable to stumble, and owing to absence of landmarks may lose their way.

When there are large numbers of wounded after a battle, the medical service may be assisted in the collection of wounded by parties of other troops, by the civil population, or by other means according to circumstances.

193. The wounded collected and dressed by the regimental medical establishments, and the wounded who have not previously received attention, must be searched for by the stretcher squads of the bearer division. When a wounded man has been placed on a stretcher by a regimental stretcher squad and is subsequently taken over by the personnel of an ambulance, he should not be moved from the stretcher on which he lies ; but the regimental stretcher squad should be provided with another stretcher and directed to return to their unit.

194. The ambulance wagons told off to act with the bearer division, or as many as are required, will be advanced at the earliest opportunity as near the area of fighting as the military situation and the nature of the country permit. They will work under the orders of the officers or N.C.Os. of the bearer division, each of whom will be responsible for directing the routes of the ambulance wagons of his sub-division or under his charge, utilizing, if necessary, semaphore, directing flags, or other means of direction fixed upon trees, walls, etc.

Each ambulance wagon is in charge of a wagon orderly from the bearer division ; a corporal in each section being in charge of one, privates of the others. Their duties are to see that the wagons keep in touch with the stretcher squads, to prepare the wagons for the carriage of wounded, to see to their immediate wants on their arrival, to attend to them on the journey, and to take charge of their kits and arms. Restoratives and dressings are carried in each wagon.

195. The officers will supervise the work of applying first-aid dressings, etc., to those wounded who have not already been attended to by the regimental establishments, and will direct the preparation of the wounded for removal ; deciding in the case of the seriously injured whether they are fit for immediate removal, and if so by what means. The main principle to be observed in directing the removal of wounded is to send off the slighter cases first, leaving those requiring hand-carriage to the last, in order that bearers may continue available for collecting wounded as long as required.

196. A stretcher squad performs its duties under the No. 4 bearer, upon whom, subject to the orders of the officer and N.C.O., devolves the general control of the squad and the rendering of such aid as may be necessary to the wounded. He directs the placing of a wounded man on the stretcher in a manner suitable to the particular injury ; first determining, in the absence of an officer or N.C.O., whether the patient is fit for removal at the time, and if so by what means. He also details bearers who may be disengaged to attend to the immediate wants of other wounded, afterwards visiting them to supervise their work. The arms and accoutrements of wounded men who are carried on stretchers will be collected and carried by the bearer detailed in Stretcher Exercises. The No. 4 bearer will detail a bearer to bring in the arms, etc., of other wounded men unable to carry them themselves.

When patients have to be carried long distances the whole squad will be required with the stretcher, in order that reliefs may be available. When the distance is short, No. 4 bearer will utilize bearers, not required with the stretcher, to assist slighter cases to reach the wagons or dressing station. Bearers should not, however, be detailed to accompany men who are able to walk back by themselves.

It usually takes about an hour for a squad to attend to a wounded man carry him back one mile, and return.

197. A specification-tally will be filled up and attached to each wounded man after first aid has been afforded, if one has not already been attached by the regimental medical establishments.

The nature of the wound (or wounds), *e.g.*, " gunshot," " shell," " bayonet," etc., its situation, *e.g.*, " chest," " neck," " right thigh," etc., and any special conditions, *e.g.* " hæmorrhage," " fracture left humerus," should be entered briefly on the tally. The man's number or name, and rank or regiment should be inserted according as such information is available from the man himself or from his identity-disc. Any precaution required in transit, and the fact of an opiate having been given and its amount will be noted. The counterfoil should be completed at the same time. Tallies of different colours, red for severely wounded, white for slightly wounded, are used to distinguish cases requiring immediate attention from slighter cases. Cases which have required the application of a tourniquet must be distinguished by a red tally, and the fact of a tourniquet having been applied must be noted on the tally.

198. The attention of a medical officer should, if practicable, be called to each severely wounded man before removal, and directions obtained from him as to the proper measures to be adopted during conveyance.

In certain cases, men very seriously wounded are best left for as long as possible where they lie, unless danger from fire or the movement of troops make it a matter of imperative necessity to move them to cover. Such cases comprise all penetrating abdominal wounds ; all cases of *severe* arterial bleeding, unless the artery has been efficiently controlled ; and cases with extreme collapse, such as wounds of the chest near or through the cardiac area.

Local circumstances must always determine whether such cases can be treated where they lie until they are fit to be brought in, or whether the risks of immediate removal must be taken. As a rule, after receiving surgical attention, they should as far as possible be protected from the weather, and left, if that can be arranged, in charge of someone, until the last possible moment, before they are eventually removed to the dressing station or other place where they may receive more complete treatment and attendance. A double move, *e.g.*, to a temporary dressing station, and then to a house or hospital, should be avoided ; the patients should be carried direct to the place where they will remain until danger from movement is past. Careful carriage by stretcher will be required.

Men with slight injuries, able to walk, should be directed to the dressing station or to the divisional collecting station appointed for the purpose of receiving such cases. (See para. 185.)

199. All stretcher squads so soon as they have carried their patients to the dressing station or placed them in an ambulance wagon, will provide themselves with other stretchers from the ambulance wagons and return to collect further casualties.

200. As each wagon is loaded it will move off in the charge of the wagon orderly to the dressing station, where it will unload and return to the front. It will carry back with it other stretchers if available from patients brought in before, and additional dressings if required.

When the work of the bearer division is prolonged, attention must be paid to watering and feeding the animals, and to the possibility of their having to be used for evacuation, or for a further advance with the troops.

201. Dressing Stations.—The dressing station or stations will be prepared by the tent sub-divisions or other dressing station parties appointed for the purpose, at the points selected. They will be in suitable buildings, if available; failing these, if shelter is required, tents will be pitched.

202. A dressing station should, if possible, be—(i) As far forward as consistent with reasonable safety. The range of rifle and shell fire and the configuration of the country must be most carefully considered; unless the ground affords adequate protection, the distance from the troops engaged is determined by the effect of the enemy's fire. Low-lying ground is more suitable than high ground as it generally affords protection, water is more easily obtained, and wounded have not to be carried uphill. (ii) Readily accessible to wheeled vehicles, and near a road close to the probable line of advance or retreat; but care must be taken not to block a road which may be required for the fighting troops. (iii) Near water if possible. (iv) Protected from gun and rifle fire. Positions in rear of troops are often subject to dropping fire. Proximity to an artillery position should be avoided. (v) On a site of sufficient space to encamp the entire field ambulance. Sites hidden in or by woods are bad, as they are difficult to find, hamper the movements of the wagons, limit expansion, and are dangerous in case of artillery fire. (vi) In suitable buildings. Such buildings should be easy of access; clean or capable of being readily cleaned and prepared for the reception of wounded; possess means of ventilation, and if possible, of lighting, warming, and cooking. Suitability for ready expansion of the dressing station is important. (vii) Where supplies of dry grass, straw, or other suitable material for the wounded to lie on are available.

203. The medical store cart will be unpacked, ground-sheets (if required), blankets and the necessary medical and surgical equipment taken out, and distinguishing flags erected; kitchens dug (if there are none suitable on the spot); and, if necessary, simple shelters erected and full provision made for the treatment and feeding of the wounded.

Every preparation will be made for the surgical treatment of such cases as demand urgent operation (which class of operation will alone be undertaken at the dressing station*), and for the thorough protection of wounds and injuries from dirt or additional injury during transit; fixation apparatus will be got ready, and material collected wherewith to improvise splints. A room for dressing and operating,

---

* In the treatment of abdominal wounds in a field ambulance, much depends on the particular circumstances of the case, and on the time and facilities for operation. The general principles are :—Avoid operation (except in urgent necessity). Avoid movement or disturbance of any kind. Give nothing by the mouth for at least 24 hours. Opium should be withheld if possible, but may be given to relieve severe pain

or the operating tent, will be prepared, instruments sterilized, and lotions and basins got ready, water boiled or otherwise sterilized, aprons and dressings put out and an operation table arranged. Restoratives, such as hot drinks and soups, and also meals for wounded men will be prepared by the cooks. Extra rations and additional medical comforts will be obtained on indent in the usual way, or if permissible, by requisition from local resources, as many of the wounded arrive exhausted and in need of a meal. If a building has been selected, it will be put in order for the reception and temporary housing of the wounded, otherwise tents will be prepared and straw or other material collected and arranged for the more seriously injured to lie upon.

Full particulars of all wounded received will be recorded according to regulations; this is a most important duty in connection with the subsequent tracing of wounded men.

204. As system and organization are of the greatest assistance in dealing with large numbers of wounded, one of the first and most important duties in forming a dressing station is to organize the station in departments, separate from one another : (*a*) for receiving, recording, and classifying the wounded on arrival and for recording their discharge or transfer ; (*b*) for severe cases ; (*c*) for slight cases ; and (*d*) for the dying.

Places should also be selected and marked out for : (*e*) cooking and the boiling of water ; (*f*) reception of arms and accoutrements ; (*g*) latrines, urinals, and the disposal of refuse ; (*h*) a mortuary ; and (*i*) a park for transport.

205. At the receiving department, all admissions will be recorded in the admission and discharge book ; only the columns necessary for the completion of Army Form A 36 will be filled in, but in all cases the instruction in the admission and discharge book for classifying wounds and injuries will be carefully complied with. In order to avoid duplication of the record in various portions of the unit, and in order that the fact of a man's having been admitted to an ambulance may be known, the designation of the ambulance and the section to which he is admitted will be marked on his specification-tally.

206. Ammunition will, when practicable, be taken from wounded men before they are sent to the rear, and will be disposed of under the orders of the divisional commander, *e.g.*, taken over by parties detailed from units of the fighting troops. Arms, accoutrement, and personal kit of sick and wounded men will be taken to hospital with the men ; and thereafter collections of arms, etc., at hospitals, not required for patients, will be periodically handed over to ordnance depots, this latter duty being usually carried out in medical units on the L. of C.

207. As regards fitness for transport, wounded men may be considered as belonging to five classes : (i) men able to walk ; (ii) men able to sit up in a wagon ; (iii) severe cases, but fit for carriage lying down in a wagon ; (iv) severe cases requiring hand carriage on stretchers; and (v) very severe cases unfit for immediate removal: these are, as a rule, penetrating abdominal wounds, which are best left for a week if the exigencies of war permit.

Transport of the severely wounded can be avoided only by bringing the clearing hospital up to where they lie, leaving them in charge of the inhabitants, or, in some circumstances, by temporarily encamping a detachment of field ambulance if one can be spared.

208. Orders regarding the disposal of the wounded from dressing stations and field ambulances generally will be received from the A.M.O. The earliest cases to be sent back should be those able to walk, who should be sent off in batches to the point indicated as soon as orders are received. Next, cases able to travel sitting up will be sent in wagons as they become available; and next, the lying-down cases. The very serious cases unfit for wagon transport, if able to be moved at all, or if it is essential to remove them, should be carried with the greatest care on stretchers or specially devised litters to the nearest place where they can be left and cared for, avoiding as much as possible change of conveyance during transit.

For loading or unloading wounded at a dressing station, personnel to assist should be obtained from the bearer division when necessary.

209. After a victory a rapid advance will be made. The divisional commander should report to general headquarters, stating the numbers and localities of the wounded not yet evacuated. The C.-in-C. may order a clearing hospital or detachment to be moved up under the arrangements of the I.G.C. to take over the wounded in the field ambulances on the spot, or that the divisional commander leave behind tent sub-divisions or other parties from the ambulances to care for the wounded until they can be removed; these parties will rejoin their units when relieved. In such circumstances bearer divisions will always remain mobile, and will be available to proceed with the troops.

210. The housing of sick and wounded may have to be arranged for. Much of the success of the undertaking, both as regards the comfort of the individuals and the maintenance of proper sanitation, depends upon an intelligent use being made of the buildings or sheds available. In selecting a building for the housing of sick and wounded (see also para. 256, Chapter XVI), special attention must be paid to its general construction and approaches, its water supply, the means of arranging for cooking and latrine accommodation.

It may be necessary, owing to the number of wounded or inability to remove them, to erect temporary shelters. Walls of turf or stones may be built up to give protection. Evacuated trenches, if large enough, clean and dry, may be used for this purpose; these can be improved by the addition of some covering to protect the patients from sun and weather.

Shelters can be constructed from wagon-covers and tarpaulins stretched over the wagon-poles; these form good shelters and can be stayed with ropes. Temporary shelters affording protection from sun and weather can be constructed from stretchers supported

on their sides or on end by means of a rifle, a piece of wood, or
branch of a tree placed beneath them. These, with the addition
of blankets or waterproof sheets hung on the weather-side, afford
serviceable protection. Shelter-tents constructed of blankets and
rifles, or of waterproof sheets laced together and supported on
sticks, afford good cover.

Stretchers, when available, make excellent beds; they can be
used either with their runners resting on the ground, or supported
head and foot by biscuit boxes or packing cases placed beneath
their handles, or on wooden trestles made for this purpose.

In whatever place sick or wounded are under treatment a Red
Cross flag should be prominently displayed.

DISPOSITION OF THE MEDICAL SERVICE WITH A DIVISION HOLDING A DEFENSIVE POSITION.

211. As in the case of attack, the A.M.O. will issue orders as to
the preliminary arrangements and the disposition of the medical
units. Greater permanence may be expected in the positions
occupied by the troops holding a defensive position, and field
ambulances allotted to areas will be able to prepare beforehand for
the reception of the wounded. Accommodation with bedsteads
should be improvised, if possible, for patients unfit for transport.

Small advanced dressing stations for the early treatment of
casualties will be thrown forward in touch with regimental medical
establishments and their aid posts. The selection of the positions
for the field ambulance encampments and dressing stations, and the
divisional collecting station or stations for slightly wounded men,
and the aid posts of the regimental medical services, should be
made after reconnaissance of the ground. More permanence may
be expected in these positions than in the case of an attack.

A proportion of the medical units or sections will be held in
reserve for the troops which may be detailed to deliver the counter
attack.

THE DISPOSITION OF THE MEDICAL SERVICE WITH A DIVISION DURING AN ENCOUNTER BATTLE.

212. When the occurrence of an encounter battle requires the
medical arrangements to be carried out unexpectedly from the line
of march, the regimental medical establishments will be guided in
the performance of their duties by the principles already described
for the attack.

213. Orders may or may not be received from the A.M.O. as to
the direction in which the field ambulances should proceed, and
there may have been no opportunity for the preparation of a
scheme of medical arrangements. The disposal of a unit will rest
almost entirely with the C.O., who will endeavour to establish and
maintain communication with the regimental medical establishments, and in the absence of orders from superior authority must
determine how near to the firing line the necessities of the military

situation permit of the approach of his unit as a whole, and where to form the dressing station. He must endeavour to prevent his transport being too conspicuous on the field : this is always important. At the same time he must avoid remaining at too great a distance from the wounded.

While arranging for the early succour of the wounded, he will not establish a dressing station until the progress of the fight indicates a suitable position. Wounded in the meantime must be left under shelter or placed in the ambulance wagons ready for removal as the situation develops.

THE DISPOSITION OF THE MEDICAL SERVICE WITH A DIVISION DURING A RETIREMENT.

214. In anticipation of a retirement, all wounded fit to travel should be sent back ; the slightly wounded should be sent off first, so as to avoid the risk of their being made prisoners of war.

215. During the retirement, if at all rapid, the formation of dressing stations will seldom be possible. The field ambulances will keep on the move as required, the bearer divisions and ambulance wagons remaining in touch with the regimental medical establishments. Cases unfit to walk will be carried in the ambulance wagons or in any transport that may become available.

During a retirement, it may sometimes become impossible to remove all the wounded, some of whom may have to be left on the battlefield to fall into the hands of the enemy. On such occasions, medical personnel with sufficient stores and equipment may, if military exigencies permit, be left in charge under the protection of the Geneva Convention.

It must, however, be remembered that medical personnel thus left in the enemy's hands will probably be lost to the army as far as the operations in hand are concerned, and that this loss may seriously interfere with the possibility of dealing efficiently with wounded or sick men who are still with the army or who may require attention in the near future.

As a normal rule, therefore, *medical personnel and equipment should not be allowed to fall into the hands of the enemy without an order to that effect from the commander of the division.*

THE MEDICAL SERVICE WITH SMALLER FORMATIONS.

INFANTRY BRIGADES.

216. When an infantry brigade is acting independently, a field ambulance, or as many sections as are required, may be allotted to it, and similar arrangements may be made for a smaller force.

The medical unit ceases, for the time being, to receive direct orders from the A.M.O., the senior medical officer becoming responsible for the medical arrangements.

ADVANCED GUARDS.

217. According to the strength of the troops employed, a field ambulance, a section, or part of a section may be detailed to accompany an advanced guard, the principle to be observed being that medical personnel is required for the collection and dressing of wounded, rather than ambulance transport for their removal.

In making the medical arrangements for any engagement which may take place, the senior medical officer with the advanced guard will be guided by the principles described for an encounter battle.

REAR GUARDS.

218. The medical arrangements for rear guards are similar to those for advanced guards, except that means for removing slightly wounded are required ; but usually no medical transport, other than ambulance transport, should accompany rear guards. Casualties will be carried in the ambulance wagons and sent on to the main body as opportunity occurs. (See also para. 215.)

THE MEDICAL SERVICE WITH A CAVALRY DIVISION.

219. As in the case of a division, the medical service with a cavalry division consists of : (i) the A.M.O. of the cavalry division and his headquarters ; (ii) the regimental medical establishments with units ; and (iii) cavalry field ambulances.

GENERAL REMARKS.

220. To appreciate the medical plans required for cavalry, it is necessary to understand the principles upon which that arm is employed in warfare, and reference should be made to Cavalry Training.

The collection and treatment of wounded cavalry soldiers frequently presents certain difficulties, mainly due to two causes : first, the greater mobility and rapidity of movement of cavalry and the distances covered ; and, second, the frequent use of cavalry on reconnaissance duties and in isolated and more or less independent detachments.

Cavalry, to be mobile, must have as few impedimenta as possible ; this tends to reduce medical personnel and equipment to a minimum, and adds to the difficulties of medical aid. The distances travelled by cavalry affect the medical arrangements because of the difficulty of keeping the regimental medical establishments and cavalry field ambulances in touch, and a halt for the collection of a few wounded men may result in the medical personnel and equipment being left behind.

In isolated and small parties, spread over many miles of country, time must elapse before medical aid can be obtained, both in sending back messages concerning men who become wounded, and in bringing them in from outlying posts, probably over difficult country. Wheeled transport cannot, as a rule, accompany patrols or scouts ; and except hand-carriage or carriage on horseback, there is little else available in the way of transport.

221. The number of wounded to be dealt with in the case of cavalry is comparatively small ; but the total while giving a low percentage for the whole campaign, may be concentrated into one or two sharp engagements. Concentration should, however, facilitate dealing with the wounded, because, after such engagements several medical units are likely to be in the vicinity.

222. Independent or strategical cavalry present more difficult problems for the medical service than protective or divisional cavalry, because the latter are in touch with the slowly moving infantry, and the distances over which wounded have to be carried before they can be properly housed and treated are less.

Patrolling and scouting work, cavalry combats, general engagements, pursuits and raids have each their own special medical problems.

223. Cavalry wounded may be classified, as far as collection is concerned, into three categories : (i) those able to walk or ride without help ; (ii) those who require help and special means of transport ; and (iii) those whom it would be difficult and dangerous to attempt to carry off the field, and whose best chances of recovery rest in their being made as comfortable as possible where they lie.

224. Cavalrymen, being employed so frequently at a distance from professional medical assistance, must depend in many instances upon their comrades for first aid, and therefore all cavalrymen should have some knowledge of that subject and the methods of carrying wounded. An extensive knowledge is unnecessary, but they should know generally what to do with the first field dressing, and, what is of equal importance, what not to do.

THE ADMINISTRATIVE MEDICAL OFFICER OF A
CAVALRY DIVISION.

225. The remarks regarding the duties of the A.M.O. of a division apply equally to the A.M.O. of a cavalry division, whose special duties are indicated in succeeding paragraphs.

THE REGIMENTAL MEDICAL ESTABLISHMENTS WITH CAVALRY.*

226. The regimental medical establishment with a cavalry regiment consists of an officer in medical charge ; N.C.Os. and men for water duties ; N.C.Os. and men for sanitary duties ; men trained in first aid ; and two orderlies for the medical officer, trained in the duties and placed under his orders, one a lance-corporal to attend and assist him in his duties, the other as driver of the cart carrying the medical equipment.

The description of the duties of the regimental medical establishments with the units composing a division applies generally to the corresponding establishments with the units of a cavalry division.

THE CAVALRY FIELD AMBULANCE.

227. The cavalry field ambulance is designed for the immediate medical assistance of the cavalry and other troops in a cavalry division or mounted brigade. Four are included in each division. They are divisional troops, under the command of the A.M.O.

A cavalry field ambulance consists of a bearer and a tent division, and is divisible, with its transport and equipment, into two sections, A and B, each section consisting of a bearer and a tent subdivision. Each section is capable of acting, or of being mobilized, independently.

---

* See " A Cavalry Regiment," in War Establishments

I

The duties of the bearer division are similar to those of the bearer division of a field ambulance, *i.e.*, to render immediate succour to the wounded and to collect them. The tent division receives the wounded, and affords them temporary treatment pending evacuation.

A cavalry field ambulance occupies 240 yards of road space when the personnel is carried in the wagons. On the line of march, they normally march in rear of the brigade ammunition columns. Medical arrangements for the line of march, etc., are similar to those described for a division.

228. Whenever rapid movements are made, or the distance is further than the normal march for infantry, the personnel will be carried in the ambulance wagons, if not occupied by sick or wounded. From the nature of their employment, the light ambulance wagons will seldom be available for the carriage of personnel : normally the heavy wagons should be used. When cavalry move rapidly, wagons that are occupied by sick or wounded may be left to follow ; or, if circumstances permit and the wagons are urgently required, the patients may be taken out and left, in charge of sufficient personnel, for subsequent collection by another medical unit, to which the necessary information must be transmitted.

THE MEDICAL SERVICE WITH CAVALRY ENGAGED IN OPERATIONS INVOLVING DISPERSION.

ADMINISTRATIVE ARRANGEMENTS.

229. Assuming that a cavalry brigade or similar formation is detached for reconnaissance duties, the A.M.O., under the orders of the cavalry divisional commander, will allot to it a cavalry field ambulance or part of one. Similarly, when a cavalry division is engaged in operations involving dispersion it will generally be advisable to allot a cavalry field ambulance to each brigade, as it will seldom be possible for the A.M.O. personally to control the medical arrangements of scattered bodies of cavalry.

230. The regimental medical establishments with strategic or protective cavalry will be assisted by the light ambulance wagons being distributed to the regiments. These wagons should be provided with material for dressings, bandages, splints, and restoratives, in charge of the wagon orderlies.

231. The cavalry field ambulance will relieve the regimental medical establishments by forming collecting posts ; receiving, treating, and carrying the casual wounded brought to these posts, and utilizing the heavy ambulance wagons, both for shelter and transport, until opportunities occur for sending the wounded back to the lines of communication.

232. Several courses are open for the disposal of a man of a reconnoitring detachment or patrol wounded during reconnaissance at a distance from the main body. If he is able to look after himself,

he may find his own way back to his detachment or his contact troop or squadron, following the line of transmission of information until he comes in touch with the regimental medical personnel, or reaches a post formed by a detachment of a cavalry field ambulance. In the case of men severely wounded, information should be sent back to the medical personnel so that means of transport may be arranged. Very severe cases should be left in any neighbouring village, house, or farm, and the inhabitants placed in charge of them.

Wounded may have to be carried over difficult and rough ground before a good road for wheeled transport is reached. In this case a suitable point should be selected on the nearest road to which wheeled transport can come up, and information sent back as early as possible to a medical officer to enable him to send an ambulance wagon to the place selected. The man must then, if he is in a fit condition to be moved, be placed in a sheltered spot or building close to the road. The message sent back should indicate where the man is to be found, the nature of his wound, etc. Remarks as to the condition of the patient are valuable, such as whether he is collapsed and unconscious, or able to attend to himself. A rough sketch to indicate the place where he lies may be useful if it saves a lengthy description.

The Regimental Medical Establishments.

233. The medical officer should, as a rule, be with the officer commanding the regiment. He will then be in a position where he is most likely to get information regarding casual wounded, and will be able on receipt of information to give instructions and arrange for bringing in a wounded man. It is inadvisable and unnecessary for him to ride off to every case ; he should judge by the nature of the information he receives what cases require immediate attention.

234. As stretchers of the usual pattern are difficult to carry on a horse unless strapped on a pack-saddle, in most cases the men trained in first aid must ride without them to the succour of wounded men.

Many improvised methods are available for the conveyance of wounded cavalrymen back to the neighbourhood of the ambulance wagons. Such are the various methods whereby a wounded man is carried on a horse, travois, or on improvised stretchers of various forms put together on the spot. For details of these see Chapter XVIII.

235. The medical officer will have at his disposal one or more light ambulance wagons, and, on receiving a message from a reconnoitring detachment or patrol, he should be in a position to detail a wagon to go forward to the place indicated, if the ground and the military situation permit. If the patient has been left at some point not actually by the roadside, the two wagon orderlies are available for bringing him to the wagon.

This method of collecting the wounded is suitable when there is no objection to a wheeled vehicle being sent forward, and where only two or three casual wounded have to be dealt with ; but when wounded are more scattered over a wide area, and where concealment of movement is desired, the first-aid men should be dispatched, mounted, with instructions to use one or other of the improvised methods referred to above.

The Cavalry Field Ambulances.

236. Collecting Posts.—A cavalry field ambulance should be with the main body of a cavalry brigade detailed for reconnaissance. The officer commanding the ambulance will select some spot for a collecting post to which the regimental medical service brings the wounded, and at which the ambulance takes them over. This collecting post may have to be moved forward or backward in conformity with the movements of the force ; the points essential are that touch must be maintained between the first and second line of medical aid, and that each regimental medical officer must be kept informed of the position selected for a collecting post from time to time. This information should be signalled or otherwise conveyed to all regiments of the brigade, so that the regimental medical service to which the light ambulance wagons are attached may bring the wounded to the collecting posts indicated.

237. A collecting post, if to provide for many casualties, may consist of a section of a cavalry field ambulance, but should usually consist of an officer with one or more stretcher squads, a few N.C.Os. and men of the tent division, with some dressings and restoratives, and one or more heavy ambulance wagons. In any case the ambulance wagons detailed must carry the personnel in case the post has to be hurriedly formed.

238. When a collecting post is advanced rapidly from one point to another, it may happen that information regarding the change of place may not have reached a unit before its wounded are sent back. If there is any doubt about this, a detachment should be left for a time at the point. In other words there should be a relay, so to speak, of collecting posts.

239. The rôle of the cavalry field ambulance when operations involve dispersion is a difficult one. Not only must it provide for the reception, care, and treatment of the wounded sent to it by the regimental medical establishments, but it must keep in touch with rapidly advancing cavalry on the one hand and evacuate wounded on the other. For touch with the regimental medical service, the light ambulance wagons will move along the roads in the direction of the reconnaissance objective, under the orders of the regimental medical officers to whom they are lent, and will bring back wounded to the collecting posts established as the force advances. The six-horsed heavy ambulance wagons will be brought up to these collecting posts as already noted. These wagons are specially constructed, not only to act as means of transport for wounded, but also to serve as a temporary shelter. In fact, the interior of the heavy ambulance wagon becomes, for the time being a four-bedded ward, so that each brigade has accompanying it a small hospital on wheels for serious cases. The advantage of this is that wounded can thus be taken on from one objective to another, until opportunities occur for sending them back towards the line of communication, or leaving them in a suitable place where they can be cared for.

Wagons or other vehicles bringing up supplies should bring back the wounded to points where they can be taken over by a clearing hospital, or to the medical units of the main force which the cavalry is covering and through them to the clearing hospitals.

WOUNDED OF CAVALRY PATROLS.

240. The principles described above are inapplicable in the case of patrols which have got behind the enemy's cavalry screen, or during cavalry raids. In these cases, sick, wounded, or injured men must either be carried on with the detachments, or they must be left in the nearest village, unless the distance does not prevent a man who is able to look after himself finding his own way back to his army.

THE MEDICAL SERVICE WITH CAVALRY ENGAGED IN OPERATIONS INVOLVING CONCENTRATION.

THE REGIMENTAL MEDICAL ESTABLISHMENTS.

241. When cavalry is concentrated for attack, the regimental medical arrangements are of a different character. Light ambulance wagons are not usually distributed to regiments.

The regimental medical personnel, immediately after the combat, should deploy over the area where the attack has taken place, affording first aid and collecting the wounded. In these conditions the first-aid men carry out the rôle of dismounted stretcher bearers and bring wounded to a selected spot to be kept temporarily under cover until the cavalry field ambulances come up.

242. Immediately the cavalry field ambulances reach the area, the personnel and equipment of the regimental medical establishments should rejoin their units as rapidly as possible.

In a pursuit, there will be much for the regimental medical service to attend to in the way of affording first aid, leaving wounded at places where they can subsequently be found by the ambulances.

THE CAVALRY FIELD AMBULANCES.

243. The chief work of the cavalry field ambulances occurs when a cavalry combat has taken place. The ambulances, no longer allotted to brigades, but retained under the orders of the A.M.O., should be, with all their transport, as near the probable area of combat as possible, prepared to push forward their bearer divisions to the area over which the combat has taken place and set the regimental medical service free. Each unit should be allotted an area over which it will operate, or have other specific duty assigned to it by the A.M.O.

244. For the purpose of concealment of cavalry movements it may not be possible to concentrate the ambulances nearer the combat area than five miles. When the order is received, the bearers should be sent forward as rapidly as possible with the stretchers in the light ambulance wagons, and might be expected to

arrive within an hour after the attack. The tent divisions should follow to establish a dressing station or stations at the nearest convenient positions for making preparations for the reception, accommodation, temporary care, and treatment of the wounded; the final duty being to evacuate to the line of communication, according to orders received through the A.M.O.

In preparing and conducting a dressing station or establishing a cavalry field ambulance encampment, the principles described for field ambulances apply.

245. A point to remember is the necessity for keeping a section of an ambulance or a whole ambulance ready to follow up any portion of the troops in pursuit. In the event of a retirement, the instructions in para. 215 regarding medical personnel and equipment must be borne in mind.

THE MEDICAL SERVICE WITH CAVALRY IN DISMOUNTED ACTION.

246. When cavalry are engaged in dismounted action, the principles and methods described for handling the medical establishments and units of a division should be followed. (See para. 215.)

THE MEDICAL SERVICE IN MOUNTAIN WARFARE.

247. While the general disposition of the medical service, and the principles upon which it is employed, are similar in mountain warfare to those for warfare in more or less level countries, operations in a mountainous country require considerable modifications in the ambulance and other transport with the medical service.

Pack-transport is usually required for the equipment; and special forms of ambulance transport such as the "tongas" and "doolies" of field hospitals in India. Riding ponies and mules are also employed for the carriage of sick and wounded. Owing to its special nature, practice in loading and the management of the transport on hilly ground is important.

248. One of the chief difficulties is that of conveying severely wounded men down steep hillsides, often under the fire of a determined enemy. Dandies and even light blanket stretchers are seldom a safe or even possible means of transport on very steep ground. On such ground advantage should be taken of some of the various means of carrying wounded men by pick-a-back or hand-seats, with puttees, etc., described in Chapter XVIII. Transport used by the inhabitants of the country should be looked for, adapted, and utilized.

WARFARE IN UNCIVILIZED COUNTRIES.

249. While the general principles already described are applicable to warfare in countries not signatory to the Geneva Convention, there is this essential difference, that sick and wounded cannot be left on the field to be cared for by the enemy. The medical units may require an armed escort, and the medical personnel may have to carry arms for the defence of the sick and wounded in its charge and for its own protection.

CHAPTER XVI.

THE EVACUATING ZONE.

250. The medical service in the evacuating zone consists of : (i) clearing hospitals, (ii) ambulance trains, (iii) advanced depots of medical stores, (iv), in certain cases, stationary and general hospitals.

The units enumerated above belong to the L. of C., and, under the authority of the I.G.C., are administered by a D.D.M.S.

CLEARING HOSPITALS.

251. A clearing hospital is a unit which is specially set apart for the evacuation of the sick and wounded collected by the ambulances. It is the pivot upon which the removal of sick and wounded turns, as it is the central point to which the collecting zone converges, and from which the evacuating zone and distributing zone diverge, and is the unit which the D.M.S. holds for establishing the channel or flow of sick and wounded between divisional ambulances and the line of evacuation.

These units are mobilized in the proportion of one to each division of the field army. Transport for them, and ambulance transport for sick and wounded, is provided when required, under the arrangements of the I.G.C.

Clearing hospitals are accommodated in suitable buildings if available, or in tents ; the camping space required is 204 yards by 190 yards when there are not more than 200 sick. The area must permit of great expansion, as a clearing hospital may be required to take in many more sick and wounded.

252. Duties in the field.—A clearing hospital only acts as a hospital in the usual sense of the term during the time it is unable to pass its patients down the L. of C. While nominally equipped for the care of 200 sick, it must be expanded when large numbers of sick and wounded are passing through from the division in connection with which it happens to be employed.

253. Normally located at an advanced base and employed between that base and the field army, the actual disposition must depend upon the movements and actions of the force which it serves. Thus, at an advanced base it may receive sick and casual wounded brought from the field medical units on the empty vehicles of the supply columns to the railway, the clearing hospital, if necessary, having sent out medical personnel to accompany them ; but if many sick or wounded are to be dealt with it may have to be advanced close up to the division, so that the ambulance wagons of field medical units, or vehicles locally collected, may bring the wounded to it ; or, if the field army is to advance, it may be sent up to the ambulances to take over the wounded in them and so enable them to go on with their division. In certain circumstances, for example, with horsed transport or water-transport, it may form a series of rest stations, with transport moving between them, constituting a column by which evacuation takes place.

254. A clearing hospital must be prepared to advance or to send on detachments at any time, and consequently its officers should be well acquainted with the surrounding country, especially the roads leading towards the area occupied by the troops in front. For the same reason the personnel should be told off as rest station parties, and as a main body. The equipment should similarly be divided into what will be required with rest station parties and what should accompany the remainder of the unit.

255. The personnel of a *rest station* will normally consist of an officer with one or more serjeants and four or five rank and file for nursing, cooking, and general duty. They will take with them a medical companion and one or more surgical haversacks with their water-bottles ; cooking utensils, medical comforts, medicines, and dressing materials according to the purpose of the rest station ; and also, if transport is available, a few blankets, mattress cases, and pillow cases. If large numbers of sick or wounded are expected, the personnel and equipment may be increased.

256. The clearing hospital or a detachment sent up to relieve ambulances, or forming a rest station on the line of evacuation will take over existing buildings and prepare them for the temporary reception of sick and wounded, and prepare food and restoratives. In a civilized country, school buildings are the most suitable : the rooms are large and airy, means of lighting and warming exist, and a water supply and sanitary arrangements are installed. As a rough estimate of the number of recently wounded men who may be accommodated in a building for one night, it may be taken that, in rooms over 15 feet wide but under 20 feet, for every yard of length one man may be accommodated ; and in rooms 20 feet wide and over, two men may be accommodated for every yard of length.

The best accommodation available and a few beds or extemporized couches should be prepared for cases of serious illness which may occur among the sick and wounded *en route*.

257. Other and smaller detachments may form rest stations principally for the preparation of food and restoratives at railway stations or along the line of route of road or water transport, but also prepared to receive cases of severe illness unfit to travel further.

258. Having relieved the ambulances, a clearing hospital must next pass the wounded on down the L. of C. so that it may not itself become clogged ; but care should be taken not to send down the L. of C. men whose condition does not prevent them from doing duty at the front. If the distance to the railway or the nearest medical unit is more than a day's journey, detachments will be sent back from the clearing hospital or brought up from another medical unit on the L. of C. to form rest stations at intermediate posts.

The transport which is used for this purpose may be either empty supply column vehicles on the return journey, supplemented by local transport collected under the arrangements of the I.G.C., or specially organized transport allotted to the clearing hospital. Medical personnel for a convoy may be required from the clearing hospital.

Ambulance Trains.

259. Ambulance trains to carry 100 sick lying down are mobilized in the proportion of one to each division. They are utilized for the conveyance of sick and wounded down the L. of C., and may, if the situation permits, be brought up into direct touch with the ambulances of the collecting zone. Methods of employing ambulance trains are described under the Distributing Zone.

Particulars of the varieties of ambulance trains and the methods of improvising ambulance railway transport are described in Chapter XVIII.

Stationary and General Hospitals.

260. Stationary and in some cases general hospitals may be within the evacuating zone when at or near the advanced base, and utilized for the reception of patients awaiting further means of transport towards the base, and also when set apart for the reception of slight cases likely to return to the front within a few weeks. They will be further described under the Distributing Zone.

Advanced Depots of Medical Stores.

261. These are mobilized in the proportion of one to every two divisions in the field, and are formed at the advanced base under the D.D.M.S. Transport is provided, when required, under the orders of the I.G.C. From these units the field medical units, and the L. of C. medical units and establishments in the vicinity, obtain replenishment of their medical and surgical equipment.

The Number and Classification of Sick and Wounded.

262. These are important factors in arranging the distribution of personnel, and in estimating the amount of transport material required. This subject, and the remaining portions of this chapter, concern the collecting, evacuating, and distributing zones.

263. As regards the sick, and the wounded from casual encounters, a fairly steady inflow occurs at all times. It is estimated for the two classes combined at about 0·3 per cent. of the force daily, but the figure may be higher or lower according to the presence or absence of epidemic disease and over-fatigue, footsoreness, etc., especially after severe marches and in the earlier stages of the campaign. In ordinary circumstances, half of these cases are of a trivial character, requiring treatment in field medical units for 4 or 5 days. Whether it is necessary or not to remove these as far as the lines of communication must depend upon the military situation at the time ; for example, an impending engagement would necessitate the clearing of the ambulances and also of the clearing hospitals, but it should seldom be necessary to evacuate such cases further than an advanced base. Rather more than a quarter (say, 30 per cent.) require treatment in L. of C. medical units for 3 or 4 weeks, while the remainder, which require longer treatment, need to be evacuated to home territory.

The most difficult problem will be the disposal of cases of infectious disease during an epidemic. The principle to follow in that case is the paramount necessity of removing and isolating these cases from the healthy troops. Supply column vehicles are not to be used for their removal, as time for disinfection is not likely to be available,

A certain proportion of mental cases may occur requiring special arrangements.

264. With regard to the wounded, the number to be dealt with after a general engagement is not likely to be more than 20 per cent. of the troops engaged or less than 5 per cent., excluding those that are killed outright and missing.*

The incidence of casualties may be such that while 20 per cent. of all the fighting troops are wounded, as many as 50 per cent. or more may be wounded in one group or small area of the field and a proportionately less number in another, and while 20 per cent. may cover the whole period of fighting, a much higher percentage may occur in short spaces of time.

265. The distribution of the total percentage of wounded in different categories is of special importance in considering the amount of transport material that has to be got ready. For this purpose, a forecast is required of the number of wounded who can find their way back on foot, who require lying-down accommodation, who can be carried sitting up, and who ought to be carried by hand or not moved from where they lie.

For working purposes the following estimate for distributing the wounded into categories for transport may be utilized :—

20 per cent. able to walk.
60 ,, ,, requiring transport sitting up.
15 ,, ,, ,, ,, lying down.
5 ,, ,, unfit to be moved by ordinary transport, and requiring careful carriage by hand, or preferably to be kept under the best conditions near where they fell.

---

* In estimating the probable number of *total* casualties after any battle, Cron, of the Austrian Army, assumes that 10 per cent. of three-fifths of the total force may be taken as a guide, the three-fifths representing the proportion of the force which will probably be engaged. Of the total casualties, it may be estimated that 20 per cent. will be killed outright (*i.e.* one killed to 4 wounded), 10 per cent. will be so slightly wounded as not to require evacuation and may be retained in the field medical units if the military situation permits, while 70 per cent. will require hospital treatment. Of those requiring hospital treatment, 70 per cent. will be suitable for treatment in L. of C. medical units, while 30 per cent. require to be evacuated to home territory,

266. But this must only be regarded as the probable proportion requiring transport* from the zone of operations to the head of the L. of C. Under normal conditions, *i.e.*, unless the army is retiring before the enemy, the more trivial cases, namely those able to walk, will probably remain at the head of the line, and the less serious cases, likely to be fit for duty after a comparatively short period of treatment, will probably be distributed to the more advanced stationary hospitals. Consequently, as the wounded go down the L. of C., the category of those fit to walk drops out altogether, and the proportion of those requiring lying-down accommodation may increase.

THE EVACUATION OF SICK AND WOUNDED.

267. The medical service in the field is based on the system of evacuating sick and wounded. The efficiency with which this is organized greatly affects the mobility and *moral* of the army, and an important duty is thrown on the administrative medical service in this connection.

The ambulance wagons of a field medical unit should not be detached to go a distance which would prevent them rejoining their unit on the same day. In considering their use for evacuation, the amount of work already performed by the horses must be taken into account, in order that the animals may be kept fit, should a further advance take place.

Under conditions of severe fighting, it would be impossible to prevent the tent divisions of the field ambulances becoming immobilized and unable to move on with their divisions, unless there is a very complete organization of sick-transport.

The following may be utilized for providing this transport in campaigns :—(i) vehicles of supply columns returning empty ; (ii) local vehicles ; (iii) permanent or field railways ; (iv) waterways ; (v) voluntary aid detachments of the British Red Cross Society or other similar body, or parties for ambulance work from among the civil population.

268. The use of supply column vehicles returning empty.— For the principles of the supply organization of an army in the field, see Field Service Regulations, Part II. No special transport is maintained for medical services with the supply columns, but the empty supply vehicles are used, when returning to the railway,

---

* To determine the amount of transport material required, or the time required with the amount of transport available, certain formulæ are of use. Taking " T " to represent the time allowed, " W " the number of sick and wounded, " t " the time taken by the material used for transport purposes to make one journey and return, " V " the units of transport material required or available—such as an ambulance train, an ambulance wagon, a country cart, etc.—and " w " the number of patients each unit of transport carries, the formulæ are as follows :—

$$\frac{W \times t}{T \times w} = V$$

i.e., the number of vehicles required in a given time to evacuate a given number of wounded to any point.

and

$$\frac{W \times t}{V \times w} = T$$

i.e., the time taken with a given amount of transport to evacuate a given number to any point.

for the conveyance of sick and wounded, supplemented when necessary by the use of local transport. Much depends on the co-ordination of the work of bringing supplies up to the troops and conveying the sick and wounded back.

During prolonged periods of halt, *e.g.*, during pauses in the operations, a system of sending the sick from ambulances to the empty supply vehicles at definite hours of the day may be arranged ; but immediately after big battles (or during them should they be prolonged over more than two or three days), the utilization of the empty supply vehicles for medical services will present many difficult problems. The supply requirements of the troops cannot be interfered with, but it may be possible to arrange that the empty vehicles of the supply column are available at a suitable hour and place sufficiently near the ambulances to permit of speedy transfer of the wounded from these units, either on foot, in ambulance wagons, or by hand-carriage.

This having been determined, the A.M.O. will issue instructions for sufficient personnel to prepare the wagons, receive and load the wounded. This detachment should collect straw, mattresses, etc., with which to prepare the wagons,* and have food and medical comforts ready for the wounded on their journey. To accompany a large sick-convoy personnel will be required, *e.g.*, from the clearing hospital concerned.

269. **The use of local vehicles.**—Information should be obtained through the Director of Transport of the number of local vehicles in each locality, and how many can be obtained for the medical service. The pressure for transport is not occasional only : there is a daily inflow of sick, and the balance between inflow and outflow must be maintained. A certain quantity, therefore, of the available local material should be assigned for the regular use of the medical service between the ambulances, clearing hospitals, and the railway. When big battles are impending the amount should be increased to the greatest possible extent and vehicles should be collected under the arrangements of the I.G.C., and of the divisional commanders if they are required to do so. The transport collected by the I.G.C. will be required to supplement the supply vehicles of the force used in evacuation, and may be sent direct to the ambulances.

270. There has been no big campaign in which this form of auxiliary transport has not been used, and therefore part of the training of the R.A.M.C. in peace is in the methods of preparing vehicles of different types in a manner suitable for the transport of sick and wounded.

The collection and registration of local vehicles for sick-transport will be carried out under instructions from the staff.

The vehicles should be classified and the various types kept separate, according to their suitability for the various classes of wounded men. As a general rule, heavy wagons are more suitable

* *See* " Preparations and Loading of G.S Wagons, Country Carts, etc.,'' paras. 338 to 341, and " By Mechanical Transport," paras. 348 to 349, Chap. XVIII.

for cases requiring lying-down accommodation, lighter vehicles for those who can travel sitting up.

271. The use of permanent or field railways.—The use of the permanent railways is obvious ; and when a line of rail, whether permanent or field, is in working order in or near the area of operations, every possible advantage should be taken of it. As much rolling stock as possible should be brought up for the transport of wounded in anticipation of a conflict, and a point selected on the line, at which the wounded can be entrained. The use of the railway line for removing large numbers by trains running at intervals is valuable during a retirement.

272. The use of waterways.*—Where suitable waterways exist, water-transport may be the best means of evacuation and is well adapted for the removal of serious cases ; canal-barges, boats, lighters, river-steamers, launches, or local craft of various sorts being converted in some of the ways described in Chapter XVIII.

Drinking water would probably have to be carried on board, and arrangements made for cooking, ablution, and conservancy at suitable stages along the route. The necessary personnel should be found from medical units on the L. of C.

273. Where there are many locks in a canal, frequent passage of boats is liable to cause lowering of the water in the higher sections, unless sufficient time is allowed for the replacement of what is lost when the lock is opened.

274. The employment of Voluntary Aid Societies, etc.— The medical service may be supplemented by Voluntary Aid Detachments. The men's detachments may be employed at rest stations for evacuation, and with sick-convoys by rail, road or water.

The women's detachments may be employed at railway stations, or at stages on the lines of communication along which sick convoys are passing by road or water.

Parties for ambulance work may be organized among the civil population, or from recognized Societies for Voluntary Aid, according to the country in which the operations are taking place.

The rules affecting voluntary assistance to the sick and wounded are laid down in Field Service Regulations, Part II, the Scheme for the Organization of Voluntary Aid, and in the Geneva Convention of 1906.

---

* *See* " Transport by Waterways," paras. 359 and 360, Chap. XVIII.

CHAPTER XVII.

THE DISTRIBUTING ZONE.

275. The medical service in the distributing zone (exclusive of sanitary units and establishments) consists of : (i) stationary hospitals, (ii) general hospitals, (iii) base depots of médical stores, (iv) convalescent depots on the L. of C., (v) ambulance trains, (vi) hospital ships, and (vii) the military hospitals and convalescent depots in the United Kingdom.

276. The units enumerated from (i) to (v) belong to the L. of C., and, under the authority of the I.G.C., are administered by a D.D.M.S. Hospital ships, when at the sea base, are also under the same administration. The military hospitals in the United Kingdom, under the authority of the G.Os.C.-in-C., are administered by the P.M.Os. of Commands, and require no further description here.

STATIONARY HOSPITALS.

277. These units are located at selected points on the L. of C., for example at the advanced base, at road posts, and railway posts where it is necessary to place a hospital but where a general hospital is not required, and also (in reserve or set apart for special purposes) at or near the base.

278. One or more should be at or in front of the advanced base for cases that are likely to be fit to return to the ranks after a short period of treatment—see Chapter XVI. The remainder should be distributed along the L. of C. as indicated above.

279. Stationary hospitals are mobilized in the proportion of two to each division in the field, and each is organized for 200 beds, but must be prepared to expand so as to accommodate a much larger number of patients on emergency.

280. The patients may be accommodated in tents ; but preferably in suitable buildings, if available. When tents are used the camping space required is 240 yards by 190 yards.

Transport is provided, when required, under the orders of the I.G.C.

GENERAL HOSPITALS.

281. The organization, personnel, and equipment of a general hospital resemble the larger military hospitals in time of peace. In addition, supplies of clothing, necessaries, and equipment are maintained for issue to patients as required, and convalescent depots are established in connection with selected general hospitals.

General hospitals are located at or near the base, or at selected positions on the L. of C., for example, at or near the advanced base, or at selected railway posts. The vicinity of a town affording facilities for obtaining supplies is an advantage ; but care should be taken that these hospitals are not so located as to interfere with one another in the matter of local supplies. Sites should be readily accessible by rail or road, and sufficiently far from activity to ensure quietness. If on the line of rail, a siding and platform for ambulance trains is an important adjunct to a general hospital.

282. General hospitals are mobilized in the proportion of two to each division in the field. Transport is provided, when required, under the orders of the I.G.C.

They are organized for 520 beds, including 20 beds for sick officers; expansion to a much larger number may be necessary on emergency. The patients are accommodated in suitable buildings, if available. If in tents, the camping space required is 550 yards by 400 yards.

BASE DEPOTS OF MEDICAL STORES.

283. Base depots of medical stores are mobilized in the proportion of one to every two divisions, and are formed at the base under the D.D.M.S. Transport is provided when required under the orders of the I.G.C.

284. Base depots supply the advanced depots of medical stores, and replenish the medical and surgical material of medical units in the vicinity.

CONVALESCENT DEPOTS.

285. These are established in connection with selected general hospitals, but are distinct in their organization. They may also be established in home territory in connection with selected military hospitals.

286. Their function both in the field and in home territory is to relieve the pressure on the hospitals, so that adequate accommodation may be at all times available for serious cases coming from the front. They receive officers and men who require no further active medical or surgical treatment, and who, although not yet fit for duty, are likely to become so in a reasonable time ; when necessary, re-clothing and re-equipping them before they return to their units.

287. Personnel, additional to that laid down in War Establishments, may be taken for camp duties from convalescents in the depot. (See also para. 151, Chap. XIII.)

AMBULANCE TRAINS.*

288. The varieties of ambulance trains are described in Chapter XVIII. In the distributing zone they are utilized in conveying sick and wounded towards the hospitals at the base or elsewhere. Empty supply trains returning towards the base are also available for conveying cases which do not require special ambulance railway transport.

289. Wherever patients are entrained or detrained, or halt on their way down the line of communication, rest stations should be established by detachments from the nearest medical unit.

---

* See " By Railway Transport," paras, 350 to 356, Chap. XVIII.

Buildings, such as sheds near the station, should be taken over and prepared with straw, mattresses, etc., for the temporary accommodation of patients awaiting entraining, or removal to hospital after detraining. Refreshments and restoratives should be in readiness, especially after a journey, as there may be unavoidable delay in removal to hospital, and it may be convenient to classify patients at the rest station according to the nature of the hospital treatment and accommodation they require.

At stations where improvised trains carrying sick and wounded halt on their journey towards the base, food should be in readiness at the time of arrival.

HOSPITAL SHIPS.*

290. In an overseas war one hospital ship is mobilized for each division of the field army.

They are equipped for 220 beds, including 20 beds for sick officers, and form a link between the base and the military hospitals in the United Kingdom to which the more serious cases and men invalided are sent.

291. Subject to sea transport arrangements, the control of hospital ships (as far as their medical equipment and readiness for the reception of invalids is concerned) rests with the D.M.S. and his representative on the L. of C.

---

* *See* " Transport by Sea," paras. 357 and 358, Chap. XVIII.

CHAPTER XVIII.

THE TRANSPORT OF THE WOUNDED.

292. Historical Sketch.—From the beginning of history we know that the human race has been engaged in fighting battles, and, though we have full accounts of their victories and losses, but little is recorded concerning their wounded. We do know, however, that the sick and wounded were carried in " litters " from the earliest times, and that at least two Roman generals transported their wounded in wagons, and also that the Roman Legions were accompanied by surgeons. It may be safely assumed that it was customary for slaves, menials, and possibly companions-in-arms to assist and help the wounded as far as they were able.

Digges, a writer in the sixteenth century, pointed out the need of a collecting station for the wounded, he says : " It were convenient " to appointe certaine carriages and men, of purpose to give their " attention in every skirmishe and incounter, to carry away the " hurt men to such place as Surgions may immediately repayre " unto them, which shall not only greatly incourage the souldior, " but also cause the skirmishe to be better maintained, when the " souldiors shall not neede to leave the fielde to carry away their " hurt men."

It was apparently the custom everywhere down to the beginning of the nineteenth century for the surgeons with their necessary appliances to remain some considerable distance in rear of the battlefields and only succour and aid such as were brought to them ; whilst those striken on the field were left to look after themselves.

It remained for those two most distinguished military surgeons, Barons Larrey and Percy, of Napoleon's Grand Army, to inaugurate a great advance and to effect far-seeing changes in the transport of the wounded in the field. The former was the first to introduce his light horsed-ambulances in the campaign against Austria, whilst to the latter we owe the organization of the first companies of stretcher bearers.

A short account of the latter may be of interest here. The men were especially selected from volunteers from the different regiments, and these " brancardiers," as they are still named in the French Army, were so equipped that when any two met they could combine, and construct anywhere in a few minutes a stout, comfortable litter. It was composed of two poles of pine-wood cut with the grain, two traverses or cross pieces, and a piece of cloth deeply hemmed on both edges ; the poles were 7½ feet long, round, with a circumference of 5 inches for 6 feet, and tapering at each end to a circumference of 3½ inches, so that they could be used as handles. The weight hardly exceeded 4 lb., with a resistance of nearly 200 lb. without bending. The poles, which were painted, served also to form a kind of halberd or pike for defensive purposes. At one end they were provided with an iron tip, and at the other

K

with a wormed ferrule on which screwed a lance-point, which was detached when on duty and worn on the left side in a scabbard attached to the shoulder belt. The brancardier passed his traverse over his knapsack, and fastened it to the centre by means of a small leather strap which bore upon an azure ground the motto : " Secours aux braves."

These companies became a recognized establishment of the Imperial Army in 1813. In was due, therefore, to the initiative of these two distinguished officers that at the present day every civilized army is provided with cadres of men belonging to the medical units, who received special instructions in the rendering of first aid to the wounded in the field and the best means of transporting them to a place of safety, and it is hardly necessary to remark that the sufferings and hardships of war have been enormously diminished in consequence.

293. Means of Transporting Wounded.—The transport of the wounded is carried out by the following means :—By men ; by conveyances carried by men ; by conveyances wheeled by men ; by animals ; by conveyances carried by animals ; by conveyances drawn by animals ; by mechanical transport ; by railway transport ; and by water transport.

294. The importance of a suitable choice, and of adequate preparation, is illustrated by the following remarks of Sir Thomas Longmore : " Every man who is rendered helpless by a severe wound naturally feels an urgent desire to get surgical aid as quickly as possible, as well as to be removed from the place of fighting, where he can no longer be of use, to a place of comparative security. But it is not merely the gratification of this longing for help that has to be thought of ; it is the more serious fact that the safety of lives and the preservation of limbs in many instances will depend upon proper means of transport being at hand. Moreover, in almost all cases the efficiency of the surgical assistance rendered will be materially influenced by the time which has elapsed before the patient is brought to hospital and the care with which the transport is conducted."*

By Men.

295. Wounded men are carried out of action either pick-a-back, by the back-lift, fireman's lift, hand-seats (see para. 405, Chap. XXII), or on stretchers, for removal to the tent division.

296. Pick-a-back.—If conscious, and able to hold on, a man can be carried pick-a-back by another. The improvised seat shown in Fig. 29 adds greatly to the comfort of the wounded man, and eases the bearer carrying him.

---

* " Treatise on Ambulances," by Surgeon-General Sir Thomas Longmore, C.B., etc. (out of print).

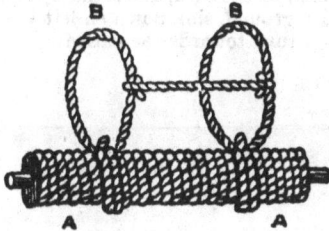

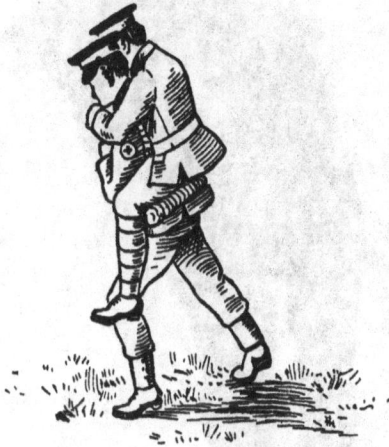

FIG. 29.—IMPROVISED SEAT, AS AN AID IN CARRYING A MAN
PICK-A-BACK.

Made of twisted straw, etc., wound round a strong stick or pole
AA. The seat.   BB. Arm-loops for bearer.

297. The Back-lift.—If able to stand, place the patient with his back to yours, slightly stoop, place your hands over your shoulders and grasp the patient under the arm-pits, bring his weight well up into the small of the back, and stand up (Fig. 30). To lower the patient to the ground, sink down on left knee, place him in a sitting posture, and turn towards the patient.

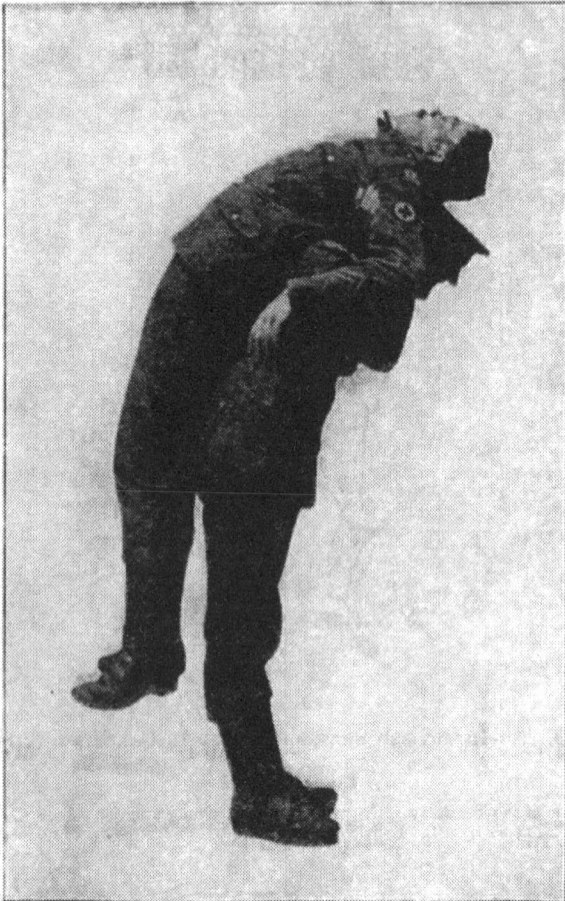

FIG. 30.—THE BACK-LIFT.

298. The Fireman's Lift.—If a patient is helpless he may be carried by means of " the fireman's lift " (Figs. 31, 32, and 33).

THE FIREMAN'S LIFT.

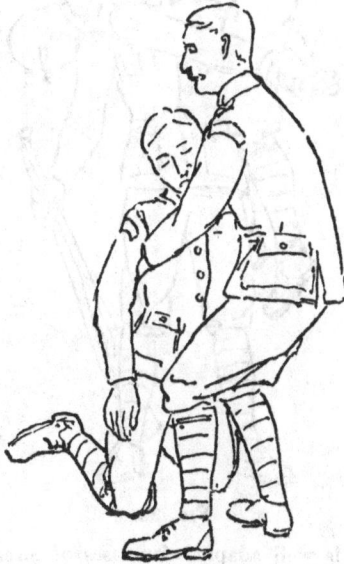

FIG. 31.

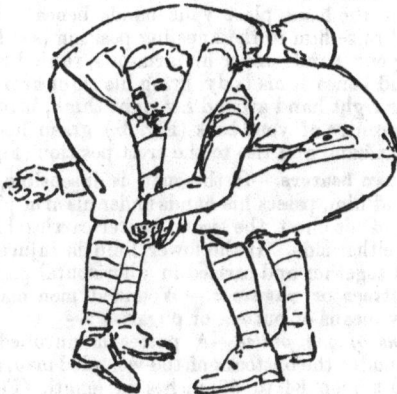

FIG. 32.

140

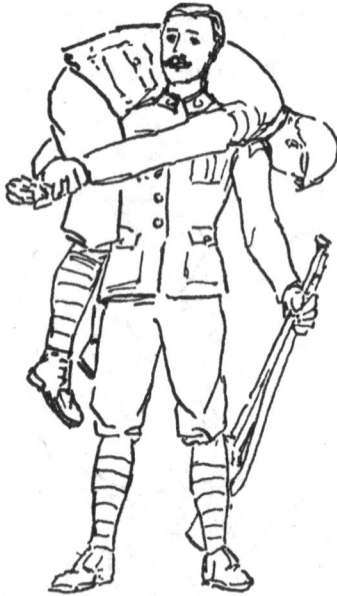

FIG. 33.

This method is well adapted for cases of insensibility, and is carried out as follows :—

(i) Roll the patient over on the face, the arms to the side.

(ii) Stand at the head, place your hands beneath the patient's shoulders, and raise him to the kneeling position (see Fig. 31).

(iii) Place your hands under his arm-pits, raise him up, stoop, place your head beneath his body, bring his right arm around your neck, put your right hand around his right thigh, bring his weight well on to the centre of your back (Fig. 32), grasp his right wrist with your right hand and rise to the erect position (Fig. 33).

299. With two bearers.—If the man is insensible, one bearer, kneeling behind him, passes his hands under his arm-pits and clasps them in front of his chest, the second bearer carries him feet first with a leg on either side. If the lower limb is injured, both legs should be tied together and carried in a horizontal position.

300. By puttees or pugarees.—Wounded men may be carried off the field by means of puttees or pugarees :—

(i) *By means of one puttee.*—A puttee is unrolled and placed well forward under the buttocks of the wounded man, and tied by a reef-knot into a loop 84 to 88 inches in length (Fig. 34). The rescuer then bends down, facing away from the injured man, and applies the loop of puttee over his own forehead, and, rising, carries off the wounded man (Fig. 35). The webbed stretcher-sling can be similarly used.

(ii) *By means of two puttees.*—One puttee is placed under the buttocks of the wounded man and over the forehead of the rescuer, as before. The second puttee is passed outside the first, round the middle of the back and under the arm-pits of the wounded man, under the arm-pits and over the front of the chest of the rescuer, and tied off at one side by a reef-knot, thus forming a loop 72 inches in length (Fig. 36).

By these means wounded men can be carried for considerable distances (one or two miles). They are especially useful for broken country and in hill warfare, but equally so on level ground, the hands of the rescuer being free.

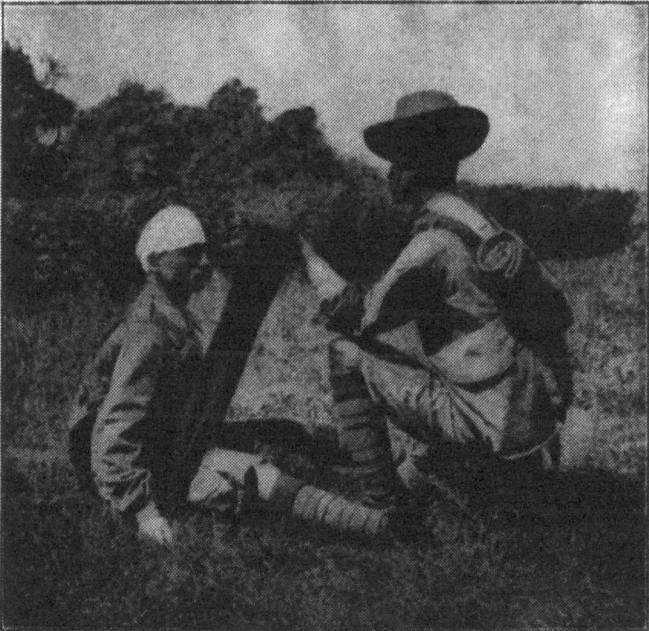

FIG. 34.   APPLYING ONE PUTTEE.

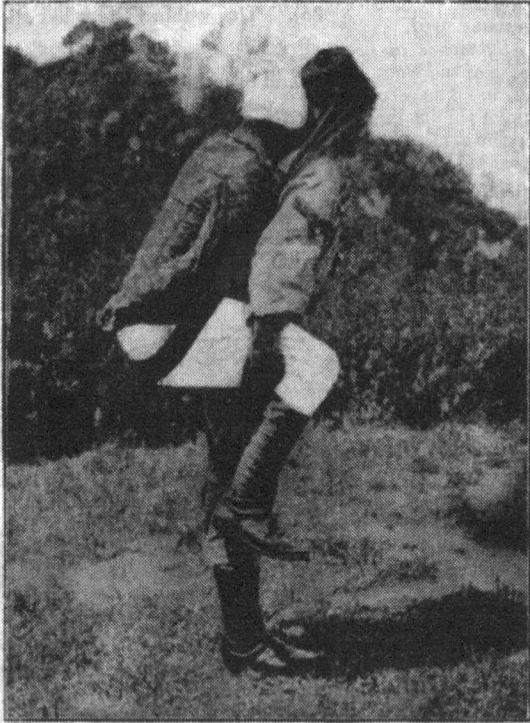

FIG. 35. USING ONE PUTTEE.

(iii) *By means of pugarees.*—Instead of puttees, pugarees may be used in the manner described above, with troops who wear this form of head-dress. The foregoing methods were devised by Captain J. S. O'Neill, I.M.S.

CONVEYANCES CARRIED BY MEN.

301. All such forms of hand ambulance transport are comprised in the general term " litter " ; but can be divided again into hammocks and stretchers, and other varieties confined to the East such as jhampans, dandies, doolies, and palkis.

The stretcher proper is composed of poles, traverses, canvas (or stout cloth), slings, and is possibly provided with feet and pillows. Every army has its own particular pattern of stretcher.

Many types of stretchers and dandies have been invented during the last half century. If the reader is interested in these various designs, as also in detailed descriptions of ambulance vehicles, he is referred to Surgeon-General Longmore's Manual of Ambulance Transport, which contains much valuable information on the subject, not obtainable elsewhere.

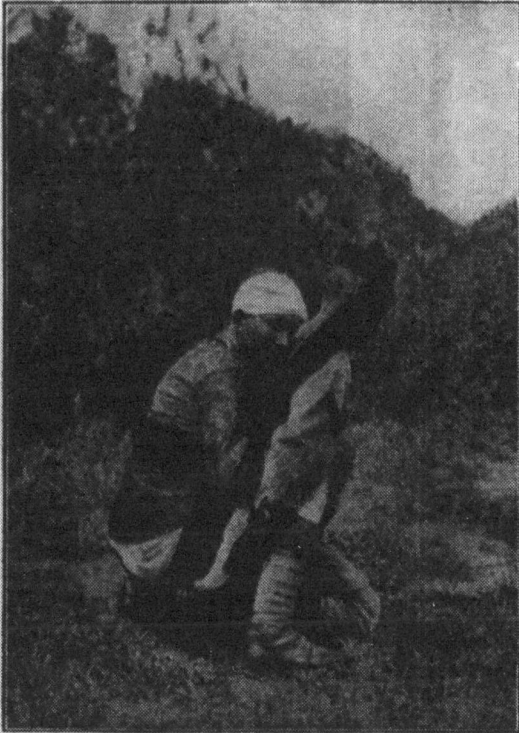

FIG. 36. USING TWO PUTTEES.

302. Dandies and Doolies.—In India, from time immemorial the doolie has been the general method of transporting the sick and wounded by litter. It consists of a canvas bed on which a man can lie full length, with frame-work and cover carried on a bamboo pole. Fig. 37 shows the Indian Army pattern dandy, used by the Army in India.

The dandy bearers are a special caste of native known as Kahars, who carry the dandies at a shuffling pace, which is neither a walk nor a run, without jolting, and which exerts an effect rather soothing than otherwise to the patient. The dandy is a comfortable means of sick-transport ; a man's equipment, food, beverages, medicine, etc., may be carried along in it, and when placed on the ground it forms a comfortable bed, and protects from the sun by day and the dew and cold by night.

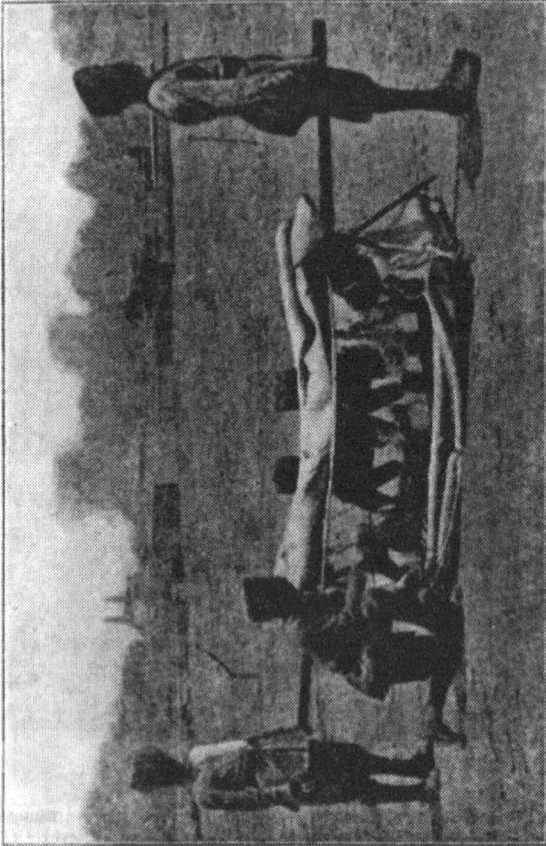

FIG. 37. THE INDIAN ARMY PATTERN DANDY.

It is, however, not always safe for transporting very serious cases over rough ground. The pole is too long for hill paths ; and the dandy and bearers can be seen a long distance off, and often draw fire in tribal warfare ; but, taken altogether, it is a most serviceable conveyance.

308. Army Pattern Ambulance Stretchers.—The ambulance stretchers in use in the British Army are those known as Mark II. Those formerly known as Mark I are being converted to this pattern as Mark I* ; a third pattern, fitted with a hood, is known as Special Mark I.

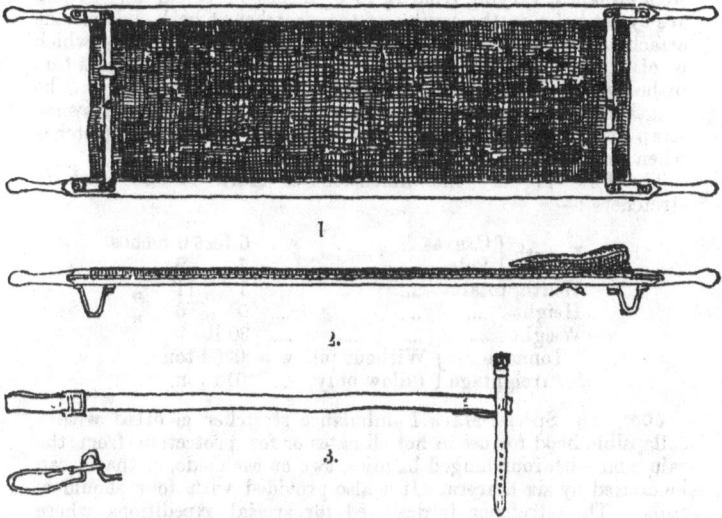

FIG. 38. AMBULANCE STRETCHERS, MARK II.

1. Plan of underside of stretcher showing traverses.
2. Side elevation of stretcher with cushion in place.
3. Sling and detail of adjustable loop in lateral view.

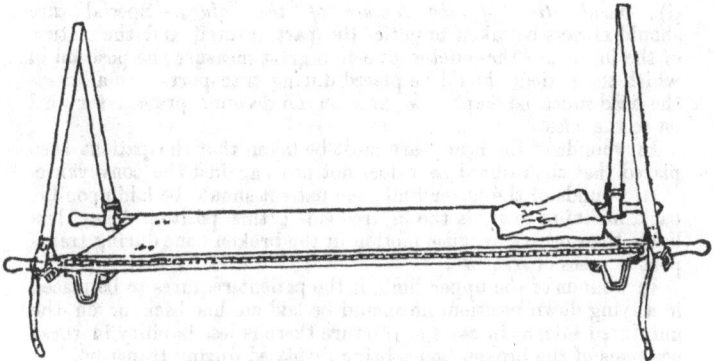

FIG. 39. AMBULANCE STRETCHER. MARK II.

304. In Mark II stretchers (Figs. 38 and 39), the canvas, which is tanned, is fastened to the pole by copper nails through an edging of leather; the poles are square and kept apart the required distance by two flat, wrought iron, jointed bars called traverses, and are fitted on the under side with steel U-shaped runners. A pillow and a pair of shoulder-slings are provided with each stretcher. The pillows are wedge-shaped, varying from $1\frac{1}{2}$ to $3\frac{1}{2}$ inches in thickness. There are eyelet holes in the canvas of the stretcher at both ends for the attachment of the pillows by thin leather thongs. The sling, which is of tanned web, has at either end a loop, one of which is furnished with a brass grip-plate, by means of which the sling can be lengthened or shortened; at the opposite end is a narrow, transverse strap fixed at right angles, which is buckled round the stretcher when closed.

The following are the dimensions of Mark II and Mark I* stretchers :—

Length { Canvas....	..	...	6 feet 0 inches.	
Pole	....	....	7 „ 9 „	
Width, total	...	...	1 „ 11 „	
Height	..	. ..	....	0 „ 6 „
Weight	....	....	....	30 lb.
Tonnage { Without pillow		·0364 ton.		
for freightage { Pillow only	....	·015 ton.		

305. The Special Mark I ambulance stretcher is fitted with a collapsible hood for use in hot climates or for protection from the rain, and with four hinged handles, two on each side, so that it can be carried by six bearers. It is also provided with four shoulder-pads. This stretcher is designed for special expeditions where natives would be employed for carrying the wounded, and is well adapted for carrying a wounded man a long distance. It weighs 8lb. more than the Mark II and Mark I* stretchers.

306. General Rules for the Carriage of Stretchers.— (i) *Consideration of the Nature of the Injury.*—Special care should always be taken to notice the part injured and the nature of the injury, as these determine in a great measure the position in which the patient should be placed during transport. In all cases the head must be kept low, and on no account pressed forward on to the chest.

In wounds of the head, care must be taken that the patient is so placed that the injured part does not press against the conveyance.

In wounds of the lower limb, the patient should be laid upon his back, inclining towards the injured side ; this position being less liable than others to cause motion in the broken bone during transport in cases of fracture.

In wounds of the upper limb, if the patient requires to be placed in a lying down position, he should be laid on his back or on the uninjured side, as in cases of fracture there is less liability in these positions of the broken bones being displaced during transport.

In wounds of the chest there is often a difficulty in breathing; the patient should be placed with the chest well raised, his body at the same time being inclined towards the injured side.

In transverse or punctured wounds of the abdomen, the patient should be laid on his back, with his legs drawn up, so as to bring the thighs as close to the belly as possible, a pack or other article being placed under his hams to keep his knees bent. If the wound is vertical the legs should be extended.

(ii) *Adjustment of Slings.*—Care should be taken at starting to adjust the slings so that the parts supporting the poles are at equal distances from the surface of the ground.

(iii) *Carriage of Patient.*—The patient is usually carried feet first, but in going up hill the position is reversed, and the patient is carried head first. To do this the bearers will lower the stretcher and turn about. If the patient is suffering from a recent fracture of the lower extremity he will, in all cases, be carried with his head down hill. The stronger and taller bearers should be down hill.

(iv) *Carriage of Stretcher.*—In all circumstances the stretcher should, as far as possible, be carried in the horizontal position, which may be maintained in passing over uneven ground by raising or lowering the ends of the stretcher.

It is an important matter for the bearers to practise the carriage of stretchers, so as to acquire skill in keeping the stretcher level on uneven ground. The bearers trained and habituated to this duty perform it with ease and dexterity, irrespective of difference in their heights, while those who have not practised it are not un-likely to cause considerable distress to the patient when they have to carry him up and down hill. Concerted action of the front and rear bearers is necessary; each must be aware what part he has to perform, and must instinctively raise or lower his end of the stretcher in order to counteract the effect of one bearer being temporarily higher or lower than the other. Facility in this can best be acquired by practising the carriage of the stretchers up and down steps, or over uneven ground.

On no account will bearers carry a stretcher with the poles on their shoulders, as it is necessary that one of them should have the patient in view. In the event also of the patient falling from such a height, owing to one of the bearers tripping or being wounded, his injuries might be considerably aggravated.

(v) *Passing a Wall or Fence.*—No attempt will be made to carry a patient over a high fence or wall, if it can possibly be avoided, as such is always a dangerous proceeding. A portion of the wall should be thrown down, or a breach in the fence made, so that the patient may be carried through on the stretcher; or, if this be not practicable, the patient should be carried to a place where a gate or opening already exists, even although the distance to be traversed may be increased by doing so. It is better to do this than risk the safety of the patient.

(vi) *Crossing a Ditch.*—On arrival at a ditch to be crossed, the No. 4 of the stretcher squad (see Chap. XXII) will select a level piece of ground near its edge where the stretcher will be lowered.

The bearers will then take up positions at the stretcher as in loading wagons. The stretcher, with the patient on it, is then lifted and carried as near the edge as possible and lowered to the ground.

The Nos. 1 and 4 bearers descend into the ditch, lay hold of the handles of the stretcher, and, lifting it, draw it forward ; the remaining bearers in succession descend and take hold of the stretcher, which is then pushed forward to the opposite side, and the front pair of runners rested on top of the bank.

The Nos. 1 and 4 bearers now climb up and guide the stretcher which is pushed forward by the other bearers until both pairs of runners rest on the ground. The remaining bearers climb up, and the whole, lifting the stretcher as in loading wagons, carry it forward clear of the ditch and place it on the ground, the bearers taking up positions as in "prepare stretchers" (Chap. XXII). The No. 4 bearer will then examine the patient with a view to re-adjusting dressings, etc., if necessary, after which the march will be resumed.

The necessary words of command for lifting and lowering stretchers, etc., will be given by the No. 4 bearer.

(vii) *Crossing a Canal or River, when no boats or bridges are available.*—In this case it is necessary to improvise a raft on which one or more stretchers can be placed. This can be done as follows :—Dig a trench 7 feet by 7 feet by 3 feet ; take a large tarpaulin, or cover of a wagon, and spread it over the bottom of the trench, leaving enough tarpaulin to fold over and bind when the trench is filled ; next fill the tarpaulin as tightly as possible with cut brushwood firmly stamped down, and cover with the spare folds of the tarpaulin. Then take it out, bind with strong ropes and fasten securely. Float the raft, and secure the stretcher to the ropes in such a manner as will keep it level when loaded. The whole can then be floated across with the assistance of the bearers.

307. The Improvisation of Stretchers, Litters, etc.—The improvisation of stretchers is not difficult, bearing in mind the principle of their construction, viz., some secure material upon which a patient can lie and be carried by men. Before any improvised apparatus is used for the conveyance of a wounded man, it must be practically tested by one of the party, in order to avoid the possibility of further injury to the patient from defective materials or construction. The materials necessary are generally to be found in the neighbourhood of operations, *i.e.*, doors, gates, hurdles, shutters, shafts, saplings, broom-handles, corn-sacks, tarpaulins, old tents, stout pieces of cloth, great-coats, hay, straw, ferns, leaves, etc., etc., all of which have their use.

A gate or door taken off its hinges, or a hurdle, are ready means of carriage, if at hand.

The hammock is the simplest special contrivance for carrying a sick or wounded man, and a soldier's blanket slung between two men, or tied to a pole carried on their shoulders offers perhaps the most primitive form.

308. By means of blankets, canvas, or sacks, an improvised stretcher can be formed with a couple of poles. A horse-blanket with two or three lances passed through several slits on each side would serve to carry a man for a short distance.

A loop may be sewn at each corner of a blanket, which is then doubled over so that the two loops at each end are brought together. A pole (preferably of cedar, pine, ash, or bamboo) is then passed through the four loops on one side, and another passed within the doubling of the blanket on the other side. This forms a secure and comfortable stretcher for a short distance.

Again, a good temporary litter can be made by laying two stout poles on the edges of a blanket, rolling the edges inwards, and finally making them fast by strong twine passed through holes cut in the blanket at intervals of about a foot along the poles and tied off strongly on the outside.

A length of blanket sewn on to bamboo poles makes a light serviceable stretcher ; but, like the preceding forms, it has no traverses, and a stretcher not so provided is unsuitable for carrying a case which might be subjected to injurious pressure when the stretcher is raised.

Two poles, each of, say, 8 feet in length, may be used, with two cross bars 2½ feet each, nailed or securely lashed on to each end of them ; the blanket being firmly knotted to the pole. A third cross-bar placed across the centre would keep the patient from falling out. An effective cover of bent boughs supporting another blanket could be arranged over the stretcher as a protection from sun and rain.

309. An addition to the blanket-stretcher has recently been invented by a German army surgeon. Stirrup-irons with the leathers attached are used as handles. The blanket is stuffed between the bars of the treads and fixed there with a sword-knot, stone, or other hard article of convenient size, thrust into the pocket so formed. The stirrup-leathers are left attached, so as to be used as slings to assist in supporting the patient's weight. The irons are fixed on to the blanket in which the patient has been placed, 2 at the head-end and 2 at the feet-end, each pair being held by a bearer. One is also fixed to the blanket on either side of the patient, and grasped by an additional bearer. Stirrup-irons can be applied to any blanket, and should be placed away from its edge and as near the patient's body as possible, leaving the free sides available for covering the patient. He can then be comfortably transported by 4 bearers with 6 stirrups, or by 2 bearers if poles are slipped through the irons on either side of the patient.

The irons and leathers may be used with 2 bearers (instead of 4) one at either end ; or used to suspend the patient in a wagon.

310. An emergency stretcher* (see Fig. 40), which takes little time to make, can be constructed with a triangular frame lashed together with yarn. (A quadrangular frame so constructed is less rigid, and more liable to collapse.)

The requisites are :—Two hop-poles or stack-props 2½ to 2 inches in diameter, not less than 9 feet long ; two lighter sticks 1 inch at

---

* Devised by Lt.-Col. H. E. R. James, R.A.M.C. (Ret'd).

Extemporized Stretcher made of hop poles & corn sacks

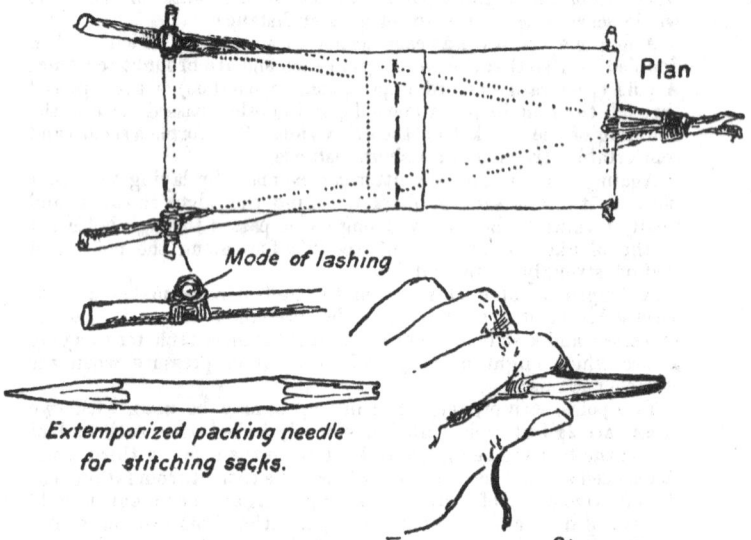

Plan

Mode of lashing

Extemporized packing needle for stitching sacks.

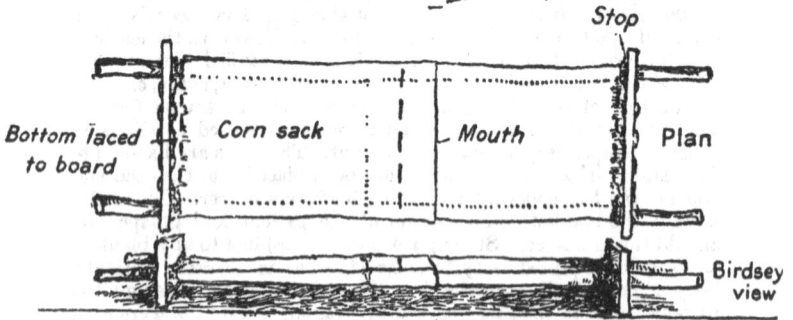

Stop

Bottom laced to board

Corn sack

Mouth

Plan

Birdsey view

Nail — Stop on pole

Twine

Extemporized stretcher for railway carriage of wounded made of 1 inch deal boards hop poles and corn sacks.

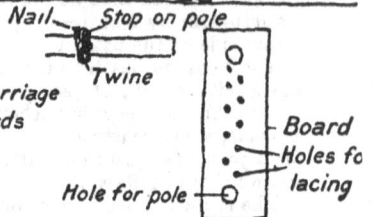

Board
Holes for lacing

Hole for pole

Scale of ½ inch to 1 ft. 3 inches

FIG. 40.

least in diameter, and 36 inches long ; two corn-sacks, 40 inches by 24 inches (ordinary size); five yards of rope yarn (tarred for choice).

The tools required are a jack-knife, and a packing needle extemporized out of a piece of stick, as shown in Fig. 40. In the case of a fractured leg or thigh it may be necessary to add transverse battens to prevent the canvas from sagging and the limb from bending over the poles (the patient's heels lie outside the poles).

The two long poles are laid together, and their smaller ends are lashed with a lashing 1½ inch wide. The larger ends are separated until, at a distance of 7 feet from the small ends, there is an interval of 28 inches between them. One of the shorter sticks is now passed through the bottom of a sack, coming out at each corner, laid over the poles, and lashed to each with square lashings at a distance of 7 feet from the end lashing.

The second stick is similarly passed through the bottom of the second sack, coming out at each corner, and the mouth of one sack is passed into that of the other until the length of the canvas so formed is 6 feet.

The sacks are now stitched together in this position by means of the extemporized packing-needle, the sharp end being used to separate the threads of the canvas, and the cleft end to push the twine through.

The centre of the bottom of the sack nearest the foot of the stretcher is now perforated, and six turns of yarn passed through the perforation, round the stick, and round the lashing at the end of the two poles, and pulled hard until the canvas is thoroughly stretched, when it is made fast.

Such a stretcher is intended only for hand-carriage and cannot be used as a bed.

311. A modification* of the stretcher used in Austria for railway transportation takes longer to make, but can be used for carriage by wagon or rail, or as a temporary bed (see Fig. 40).

The materials required are :—Two pieces of planking 3 feet by 10 inches by 1 inch, if of deal, thinner if of hard wood ; two poles 2 inches in diameter, tapering to 1¾ or 1½ inch ; two grain-sacks 40 inches by 24 inches ; 6 yards of stout twine or tarred rope-yarn ; four 1½-inch wire nails. The tools necessary are a saw, a gimlet, a centre-bit (if possible 2 inches) and brace, an extemporized packing-needle, a hammer, and a knife.

The boards are perforated by means of the centre-bit, the holes being made large enough to pass the poles through, and their outer edges being 24 inches apart ; they are made in the middle line of the length of the boards, their centres 5 inches from either edge. Other holes are made in the boards with the gimlet large enough to pass the twine through easily ; ten holes are enough, alternately above and below a line passing through the centres of the larger holes, the two rows of five being 1 inch apart. Holes are made in the corners of the two sacks large enough to allow the poles to pass through. The two poles are now passed through one of the boards, and one sack is drawn bottom first over them, the poles being

---

* Devised by Lt.-Col. H. E. R. James, R.A.M.C. (Ret'd).

passed first through the holes in the corners of the sack so as to be inside it.

The second sack is now passed over the poles, mouth first, and the poles are passed through the holes in its corners, and then through the holes in the second board.

The boards are now adjusted so that they are square with the poles, and parallel with one another at 6 feet 2 inches distance. The poles are marked with chalk or pencil where the inner edges of the board cut them, and at this point a nail is driven for half its length, and twine is wound round to form "stops" which may be further helped by wedging to keep the boards apart. The spare ends of the poles are now cut so that they project 9 inches beyond the boards. The mouth of one sack is now drawn over that of the other, so as to form a continuous canvas of 6 feet long, each end formed by the bottom of each sack being 1 inch short of touching the board. Stitches of twine are passed through both thicknesses of both sacks to keep them in this position. Finally, a lacing is made to fix the bottoms of the sacks to the boards, the twine being passed through the holes in the boards and through two thicknesses of the sack's bottom.

The stretcher so formed is not perfectly rigid, and, owing to the poles being round, the boards may twist upon them if the stretcher is not evenly carried, but, if properly stoppered and wedged, this will not be found troublesome, and the lacing at the head and foot keeps the frame square. The only thing that may present difficulty is making the holes in the boards. With a small-sized bit three or four holes may be cut and made into one, and this may be enlarged by means of a red-hot iron.

312. Stretchers can be improvised with rifles and puttees, pugarees, etc., *e.g.* :—(i) Two puttees are applied to two rifles, forming nine bands from muzzle to butt (Fig. 41). The cartridges are withdrawn. The two rifles are placed with their trigger-guards uppermost, the two puttees being knotted to the rifles so as to form nine cross-bands uniting the rifles.

The first cross-band passes from the muzzle of one rifle to the piling-swivel of the other ; the second cross-band from the piling-swivel of one rifle to midway between the "upper band" and the "lower band" of the other ; the third cross-band from midway between the "upper" and the "lower band" to the "lower band"; the fourth cross-band from the "lower band" to the hand-guard ; the fifth band from the hand-guard to the front of the magazine. The second puttee is then knotted to the first. The sixth cross-band runs from the front of the magazine to the small of the butt ; the seventh band from the small of the butt of the one rifle to the small of the butt of the other rifle ; the eighth cross-band from the small of the butt to the butt-swivel; the ninth cross-band between the two butt-swivels. The puttees are applied to the rifles by a simple hitch, and fastened to such parts of the rifle as will prevent slipping. The stretcher thus formed by the puttees has a length of about 44 inches and a breadth of about 15 inches.

This method* of carrying wounded by means of rifles is useful where men are seriously injured. The head can be kept level, being at the butt-end, and the legs allowed to hang down at the muzzle-end of the rifles. The slings of the two rifles can be tied over the chest of the wounded man by means of a piece of bandage, etc.

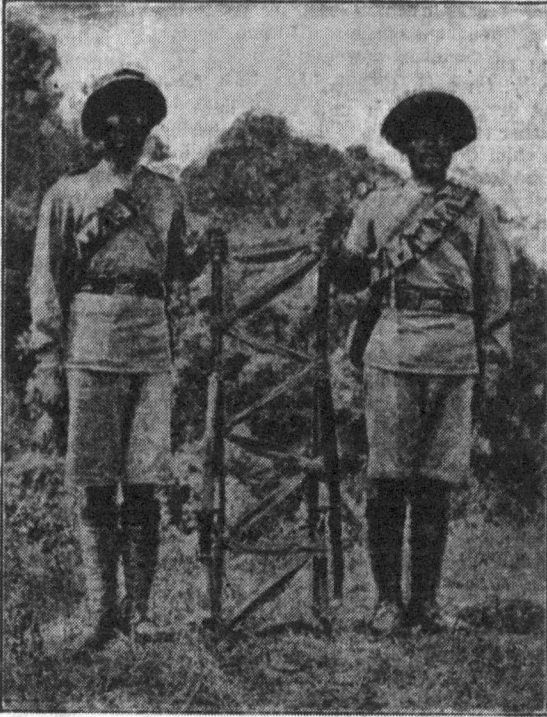

FIG. 41.—RIFLE AND PUTTEE STRETCHER.

(ii) Satisfactory results were obtained on several occasions during the siege of Ladysmith in the South African war by tying waterproof sheets to rifles by means of pugarees taken from the men's helmets. The sheets must be in good condition.

313. Perhaps the most comfortable of all litters is that formed by one or two poles passed through a strong net. This mode of carriage is adopted by aboriginal tribes in Africa and New Zealand, and the North American Indians also use a net in their "travois."

The ordinary string or grass hammock terminates at either end in several small lines looped together at their extremities, or formed

---

* Devised by Captain J. S. O'Neill, I M.S.

into lines, so that it can be supported between 2 solid supports by means of hooks, etc. In a sailor's hammock, on board ship, these lines are called "clews" and they meet at each end in an iron ring called a "grummet"; such can be readily suspended from a single long pole and made to serve as a useful litter.

314. In hill warfare there is often great difficulty in removing wounded men by means of the ordinary stretcher, or dandy as used in India, and small detached parties often find themselves without these, or without sufficient of them, or else it is impossible to attempt the removal of wounded by them. It is generally safer, especially on a steep hillside, to carry a wounded man down in a blanket or greatcoat, or improvised hammock such as a transport net, rather than attempt to use a stretcher or dandy if available.

The chief desiderata for hand-carriage in hill warfare are :—(1) The total length of the litter, including bearers, should be short to allow of zig-zagging amongst rocks ; (2) it should be well above the ground to avoid irregularities during ascents and descents ; (3) it should be so constructed that the patient cannot fall out ; (4) it should be very light and easily carried when not in use, so that detached parties may be provided with means of removing their wounded without being encumbered with extra weight, or even with special bearers.

315. The hammock devised by Lieutenant-Colonel A. R. Aldridge, R.A.M.C., for use in hilly country is made of canvas and supported by canvas bands arranged at suitable positions to carry the weight. The following sketch (Fig. 42) shows how it is constructed. A piece of canvas 7 feet long and 3 feet broad is folded lengthwise in the centre and cut as shown by the dotted lines. The two edges along these lines are sewn together, thus forming a boat-shaped hammock.

Supporting straps of double canvas, 2½ inches broad, are sewn round the hammock in the positions indicated, the length of these

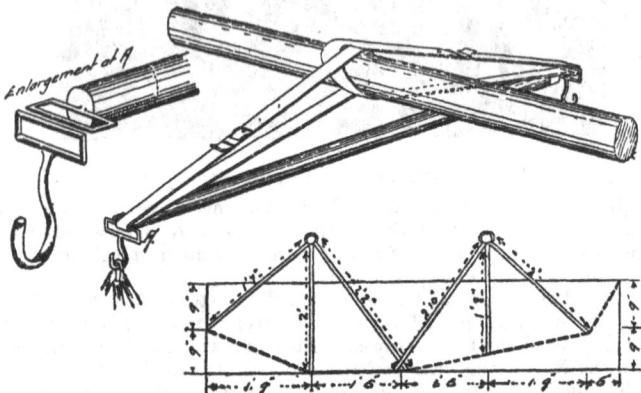

FIG. 42.—THE "ALDRIDGE" HAMMOCK.

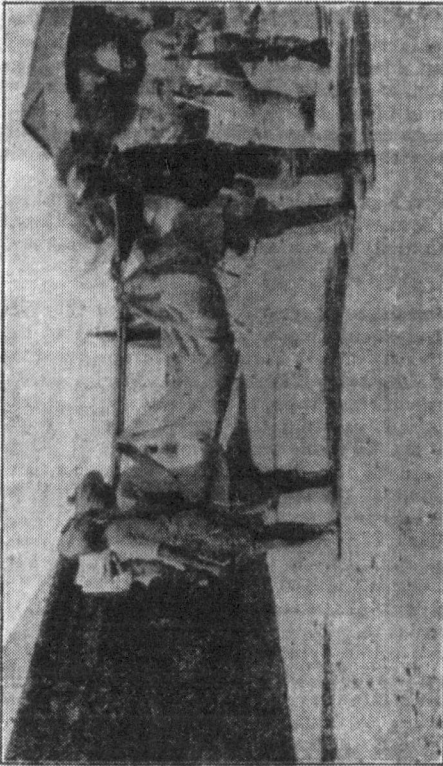

FIG. 43.—THE "ALDRIDGE" HAMMOCK.   (LOADED.)

being double that shown in the sketch, which represents one side only. The free ends of these straps are joined up to two 2-inch iron rings on each side of the hammock ; each ring having three straps sewn to it.

Four stout leather straps, 27 inches long, with buckles at one end, are required for suspending the hammock from the pole or poles, also two wooden traverses, 1½ ft. long, with wire slots at each end for the straps to pass through (A of Fig. 42). These are to keep the sides of the hammock apart. The straps are attached to the hammock by means of hooks ; but if these are not obtainable the straps can be looped through the rings.

For carrying with one pole, the two straps on one side are loosely looped through the corresponding ones on the other side and the buckles fastened ; the pole is placed through the double loop so formed (Fig. 18). For carrying with two poles all the straps are shortened up, leaving room for one pole to pass through the two straps on each side of the hammock. The poles should have leather stops nailed on, to prevent slipping of the hammock when going up and down hill (Fig. 43).

The hammock can also be carried with a patient at full length by four bearers with two rifles, or with the patient sitting, by two bearers.

The complete hammock has jointed poles, hood, and leg-boards to support the lower limbs in cases of fracture. When folded, the hammock can easily be carried slung over the shoulders.

CONVEYANCES WHEELED BY MEN.

316. Opinions vary as regards the utility of this form of hand ambulance transport, though it is on record that at the battle of Bautzen in Saxony in 1813 Baron Larrey transported two-thirds of his wounded a distance of thirty miles in hand-carts.

Conveyances of this nature, to be of real use, must take the army pattern stretcher, and admit of its being securely mounted and dismounted. On the whole they are not very well adapted for field service, but can be utilized with advantage where there are good level roads, and in transporting cases in a general hospital, etc. The pattern approved for the Army is the "Carriage, Ambulance Stretcher, Mark I."

There are possibilities in the cycle-stretcher and the subject is receiving attention and study by several nations, but a satisfactory arrangement which has stood the test of time and service has not yet been arrived at.

Among the various types may be mentioned Furley's "Ashford Litter," Luce's Portable Trolley, and the Simonis Combined Cycle and Ambulance Litter.

317. Carriage, Ambulance Stretcher, Mark I.—This consists (see Fig. 44) of an under carriage built up of two light wheels with steel spokes, rims with rubber tyres, and ball bearings ; on the axle are two light elliptic springs, to which is attached a transverse seat for the stretcher-carrier proper, which takes an army pattern stretcher. The carrier is securely bolted on to the seat and consists of two pieces of hard wood, suitably worked and forming an angle frame. On the bottom side the stretcher-poles rest, and the sides of the "L" formed by the carrier proper prevent effectually any jerking or turning of the stretcher when once it has been laid in the carrier. The carrier is about 30 inches long, but can be increased to any length desired. It has been found that this length is suited for most purposes. To prevent any lateral or upward movement of the stretcher, two buttons with tightening screws are attached to the top of the carrier on each side. When the stretcher is laid on the carrier the screws are tightened and the stretcher is held rigid.

Two iron supports are provided, one at each end and on opposite sides of the carrier. These are lowered when it is desired either to place the stretcher on the carriage or to remove it, actions which can be effected rapidly. The carriage meanwhile remains perfectly still.

When the carriage is in motion the iron supports are turned up and lie along the respective sides of the carrier, where each rests in a small clip. The object of this stretcher-carriage has been to obtain mobility, strength, and lightness, combined with efficiency, and a ready and easy means of transport for sick and wounded no matter where a patient has to be transported from.

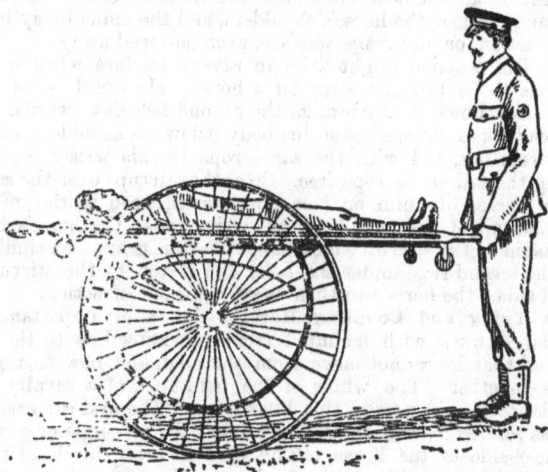

FIG. 44.—CARRIAGE, AMBULANCE STRETCHER, MARK I.

The loaded stretcher and wheeled carriage can be readily handled by one man on good roads, and by two men in rough country. The springs prevent any jar from being felt by the patient on the stretcher.

BY ANIMALS.

318. The removal of a wounded comrade by mounted men is a useful practice in all mounted corps.

A man can be brought out of action on a horse without any special contrivance for carrying him, other than the saddle. If only slightly wounded, he may be able to ride off unaided, or he may be assisted out of action by a comrade sitting behind him, or by one walking on either side of his horse. If dismounted, he may be given a stirrup and assisted to mount behind the rider ; or, if unable to mount in this way and another horse is at hand, the comrade may dismount and help him up. If badly hit the comrade should place the wounded man in front of him facing the horse's tail, and hold him in his arms, the wounded man, if able to assist, holding on to the cantle of the saddle with both hands ; or he may be laid across the saddle face downwards, supporting himself with one foot in a lengthened stirrup, while the horse is led by a comrade.

To carry an insensible man on a horse, make, if possible, a pad with a horse-blanket or sack on the saddle, place the man astride over the horse's withers, his body lying on the saddle face down-wards, his head toward the horse's tail ; cross the stirrup leathers over the man's back, and secure the stirrup-irons by the head-rope from the off to the near-side under the horse's belly. The man's legs hang clear of the horse's shoulders, and the animal may be led out of action, or, in savage warfare, even galloped away.

819. The occasion might arise in savage warfare when a dead man has to be brought away on a horse. He could be securely tied on as follows :—Lay him on the ground face downwards. Get two head-ropes, tie one round his body below his shoulders, stretch both arms out, and with the same rope tie his wrists together, leaving the tail of the rope free. Cross the stirrups over the saddle of the horse, lift him on face downwards, head to the off-side. Pass the tail of the rope from the wrist under the horse's belly, and fasten to the stirrup which hangs over the near-side ; similarly, pass the second rope under the belly and fasten to the stirrup on the off-side ; the horse can then be galloped out of action.

320. Tying and Coupling Horses.—It is of importance in ambulance work with mounted troops to know how to tie up a horse so that he cannot move from the spot, and how to tie two horses together. The whole of the personnel of a cavalry field ambulance should possess this knowledge. The first can easily be done as follows :—Pass the bit-rein under the surcingle or girth on the near-side of the horse, taking care to bring his head round quietly, without jerking, so as to shorten the rein ; then pass the stirrup-iron and leather through the loop thus formed and draw taut.

Another method is to unbuckle the near stirrup-leather and pass one end of it through the ring of the bridoon on the near-side, and rebuckle. At the same time the stirrup-iron should be run up to the flap of the saddle.

Horses can be securely coupled by turning them head-to-tail, and tying each with the bridoon-rein to the off back-strap or arch of the saddle of the other, taking care that the rein when tied is not more than six to eight inches long.

321. To Remove a Wounded Man from a Horse.—Three bearers are enough, but a fourth can hold the horse's head. First of all the man's spurs must invariably be taken off whatever the injury may be, and if the horse is restive hold up one foreleg with the knee bent. In the case of an injured lower limb, Nos. 1, 2, and 3 approach on the wounded side. On the word "*Lay-Hold*" (given by No. 1), No. 1 from behind takes hold of the pelvis and sound leg, No. 2 is held round the neck and shoulders by the wounded man, and No. 3 holds the wounded limb. On the words

" *Ready, Lift-Off,*" the patient is taken off and held over the stretcher placed alongside, and on the word " *Lower,*" is laid on it. In the case of injured upper limb the wounded man is approached on the sound side. No. 1 supports the pelvis and leg, No. 2 is held round the neck by the patient's sound arm, and No. 3 supports the wounded limb. Words, same as before.

CONVEYANCES CARRIED BY ANIMALS.

322. To this the name of Pack Ambulance Transport is given. The animals used are the camel and the mule, and their employment is restricted to mountain and desert warfare in Asia and Africa.

323. In India, up to the time of the Mutiny, the camel was one of the chief means of transporting the wounded and reinforcements of fighting men, notably in the Campaigns of the Punjab and during the Mutiny ; however, the development of the railways and roads since then renders the use of camels unnecessary in ordinary circumstances.

Men were carried on camels in what are called *kujawahs*, which are of various patterns. The kujawah-litter was a framework of wood, with the sides and bottom filled up with laced rope or strong canvas. Iron rings were fixed to the edge of the framework, through which ropes passed to secure it firmly to the camel. The conveyance was furnished with legs, so built as not to interfere with the progression of the animal. A pair of kujawahs was borne by each camel and the patients sat back-to-back.

Another type was a kind of box in which the men sat in a half-doubled up position. Litters and crates were also employed by which men could lie down full-length.

The load of a camel is 400 lb. and his average pace is from $2\frac{1}{2}$ to 3 miles an hour. This of course does not apply to the riding camel which can cover ten miles an hour easily.

324. The best improvised litter for a camel is a native bedstead such as the Indian *charpoy* or the Egytian *angareeb*, the bedstead turned upside down, and the legs laced with stout rope, so as to form shut-in sides to it. In Egypt an angareeb is strapped on crossways to the animal's back and the patient is secured on, face downwards, the legs of the bed being secured under the animal's belly ; or cacolets similar to those used with mules are employed.

325. Figure 45 shows an improvised litter carried by two camels, and by which a sick officer was actually carried two hundred miles through the Soudanese desert without a mishap. It consists of a bed supported on each side by a couple of long poles (telegraph poles were used), which form a pair of shafts secured to the saddles of the camels. An important point to remember is that the shafts for the rear camel must be twice as long as those for the leader. The legs of the bed are prolonged upwards, forming supports for an awning formed by blankets folded double, the side opposite to the sun being rolled up to give plenty of air. Four blankets are sufficient to form the awning ; two form the roof, meeting in the centre and the ends are left hanging over to protect the head and feet from the sun, if

necessary. A bar at each side of the litter above the poles provides against the patient rolling off ; the sides are furnished with a " gate " in the centre for exit and entrance.

The camels must be made to rise and kneel together, so as not to cause inconvenience to the patient when loading or unloading. With carefully selected and trained camels the man need never leave his bed and sound sleep can be procured. Each camel is led by its respective attendant.

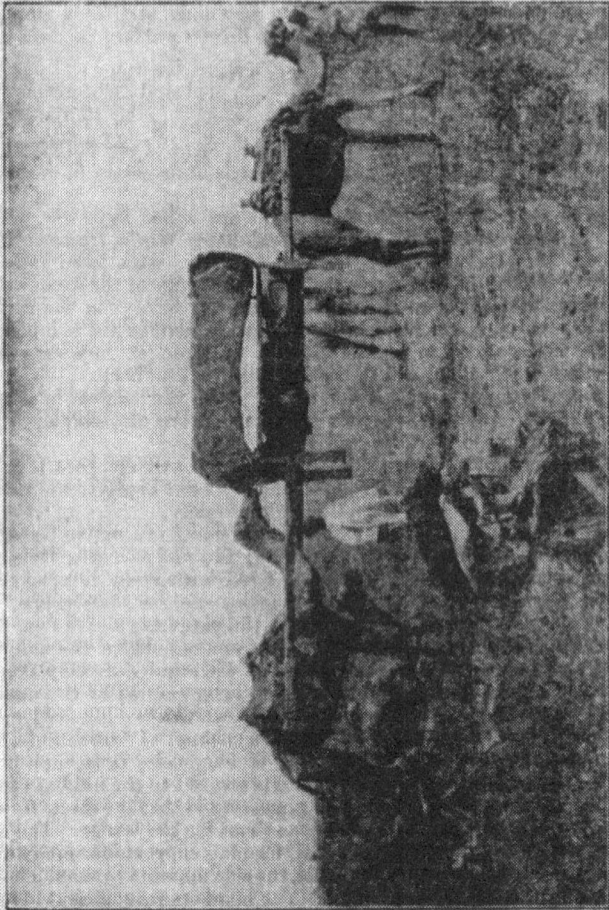

FIG. 45.—EGYPTIAN CAMEL LITTER.

326. The cacolets used with mules consist of folding chairs which are hooked in pairs to the sides of a pack-saddle ; the patients sit on each side facing the direction of the animal's head This form of transport has been much used by the French in Algeria and proved a success. It is, however, fatiguing for the animals. The weight of a pair of army cacolets is 56 lb., and the pack-saddle, with accessories, weighs 53 lb. The authorized load of a pack-mule is 160 lb., so that it would be impossible to transport a couple of men any long distance, unless the strongest type of mule is available.

327. Mule-litters, each carried by two mules, were used by the Russians in the war in Manchuria with successful results.

The litters consist of two strong poles about fifteen feet long connected in the centre by two cross-pieces ; netting with a sheet sewn above it is fastened on between them. The cover is formed of two arches of bent wood with cloth stretched over them, and covered with tarpaulins if necessary. A mattress or improvised bed is placed on the netting, or, if these are not available, a great-coat or blanket. The free ends of the poles are fastened to the pack-saddles. The weight of the litter with two pack-saddles is about 108 lb., so that counting the wounded man's weight at, say, 144 lb., the weight on each mule comes to about 130 lb. The litter is only about $3\frac{1}{2}$ feet from the ground and can be easily loaded and unloaded. It can be taken off and used as a hand stretcher over any especially dangerous part of the road. Such a litter can be brought nearer the fighting line than a wheeled vehicle, and can be repaired easily if broken.

328. The Arabs strap a bedstead across the back of a mule, in a manner similar to the Egyptian method of angareebs with camels. It has been found a comfortable mode of carrying wounded.

CONVEYANCES DRAWN BY ANIMALS.

329. In every country, where the roads permit of wheeled ambulance transport, vehicles of varying design, drawn by horses, ponies, mules, or oxen, form the chief means of transporting sick and wounded.

330. Army Pattern Ambulance Wagons.—The vehicles which are designed expressly for the conveyance of the sick and wounded are called ambulance wagons, and each country has its own pattern Those in use in the British Army are the Mark V*, Mark VI, and Mark I (light). For the dimensions of army pattern vehicles, used by the medical service, see table at the end of this chapter.

331. *Mark V*, Ambulance Wagon.*—This wagon (Fig. 46) is a conversion of the former Mark V. It is constructed to accommodate 4 patients on stretchers (2 stretchers on the floor and 2 on the rails which fold down on the forward seats), or 12 patients sitting (6 on each side), or 2 on stretchers on the rails resting on the seats, and 4 sitting on the seats at the rear end,

Lockers, "Medical" and "Drivers," are formed under the driver's seat, and are closed by doors opening outward below the footboard. Three lockers are also provided at the front end of the interior, one on each side of the floor, and a narrow one for medical comforts and restoratives immediately beneath the centre of the driver's seat. Fittings are also provided to carry thigh-splints above the front lockers.

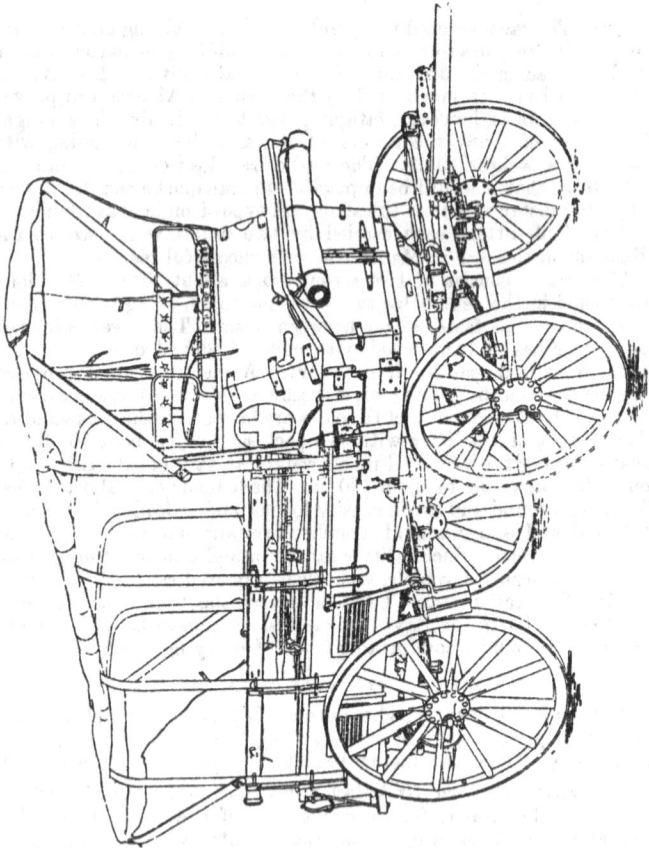

Fig. 46.—Wagon, Ambulance, Mark V*.

Two stretchers are placed on the floor of the wagon, the runners resting on rubber pads to prevent slipping, and two on the lifting seats, which are supported on iron brackets. Above the lifting seats are rails (one long in front and one short behind on each side), folding down to take a stretcher on each side, the ends of the stretcher-poles, when pushed home along the rails, passing through the heel board on the driver's seat. The surfaces of the long rails, uppermost when folded down, have bevelled pieces of wood with indiarubber pads in which the runners of the stretcher rest to prevent slipping. The vehicle is fitted with a perch and a "Jacob's" lock fore-carriage, which reduces the strain on the body in travelling, and admits of large front wheels being used so as to minimize the pull on the horses. It is also fitted with a pole and swingle-trees for long-rein driving. There is a sliding step to the back of the wagon, which, when not in use, can be raised and pushed close up to the tail-board in guides fixed along the bottom for that purpose.

The sides are fitted with ventilators, staples for the bale-hoops, and standards for the back-rails. Fittings are attached to the back-rails under the seats for carrying rifles, and there are two straps attached to the back-rails for the safety of the patients. Sockets are fixed to the sides for supporting the lamp-brackets.

A wooden ladder, strapped to the underside when not in use, is carried to assist the patients in mounting.

A water-cask, capable of carrying 10 gallons, is secured under the rear by iron bands, and a small tackle is fitted just above it with which to lift it into position when required. This water-cask will eventually be replaced by an iron tank.

The splinter-bar is arranged to allow a vertical play to the pole ; and spiral "draw-spring," through which the loops for the swingle-trees pass, are fixed at the rear of the bar. These are intended to ease the strain upon the horses, especially at starting.

The wagon is fitted with a brake which acts on the front of the hind wheels, and is applied by the driver by means of a hand-lever. A rack keeps the brake on when it is applied. The wagon is fitted with bale-hoops and a canvas cover, a leather apron for the driver, cranked guard-irons, a drag-shoe, and grease-tin.

332. *Mark VI, Ambulance Wagon.*—This wagon (Fig. 47) is constructed to carry 4 patients on stretchers (two stretchers on the floor, and two on rails resting on the seats), or 12 sitting (on the seats), or 6 sitting at the rear end and 2 on stretchers on the rails.

The vehicle consists generally of a body, with a roof, fore-carriage, brake-gear, springs, axletrees, and indiarubber-tyred wheels. The body, which is supported at the front by the fore-carriage, and at the rear by two cross-springs and two side-springs on the hind axletree, is fitted with six movable standards (three on each side) to support the roof, ventilators along the sides, travelling lamps, and curtains of waterproof canvas.

The interior is provided with seats, lamps, hand-straps for the convenience of the lying-down patients, fittings to carry six rifles, a seat between the stretchers for an orderly, and a compartment on each side for medical comforts.

Under the body four lockers and a compartment for a water-tank are fitted, the former for surgical appliances, dressings, etc., and the latter for a 10-gallon water-tank.

At the front of the wagon two lockers are formed, over which is constructed a driving seat fitted with guard-irons ; immediately under the seat, in the centre, a small locker is formed. The seat is provided with a seat-box for the driver, and is protected with a hood of waterproof canvas with curtains at each side. A waterproof apron is attached to the footboard for the protection of men riding on the seat. The brake, which acts on the front of the hind wheels, is applied by the driver.

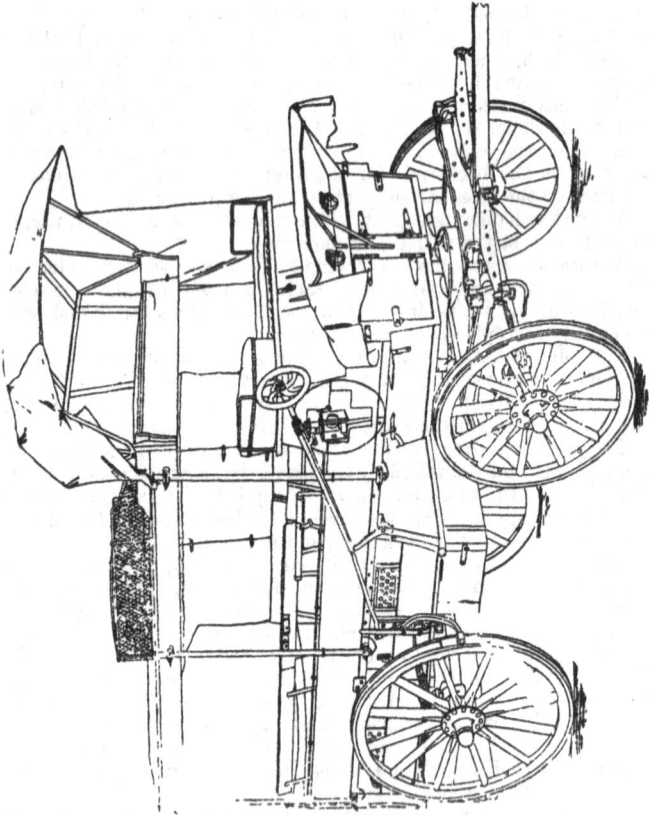

Fig. 47.—WAGON, AMBULANCE, MARK VI.

383. *Mark I, Light Ambulance Wagon.*—This wagon (Fig. 48) is constructed to carry 2 patients on stretchers ; or 8 sitting, 6 inside and 2 outside.

The vehicle consists geneially of a body, fore-carriage, brake-gear, cover, axletrees, and four wheels.

The body, which is supported at the front by the fore-carriage and at the rear by the two side springs on the hind axletree, consists principally of an oak frame, with sides, floor, and tail-board ; the interior forming a well for the stretchers and seats. The front portion consists of a footboard and lockers ; the top of the lockers forming the driver's seat, which is provided with guard-irons, back-rests, and driver's seat box. The interior is provided with two removable arm-rests and three hinged seats on each side, which may be tuined upwaids and secured to a back-rail. The floor is fitted

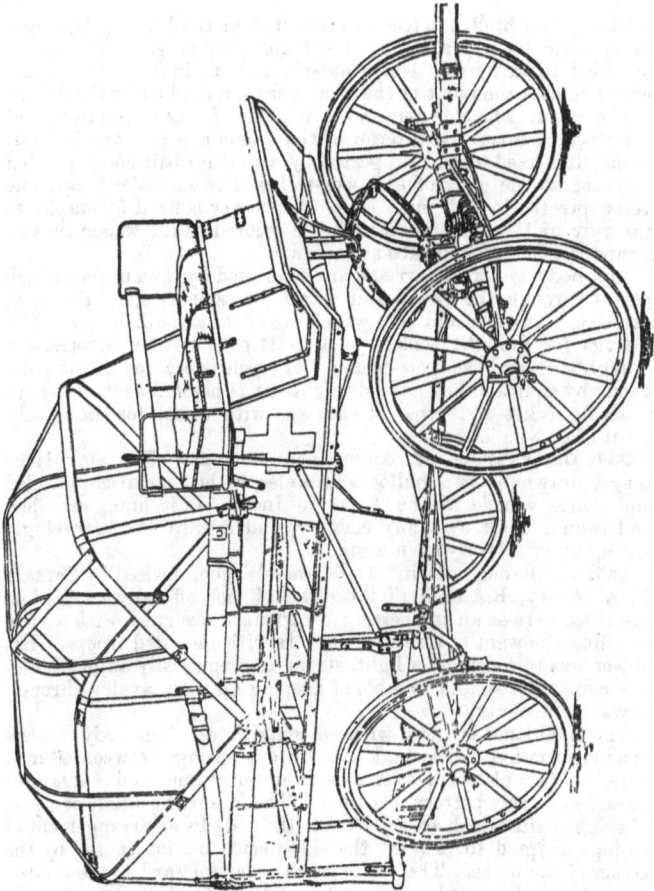

Fig. 48.—Wagon, Ambulance, Light, Mark I.

with indiarubber pads for the stretchers, which are secured by leather straps. The tail-board, which is hinged to the floor, is fitted with a folding step. A compartment to carry an aluminium water-tank is formed under the floor at the rear. A leather guard-strap is attached to two standards at the rear to protect the sitting patients. One of the lockers under the driver's seat is accessible from the interior and is closed by a door; another, with two compartments and a tin-lined box, is accessible from the footboard.

The front part of the body is supported over the fore-carriage by two bolsters (one upper and one lower) separated by transverse springs, a sweep-plate being fixed to the under side of the lower bolster. The hind axletree is connected to the lower bolster and sweep-plate by a perch with front and rear stays. Fittings are provided to carry two lamps outside and one inside. The brake, which acts on the front of the hind wheels, is applied by the driver.

The cover, which is removable, is made of canvas and duck and is formed to cover the interior of the wagon and give ample head-room ; it is fixed to, and supported by, two main bail-hoops pivoted together at the ends of each side-rail, and two smaller hoops, one being pivoted to each main hoop. The cover is fixed by staples to the rear of the driver's seat, and is secured to the wagon by two straps at each end and tabs at each side.

The body and fore-carriage are connected by a main pin, which passes through the sweep and wheel plates in front of the front axletree. The fore and hind wheels are of the same diameter. The fittings for draught consist of a draft-pole, two swingletrees, a draught-bar, and two pole-chains. The pole is secured to the pole-socket by a pin and key ; the draught-bar is pivoted at its centre to the pole-socket and fitted at each end with a hook for the attach-ment of a swingletree.

334. Other types of Ambulance Wagons.—The ambulance tonga, drawn by two bullocks or mules, is the regulation wheeled ambulance vehicle in the Army in India. It is hung very low and cannot upset over any country, and is capable of carrying 4 sitting-up or 2 lying-down cases.

335. A " Rapid Transit " Ambulance Wagon, devised by Captain L. A. Avery, R.A.M.C. (T.F.), although not officially adopted, is described here as an interesting contrivance designed with a view to filling the want of stretcher bearers with mounted troops. His object was to construct a light, strong carriage easily adjustable to any riding horse, and capable of keeping up with cavalry through any sort of country.

The ambulance is a two-wheeled contrivance. The body consists of a platform fixed to a crank-axle by long springs between 46-inch wheels. This platform is 2ft. 3ins. from the ground, and is arranged to carry an army pattern stretcher. The fore part consists of a pair of short shafts which are attached to the body by an arrangement of springs adapted to prevent the side-to-side motion caused by the action of the horse. The shafts reach as far forward as the saddle-flaps, where they are held in position by a girth-strap, breast-plate, and belly-band (see Fig. 49). The body is covered by a canvas hood. The weight is about 3 cwt. Length over all, 12ft. Track, 4ft. 1in. Surgical dressings, splints, water-bottle, etc., are carried.

The driver, having placed a wounded or helpless man on a stretcher, is able to transfer him from the ground to the platform of the carriage single-handed.

An apparatus (not officially adopted) for fixing to an ambulance tonga has been devised by Colonel H. G. Hathaway. It consists of two " H "-shaped frames ; when these are superimposed the cushions are arranged for four men to sit in the tonga, or when the upper " H " is turned at right angles (see Fig. 50) and bolted into position, three men can be carried lying down, on army pattern stretchers.

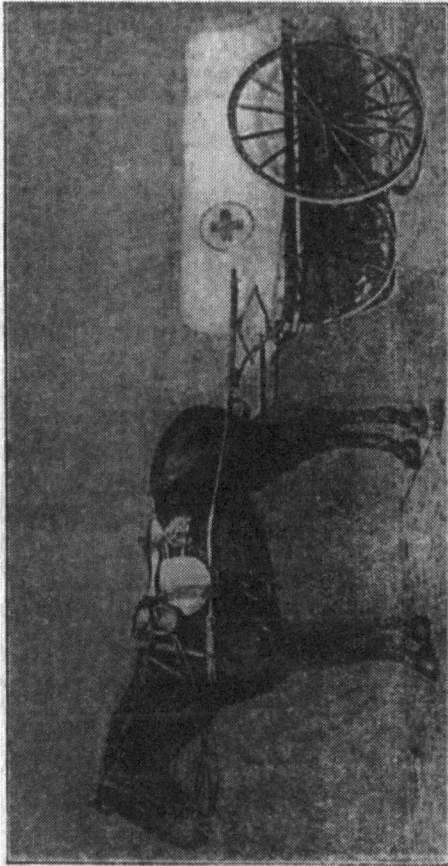

Fig. 49.--Avery's "Rapid Transit Ambulance Wagon."

336. General Service Wagons and Conveyances from Civilian Sources.—A general service wagon holds 6 patients sitting up, with their arms and accoutrements, to which may be added 2 patients able to walk and ride by turns; or 2 patients lying, without stretchers. Three may be carried lying down if their injuries permit of it, two with their heads one way, the third with his head the opposite way.

(B 10977)   M

337. In all countries where war is being waged on an extensive scale, vehicles of all descriptions available from local resources (see paras. 269 and 270, Chap. XVI) will be required for the transport of the sick and wounded.

In Europe, furniture vans, farm wagons and carts, delivery vans, char-à-bancs, open brakes, omnibuses, cabs, gigs, etc., etc., would all be obtainable.

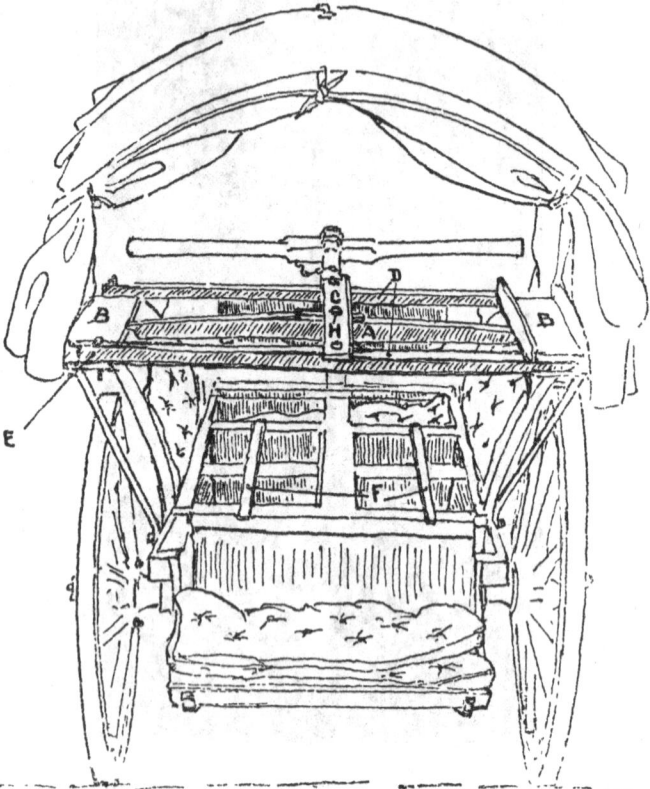

Fig. 50.—Hathaway's Apparatus for Ambulance Tongas.

The tonga ready to carry three stretchers. The upper "H," formed by C, D, D, is turned on the bolt H to a right angle with the lower "H" formed by A, B, B; the ends of D D rest on the sides of tonga B B and are bolted at E. There is a rail on the bar C and off-side of tonga B, so that a stretcher is run in on the off-side of tonga, then lifted to near-side of frame; the second stretcher is run in on off-side and remains there. The third stretcher is run in below on the rails F F.

Similarly, in India, the ekka, the hackery, the bandy, and country carts of all shapes and sizes might be utilized.

The trek ox wagon was used extensively in South Africa. It is 18 to 20 feet long and 4 feet broad, and can easily carry 4 men lying down or 16 sitting up. It has no springs, but owing to the great length of the body it is comfortable to travel in. It is drawn by a team of 16 oxen. A smaller wagon in South Africa drawn by mules carries a dozen men. Cape carts may be fitted up to take the regulation stretcher by having the seat removed.

338. Preparation and loading of G.S. Wagons, Country Carts, etc.—Before vehicles from civilian sources are accepted for the conveyance of sick and wounded they should be thoroughly overhauled, special attention being paid to the working of the brakes, condition of the axles, and lynch pins where these are used.

When patients who are seriously wounded or dangerously ill have to be carried, heavy wagons are recommended for the purpose in preference to vehicles of light construction.

If possible all wagons and carts prior to their being taken into use, should have covers fitted to them, to ensure at least a partial protection from the sun and weather.

339. Patients may be carried on stretchers in the vehicles or lying on some springy material on the floor. In the latter case a plentiful supply of straw, hay, dried leaves, or bracken should be strewn over the floor and sides, about 15 lb. of the material for each lying-down case, some of the material being tied up in bundles as pillows. If mattresses and bedding are available, they should be laid on the top of the straw. In loading and unloading G.S. wagons or country carts of similar construction, so prepared, stretcher squads will act as detailed for Ambulance Wagon Exercises (Chap. XXII). In loading, however, the Nos. 1 and 4 of each squad, after the end of the stretcher has been placed on the floor, will get into the wagon, and, with the assistance of the other bearers on the ground, lift the stretcher into position, unload it, and remove it. The patient should be placed in the most comfortable position, special care being taken to support the injured part and prevent its movement during transit. No. 4 gives the necessary instructions for the careful handling of the patient and removal of the stretcher.

This method, suitable for seriously injured cases, requires that there should be sufficient space in the vehicle for its accomplishment. After one or more patients, according to the size of the vehicle, have been placed on the mattresses, etc., others, less seriously injured, may be carried or assisted in without the use of stretchers.

Sometimes lying-down cases have to be put into the wagons without stretchers, none being available. When this happens the bearers, following as far as possible the instructions given for lifting wounded in Stretcher Exercises (Chap. XXII), will lift each wounded man and carefully carry him to the wagon. On arriving at the back of the wagon, No. 4, or a bearer directed by him, will get in, and, supporting the patient under both shoulders, will lift him in, being assisted by the other Nos., who will subsequently get into the wagon and help to place the man in the most comfortable position. In unloading this proceeding is reversed.

340. Occasionally it may be necessary to dispatch a patient on a stretcher in which case the stretcher will be carefully lifted into the wagon, as described before, and secured by means of straps, rope-lashing, etc.

Various means have been improvised for this purpose with the object of minimizing the jolting of springless vehicles. The principle usually adopted is that of fixing poles or branches across the wagon secured to the sides, and slinging the stretchers from the poles by means of ropes. Material for the purpose can generally be found in farms and villages and with a little ingenuity and skill in carpentry satisfactory fixtures can be constructed.

A suitable method of adaptation,* as applied to a Scotch haycart, with a view to forming extemporized springs, is illustrated in Figs. 51 and 52. The value of it is that it can be applied to almost any large vehicle, and the requisites for its use can be found in most farmyards. The suspensory apparatus consists of four poles, in two pairs, which are crossed about their centres, and rest upon a transom across the top of the cart's body, which takes the downward thrust. The lower ends must pass under, and are lashed to the projecting ends of the lower transoms at the ends of the cart, which take the upward thrust. Lighter transverse poles are lashed to the upper surfaces of the crossed poles, the distance between them in plan being 6 feet. Looped stretcher-slings and rope (see Fig. 58) are placed round the transverse poles (four on each), and the stretchers are suspended from them. In this case, for each stretcher, two loops are formed from stretcher-slings and two from ropes. Square lashings are used. The loops are secured from slipping by lashings passed above the handles, and below and behind the runners of the stretchers.

For the suspensory apparatus are required two stretchers with slings, 20 yards of $\frac{3}{4}$-inch cord (often to be found in stack-yards), four stack-props, which are larch poles 10 feet 6 inches by $3\frac{1}{2}$ inches tapering to $2\frac{1}{2}$ inches, and two lighter poles of $2\frac{1}{2}$ inches in diameter and not less than 5 feet 6 inches in length, which should be cut to length after lashing.

For the floor of the cart are needed four sacks of about 3 feet 6 inches by 2 feet, and 48 pounds of straw. To cover the wounded, a tarpaulin of about 8 feet by 12 feet.

The tools required are a yard-measure, a tenon-saw or billhook, and a jack-knife.

The amount of spring given by the crossed poles, transverse poles, and stretcher-handles combined is sufficient to absorb any ordinary shock. The floor can be used for two slightly wounded patients. One of these carts would thus carry four wounded men.

The method of loading is as follows :—The wounded on stretchers are first loaded ; four bearers are necessary. The shafts should be propped, and the suspension-loops should be adjusted so that the stretcher is horizontal. The stretcher has to be raised to a con-

---

* Devised by Lt.-Col. H. E. R. James, R.A.M.C. (Ret'd.).

siderable height (the top of the body of the cart), where it is rested, and subsequently lifted until the handles can be put into the loops.

No. 1 bearer gets into the cart, while the remainder raise the stretcher and place its handles upon the upper back transom of the body of the cart.

No. 1 takes the handles, and, assisted by the remainder, eases the stretcher forward until its front handles can be supported by the upper forward transom.

No. 3 now gets into the cart, No. 4 keeping the rear end of the stretcher raised, and Nos. 1 and 3 raise the stretcher to a level with the loops. No. 2 now gets up, and places the loops over the handles.

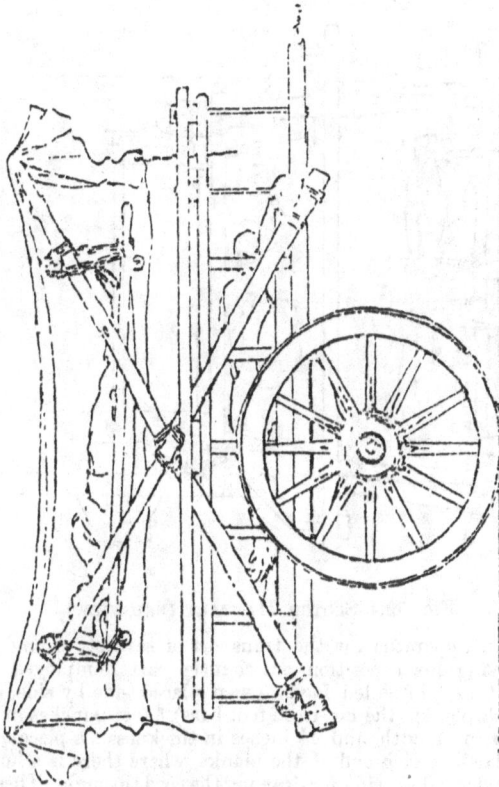

FIG. 51.—SCOTCH HAYCART.

Fig. 51.—Scotch haycart (lateral view), adapted to the transport of wounded. Two on stretchers suspended; two on sacks of straw on bottom of cart. Scale ¼ inch to 1 foot.

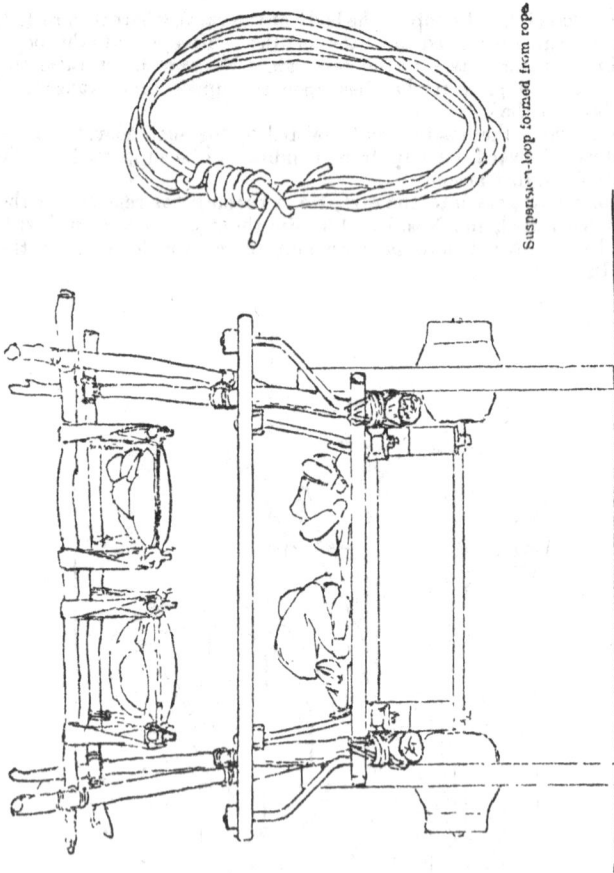

Suspension-loop formed from rope.

FIG. 52.—SCOTCH HAYCART (END VIEW).

341. An apparatus for the transport of severely wounded men in the lying-down position on country carts, employed on the Continent, and intended for two men placed side by side, consists of two ash planks (the head and foot bars), 5 feet 9 inches in length, $2\frac{3}{5}$ inches in breadth, and $1\frac{1}{2}$ inches in thickness : a piece of hemp cord is fixed to each end of the planks, where there is a hole, and, on the under side, a ring for drawing the cord through. These cords serve to lash the planks across to the side beams of the *Leiter-wagen* or "Ladder-wagon," a common wagon on the Continent. The body of the litter, or stretcher, consists of two pieces of canvas, about 6½ feet long, provided with loops at both ends, through which the planks are passed. To the outer edges of the canvas are attached three short cords for tying to the side-beams of the wagon ; the inner edges are strengthened by binding and a sewn-in cord. The head part of the canvas is double, forming a pocket opening behind, which can be filled with straw, etc., to form a pillow. Two covers of tent-cloth are provided, which serve as a waterproof protection when the litter is rolled up, and as a protection for the patients when in use.

The litter can be used with any wagon with side-beams and capable of holding two men side by side in the recumbent position at the level of the beams. For use it is placed transversely on the wagon, the ends of the planks resting on the sides to which they and the outer edges of the canvas are lashed. The weight of the litter is about 30 lb.

Wheel-less Conveyances.

342. Travois.—In addition to horse-drawn vehicles the United States Army use what are known as " travois." Several patterns of these have been invented ; perhaps the best known being the Greenleaf travois (see Figs. 53, 54, and 55). This travois, perfected by Surgeon-General Greenleaf, U.S. Army, is a vehicle primarily intended for transporting the sick and wounded in countries, or under conditions, where wheeled vehicles cannot be used. It consists of a frame having two shafts, two side-poles, and two cross-bars, upon which a stretcher or litter may be rested and partly suspended. When in use a horse or mule is yoked between the shafts and pulls the conveyance. The rear ends of the poles drag on the ground, and the poles make admirable springs for the litter, as any jar communicated to them is well distributed before it reaches the patient. One pole is always cut slightly shorter than the other, in order that when passing over any obstacle the shock may be received successively by each pole and thus be reduced by about a half. It is made of wood with attachments of malleable iron, and weighs 50 lb.

The travois may be used with two horses, the free ends of the poles being fixed to the saddle of the second horse in a similar way to the mule-litter previously described.

Improvised travois may be constructed ; an example is shown in Fig. 56.

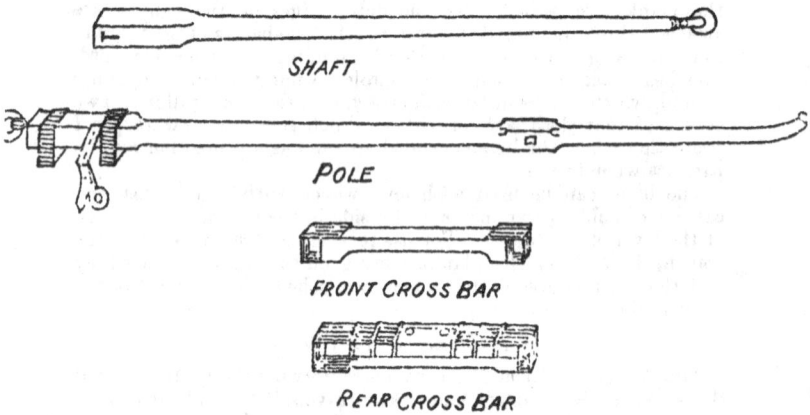

SHAFT

POLE

FRONT CROSS BAR

REAR CROSS BAR

FIG. 53.—GREENLEAF'S TRAVOIS.—SCALE 1½" = 1'.

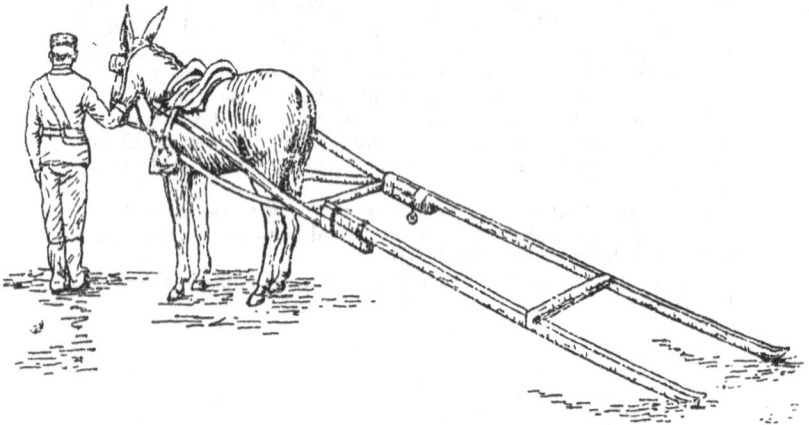

FIG. 54.—GREENLEAF'S TRAVOIS.   (PREPARED.)
(Figs. 53—56 are reproduced by permission of the Association of Military
Surgeons, U.S.A.)

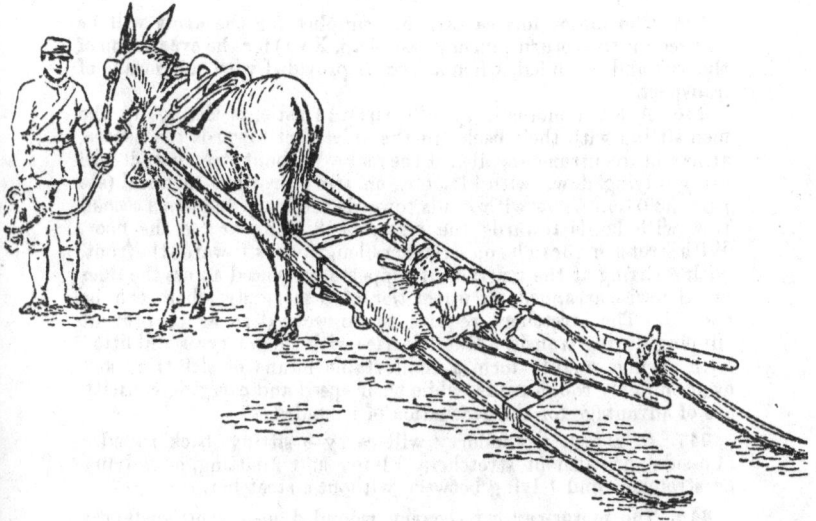

FIG. 55.—GREENLEAF'S TRAVOIS. (LOADED.)

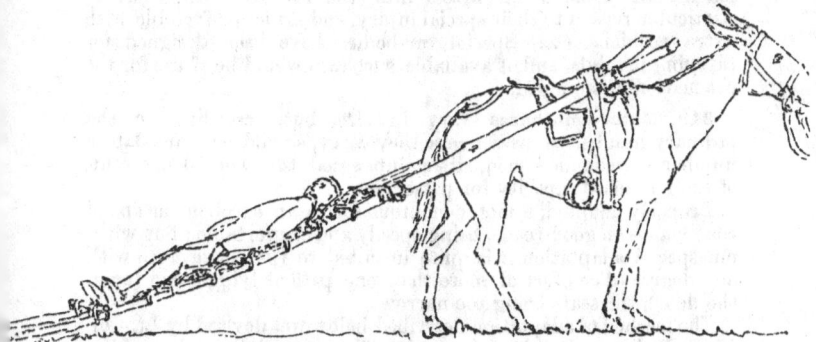

FIG. 56.—IMPROVISED TRAVOIS.

BY MECHANICAL TRANSPORT.

343. When petrol-driven conveyances are used for sick or wounded, the danger arising from the possibility of the vehicle taking fire should not be lost sight of.

344. Motor ambulance wagons are in use in the British Army at various home stations, built to accommodate patients lying down or sitting up.

345. The motor lorries carrying supplies for the army will be utilized on the return journey (see Chap. XVI) for the evacuation of the sick and wounded, when a force is provided with this means of transport.

346. A 3-ton motor-lorry will carry 14 patients sitting up, the men sitting with their backs to the sides, feet towards the centre, arms and accoutrements piled at the rear. Without stretchers, it will carry 8 lying down with kits, etc., on straw or other material (see para. 339) 4 in a row with heads towards the front and 4 in a second row with heads towards the rear; or 8 lying across the floor. With stretchers, 3 can lie on stretchers, lengthways, towards the front, with 4 sitting at the rear; or, if supports are placed across the sides or otherwise arranged, an upper tier of 3 more stretchers can be carried. The stretchers require to be secured so as to prevent slipping during transit. Motor-lorries with rubber tyres and fitted with springs readily form a comfortable means of sick-transport even on fairly rough roads, while their speed and carrying capacity are of advantage for the evacuation of wounded.

347. A 30-cwt. motor-lorry will carry 8 sitting, back to sides (4 a-side), or, without stretchers, 3 lying and 2 sitting, or 2 lying on stretchers and 1 lying between without a stretcher.

348. The motor-car can convey wounded men long distances with speed and comfort. The ordinary-sized car will carry three patients, but not in the recumbent position. Patients should be assisted or lifted into the car with care, having particular regard to their special injury, and made comfortable with extra cushions, etc. Special car-bodies have been designed for carrying invalids, and, if available, such cars would be of use for the evacuation of wounded.

349. Motor-omnibuses vary in size, but, according to the ordinary number of passengers they carry, should accommodate a number of wounded men, sitting up, equal to 70 or 80 per cent. of their licensed capacity for passengers.

Properly adapted, a motor-omnibus forms an excellent means of conveyance on good roads, being speedy and comfortable; but without special adaptation it is quite unsuited to the conveyance with any degree of comfort of more than one patient lying down (upon the floor), the seats being too narrow.

The method of adaptation described below was devised by Lt.-Col. H. E. R. James, R.A.M.C. (retired). The internal dimensions of the type of motor-omnibus for which the directions are given are as follows: Length, 11 feet 3 inches; width at level of seat, 4 feet 6 inches; width half-way between seat and roof, 5 feet 6 inches; height (approximate), 5 feet 8 inches; width of door, 2 feet; width of seat, 1 foot 4 inches. An arm half-way along each inside seat forms an obstruction, and the hand-rail to the steps leading to the roof is also an inconvenience to carrying in stretchers. The seat and back are usually cushioned in two sections on each side.

The structural alterations required are the removal of the arms which divide the seats, and possibly the removal of the hand-rail to admit the stretchers.

In addition to four stretchers with slings, the apparatus necessary for the adaptation of an omnibus of the dimensions given above is :—
(1) Four battens or bars of ash, or oak : two of 4 feet 6 inches by 2½ inches by 2 inches, two of 6 feet by 2½ inches by 2 inches ; (2) eight 2-inch by ¼-inch iron screws ; (3) twenty yards of ¾-inch cord for lashings.

The tools required are a screw-wrench, a screw-driver, a $\frac{3}{16}$-inch gimlet, and a jack-knife.

In applying this method to omnibuses of different dimensions or to other vehicles of a similar nature (e.g., a tram-car), the measurements of the apparatus must be varied to suit.

The method of adaptation (see Fig. 57) provided for is :—

(a) Suspending two stretchers from transverse supporting battens, or bars, whose ends pass through the ventilating apertures and rest upon the frames of the apertures. The weight to be carried is two stretchers, each 30 lb. = 60 lb. ; two patients, say, 170 lb. each = 340 lb. (400 lb.). This weight is distributed over four frames, each taking 100 lb. The frames are of 1-inch square ash, and strongly mortised into the uprights.

The two end ventilators on each side are opened, the restraining straps being detached. The two longer battens are thrust through the apertures and rest on the frames near the uprights. A screw is driven (leaving 1 inch projecting) into the underside of each batten at each end, half an inch from where it cuts the outer edge of the aperture. The eight slings of the four stretchers are made into closed loops, four round each batten, by the method shown in Fig. 58, or supplementary loops may be formed from ¾-inch rope.

(b) The two remaining stretchers are laid upon two transverse battens whose ends rest upon seat-cushions laid across the seats. Screws should be driven half their length into the upper faces of the batten to stop the stretchers from slipping inwards.

Lashings should be used as necessary. In applying them to steady the upper stretcher, the point of purchase should be taken from the strap-rails ; and, to prevent the lower stretchers from slipping lengthways, a purchase may be taken from the stanchion that supports the seat. Enough rope is allowed in the detail of apparatus to form suspension-loops in case slings should be wanting ; four thicknesses are considered sufficient to support each pole.

The method of loading is as follows :—The upper battens are placed in position first, and suspension-loops formed. Next, the lower battens are laid across the seats beneath the upper ones to form a temporary support for the stretcher. The upper tier is first loaded commencing with the near-side.

Four bearers are necessary. When the stretcher has been brought up to the omnibus opposite to the centre of the door, and with its long axis in continuation of that of the omnibus, Nos. 2 and 4 turn inwards, and, with No. 3, take the weight of the stretcher ;

No. 1 mounts the platform. Nos. 2, 4, and 3 raise the stretcher, keeping it level, and with its long axis in the long axis of the omnibus until it clears the hand-rail (if the hand-rail has not been removed),* No. 1 steadying it in this position while No. 3 disengages and mounts the platform. No. 1 now takes both the poles, and, assisted by the remainder in supporting the stretcher, backs into the omnibus; No. 2 mounts the platform and the stretcher is lifted in until the rear ends of the poles clear the rail, when Nos. 1 and 3 bring it completely in and lay the poles upon the lower battens, No. 1 stepping over them as he backs up the omnibus. No. 2 now enters. Nos. 1 and 3 mount the seats, and raise the stretcher till its handles come opposite the prepared loops. No. 2 passes the loops over the handles and a lashing is placed under the runners and over the handles so as to secure the loop from slipping.

The off-side upper-tier stretcher is next loaded.

When this is done the lower battens are placed in their proper positions (as in Fig. 58) on the two cushions laid across the seats, the foremost one being 9 inches from the front end of the interior of the omnibus, and the hindmost one 6 feet in rear of the first. The near-side lower stretcher is loaded first, and finally the off-side one. Some nicety of manipulation will be required in introducing the last stretcher.

Room is left in the body of the omnibus for one sitting-up patient in addition to the wagon orderly. The kits and rifles can be placed on the floor between the seats.

The top will accommodate probably ten sitting-up cases, each omnibus carrying fifteen patients in all.

---

* *Note.*—The loading will be greatly facilitated by the removal of the hand-rail. This is mounted on stanchions secured to the steps by square-headed screws. These can be unscrewed with the screw-wrench; and, the bolts which connect it with the top rail having been unscrewed, the whole comes off in one piece without damage to the vehicle.

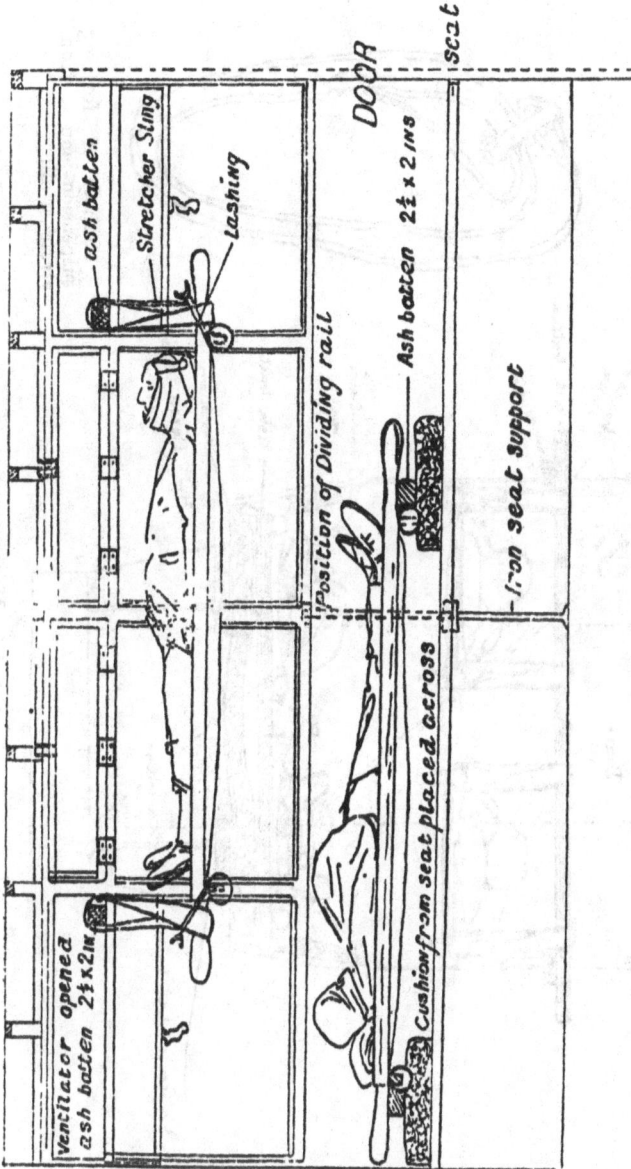

FIG. 57.—MOTOR-OMNIBUS. TRANSVERSE VIEW.

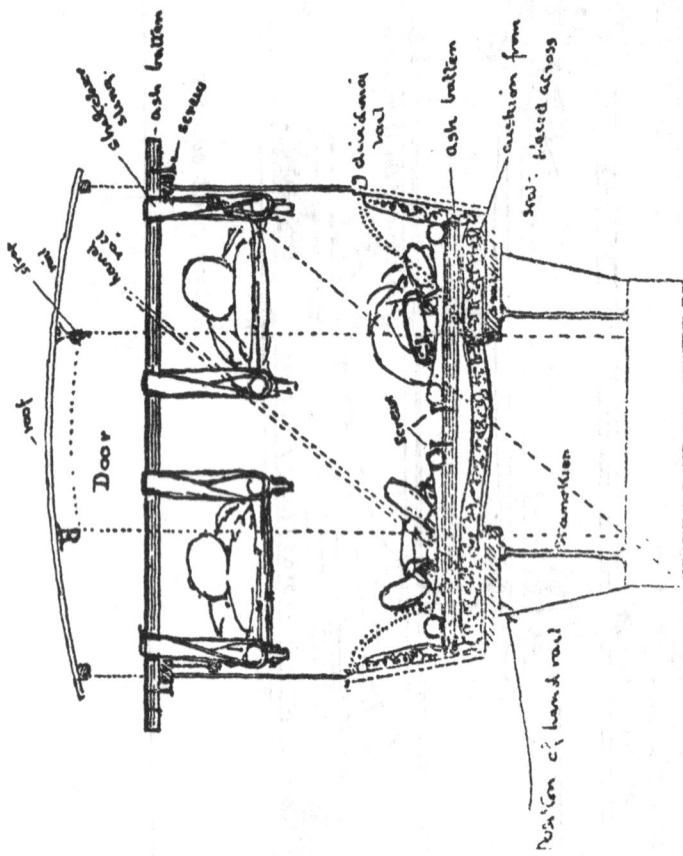

Method of forming suspension-loop from stretcher-sling.

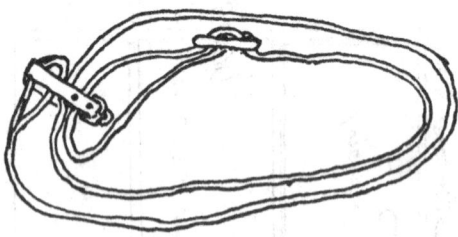

Fig. 58.—MOTOR-OMNIBUS.

Longitudinal view of interior of motor-omnibus adapted to carry four patients lying down on stretchers.
Scale ¼ inch to 1 foot.

By Railway Transport.*

350. The transport of the sick and wounded from the seat of war by railway is undoubtedly the best means of speedily evacuating the field medical units, and should be adopted whenever feasible.

Ambulance trains are divided into three categories :—

(1) Permanent ambulance trains, *i.e.* ambulance trains properly so called. These are trains built for the purpose and are for transporting serious cases. They consist of special ambulance coaches fitted with tiers of cots, coaches for the personnel, dispensary, pack-stores, supplies, kitchens, etc., and have corridor communication throughout. The coaches for the sick are so constructed as to enable patients on stretchers to be taken in and out with ease. Such trains, in fact, constitute well-equipped rolling hospitals.

(2) Temporary ambulance trains which are made up of the ordinary vehicles equipped with some arrangement for carrying sick and wounded, such as vans fitted with the Zavodovski or other apparatus, and which, when once so fitted, are kept for this special purpose during the progress of hostilities. They are intended for the conveyance of the seriously wounded, and to supplement the permanent ambulance trains.

(3) Improvised ambulance trains composed of vehicles which have brought up troops or stores to the front, and are improvised on the spot for the transport of sick and wounded on the return journey. After disposal of the casualties the vehicles are used again for the transport of troops and stores.

351. With British rolling stock, on an average, there are six compartments to each passenger coach ; each compartment can accommodate six slight cases, but it would be better to put in only five as then three men could sleep at a time. Two serious cases could be accommodated lying down in each compartment. Kits should be carried in a separate carriage.

In India, each 1st class railway carriage has accommodation for eight or twelve beds and is always provided with a lavatory and very often with a shower-bath. A disadvantage, however, is that there is no corridor communication between the coaches.

In the United Kingdom the larger railway companies possess sleeping-cars and a certain number of invalid-coaches, the doors of which are wide enough to permit of the entrance of stretchers. They also possess practically unlimited quantities of bedding-material, so that if the emergency should arise suitable trains could be fitted up. Through, end-to-end, communication is almost a necessity in an ambulance train, and every endeavour should be made to secure it.

352. There are various specially devised fittings for converting railway vans into ambulance coaches, such as the "Bréchot-Desprez-Ameline," and the "Linxweiler," which allow of a large number of patients being carried in each wagon. There are also systems by which, with ropes, blocks, poles, etc., the end can be obtained in a more rough and ready, but at the same time, serviceable manner—systems, moreover, for which means should be readily available in the field.

---

* *See* "Ambulance Trains," para. 259, Chap. XVI, and paras. 288 and 289, Chap. XVII.

353. Of these latter the "Zavodovski" is described in Chap. XXIII. It is practical and expedient, permits of the stretchers being placed in position without lifting the patient off them, and all large postal, goods, fish, and fruit vans, etc., could quickly be so fitted. The majority of these vehicles could take from eight to ten stretchers.

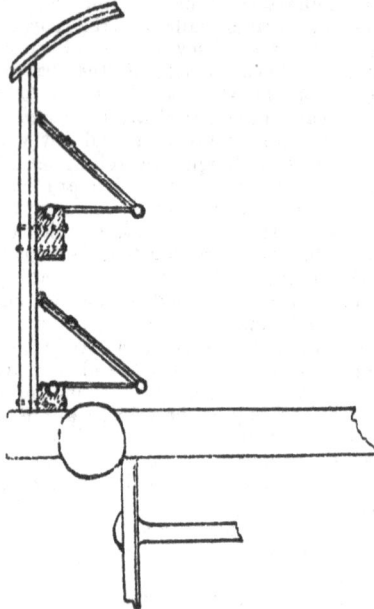

FIG. 59.—AUSTRIAN METHOD OF PREPARING RAILWAY VANS.

354. An Austrian method, with a similar advantage, is to fix blocks to the sides of vans, with a rounded notch at the top of each block to take the inner handles of stretchers ranged along the sides. The outer handles (see Fig. 59) are supported by buckled straps fixed to the sides higher up.

355. Port's method is rapid, simple, and economical. The principle is to fix poles, in pairs across the interior of a van and to lash the stretchers to these. One pole of each pair is placed at the ends of the car, and the second about 6 feet from the first, towards the centre. Stout blocks of wood, with V-shaped notches at the top (similar to those for the preceding method), are fastened by large screws to opposite sides of the car. Pinewood poles, the exact width of the interior, are laid across the car, resting in the "Vs." Three stretchers are lashed, lengthways to the car, underneath each pair of poles. The poles and lashings act as springs.

Other stretchers may be placed on the floor, which should be prepared in some of the ways described below.

356. If the wagon cannot be arranged according to any of the above plans, the best method is to fill sacks with straw or hay, and lay them on the floor, three together, with their longer sides touching. Each set of three sacks forms a comfortable bed, across which two men can lie. Failing sacks, straw, hay, ferns, brushwood, etc., may be tied in bundles and arranged as couches. Mattresses, if available, may be placed over these. If stretchers are procurable they should be laid on stout trusses of straw, etc.

The advantage of using sacks, or making bundles of the material is that the springiness of the straw, etc., is not lost through its being displaced by the weight of the body, as is apt to happen if even a thick layer of straw is laid down loose. Further, they are more easily dealt with in case of accidental fire.

By Water Transport.

357. Transport by Sea.*—The ships used for the conveyance of sick and wounded from campaigns over seas are known as hospital ships, and have the personnel, stores, appliances, fittings, etc., necessary for such floating hospitals.

358. The wounded may be embarked or disembarked from the wharfs direct, or from lighters, according to the nature of the harbour. In the latter case, although many ships are fitted with "cargo-ports" through which men can be carried direct to the hospital deck, difficulty may be experienced in getting the patients up the ship's side. Wounded who can sit up for a short time can conveniently be carried up a ship's companion by means of an arm-chair having two handles projecting from the seat in front and two from the top of the back, thus permitting carriage of the patient without tilting.

Another appliance is an oblong, open box of a size to take a naval hospital cot, with four stays attached to the sides meeting above at a central ring.

Various ambulance lifts or cots have been invented. That of Surgeon Macdonald, R.N., is shown in Fig. 60. Another, invented thirty years ago by Medical Director Gihon, of the United States Navy, is shown in Figs. 61 to 63. This consists essentially of an oblong piece of stout canvas, $7\frac{1}{2}$ feet long and $2\frac{1}{2}$ feet wide, with the sides and ends doubled and sewn to take the frame. The sides take two stretcher-poles, which pass through metal rings at the ends of the traverses; the ends of the poles are rounded as convenient handles. A canvas band 12 inches wide, securely sewn to the bottom of the canvas, is used to fix the chest and is attached to the cot-sides by cords fastened on opposite sides. Two femoral bands are sewn on diagonally to envelop each thigh and are likewise fixed to the frame at the side. They sustain most of the weight of the body when the cot is elevated perpendicularly. Two narrow bands 5 inches wide confine the legs; a canvas hair-pillow, loosely secured, completes the apparatus. The patient can be swung over the ship's side or lowered down a hatchway. The whole device is simply an ordinary stretcher with these additional bands sewn on.

---

* *See* "Hospital Ships," paras. 290 and 291, Chap. XVII.

N

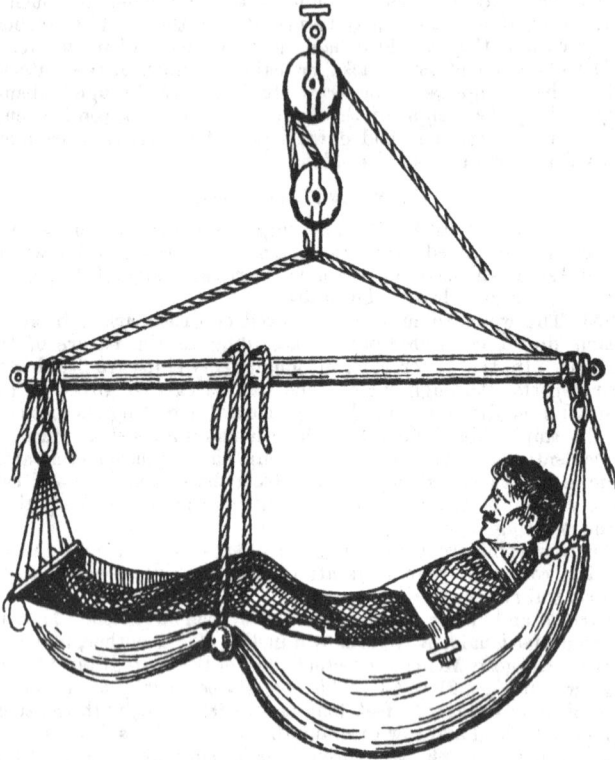

Fig. 60.—Macdonald's Ambulance Lift.

An extemporized lift can be made from an ordinary life-buoy, which is passed up close to the arm-pits (see Fig. 64). A couple of stays support the seat, and two or three more are attached to a block and single rope working over the block at the end of a spar.

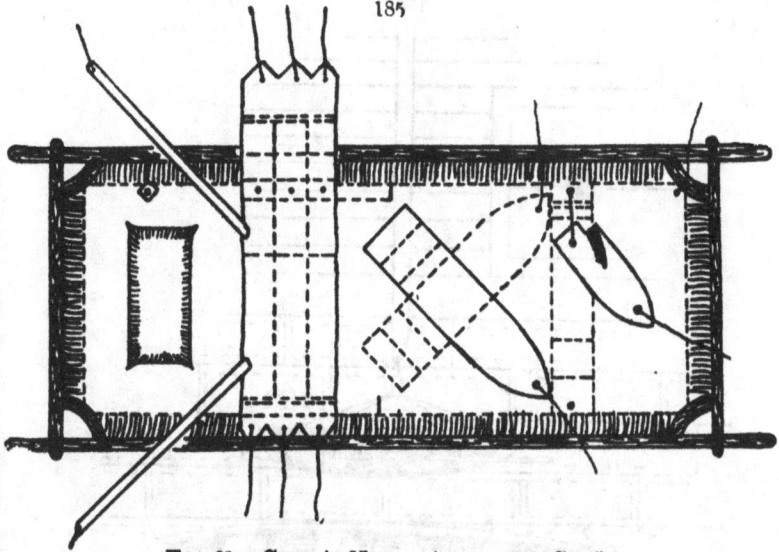

FIG. 61.—GIHON'S NAVAL AMBULANCE COT.*

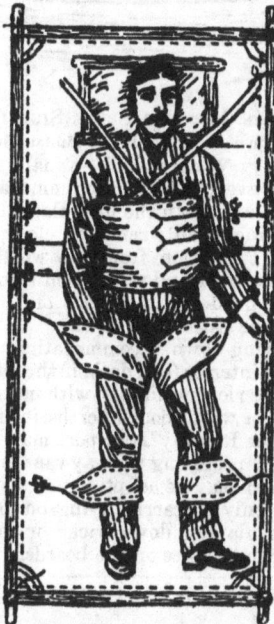

FIG. 62.—PATIENT SECURED FOR REMOVAL.*

* Reproduced by permission of the Association of Military Surgeons, U.S.A.

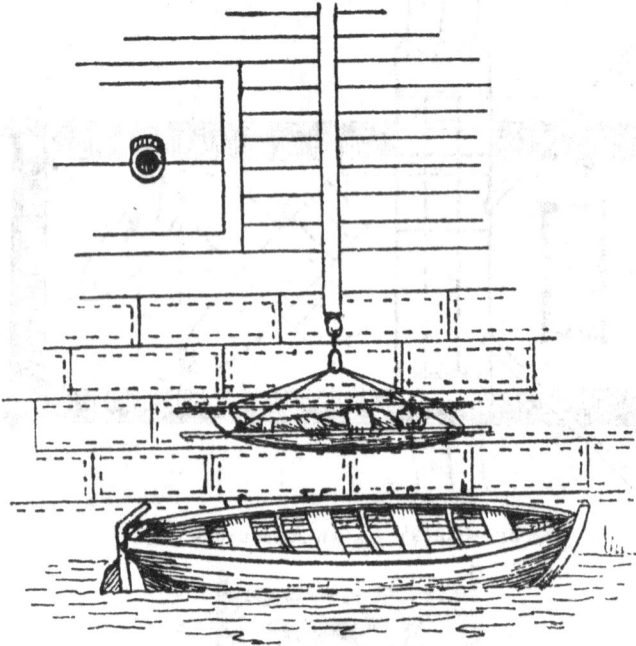

Fig. 63.—Swinging Cot over Ship's Side into Boat.
(Reproduced by permission of the Association of Military Surgeons, U S A)

359. Transport by Waterways.*—Canal barges, boats, lighters, etc., may be converted for the accommodation of sick and wounded in a variety of ways. In the first place the vessel must be clean, or capable of being readily rendered clean, and suitable for the purpose in view. Protection from the weather by awnings, screens, etc., must be provided, and ventilation if lower decks are to be used. If there are no decks, platforms of boards can be laid across the interior for the patients to lie on.

If space permits, lying-down accommodation can be suitably arranged by fitting the interior (and deck, if the climatic conditions are favourable or the interior unsuitable) with naval hospital cots or similar fixed bedsteads, or with wooden berths, in tiers. The special fittings mentioned under Railway Transport may be set up, or any of the other systems for preparing railway vans for the conveyance of wounded on stretchers may be adopted.

If the wounded can only be carried lying on the decks, couches should be prepared by laying down sacks or bundles of straw, hay, etc., or spreading mattresses on the boards.

---

* See " The use of waterways " paras. 272 and 273, Chap. XVI.

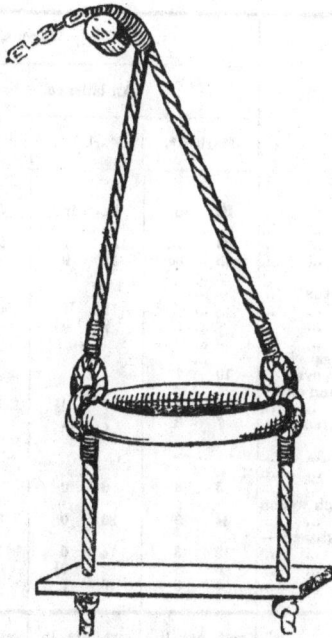

Fig. 64.—Improvised Life-buoy Lift.

360. The conversion of river-steamers, launches, and other craft of that nature into suitable vessels for the conveyance of sick and wounded, while it can be carried out on emergency on the principles above described, is properly a question of ship or boat building, directed by medical requirements.

TABLE SHOWING DIMENSIONS, TONNAGE, WEIGHTS, MEDICAL

	Wagons.			
	Ambulance.			G.S.
	Mark V*.	Mark VI.	Light.	Mark X.
Dimensions.	ft. in.	ft. in.	ft. in.	ft. in.
Length :—				
With shafts	...	...	...	...
With pole	23 1a	23 1	22 4	23 0
Without pole	13 8a	13 9	12 6	13 6
Height —				
With filtering apparatus ...	...	...	...	...
With hood	...	11 1	...	...
With hood lowered	...	9 5	...	...
With seat	...	...	...	7 0
Without seat and raves ...	...	...	...	4 10
With bale-hoops and cover ...	10 7	...	8 9	...
Without bale-hoops and cover	7 8	...	7 2	...
Width	6 3	7 0½	6 3	6 2½
Distance between axletrees ..	7 3	7 11	7 3½	7 0½
Floor Space.—				
Length	...	...	...	9 1¾
Width	...	...	...	3 2
Track	5 4	6 0	5 2	5 2
Minimum space in which wagon can turn	34 3	26 0	34 0	34 0
Space occupied for freightage —				
Length	13 3	14 0	12 8	14 6
Breadth	6 3	7 0½	6 3	6 4
Height	6 3	6 7	6 0	4 0
Weight.	cwt. qrs. lb.	cwt. qrs. lb.	cwt. qrs. lb.	cwt. qrs. lb.
	...	23 2 8b	...	...
Vehicle without load or equipment	...	24 2 7c	...	...
	23 0 16	...	15 2 23d	...
	...	...	16 2 23e	...
	...	...	...	15 2 21
	tons.	tons.	tons.	tons.
Tonnage or freightage	12 939	16·225	11·875	9·183
wheels	...	...	...	...
shafts	...	...	...	...
Capacity { of tank	...	10 galls.	5 galls.	...
{ of cistern .. .	...	...	...	...
Rate of filtering per hour ..	...	...	...	...

(a) With rear step down ; with rear step folded up, 6 inches less.
(b) With rubber-tyred wheels Nos. 48 and 204.
(c) With steel-tyred wheels, Nos. 159 and 200

ETC., OF ARMY PATTERN VEHICLES USED BY THE SERVICE.

Carts.				
Forage.		Water Tank.		
Mark I.	Mark II.	Mark IIA.	Mark IIB.	
ft. in.	ft. in.	ft. in.	ft. in.	
14 9	14 9	13 11	13 11	
...	...	..	...	
...	...	...	...	
...	...	5 3½	5 3½	With shafts resting on ground 5 ft. 9 ins.
...	...	..	.	
...	...	.	..	
...	...	...	...	
...	...	...	..	
7 9f	7 9f	...	...	
5 4†	5 4†	...	...	† Also without raves.
6 1	6 1	6 1	6 1	
...	..	...	...	
...	...	...	...	
5 2	5 2	5 2	5 2	
...	..	...	..	
14 4	14 4	7 0	7 0	
6 1	6 1	6 1	6 1	
1 7	1 7	3 7	3 7	
cwt. qrs. lb.	cwt. qrs. lb.	cwt. qrs. lb.	cwt. qrs. lb.	
...	...	12 2 21	12 2 21	
...	...	..	...	
...	...	...	...	} Including bale-hoops and cover.
...	...	...	...	
8 0 14	8 1 14	...	...	Not including bale-hoops and cover.
tons.	tons.	tons.	tons.	
2·712	2·712	3·8147	3·8147	
...	...	·7486	·7486	
...	...	·0914	·0914	
...	...	113 galls.	113 galls.	
...	...	7 „	7 „	
...	...	180 „	270 „	

(d) With rubber-tyred wheels No. 46.
(e) With steel-tyred wheels No. 159.
(f) With wheels 4 ft. 8 ins diameter.

CHAPTER XIX.

THE GENEVA CONVENTION.

361. The Geneva Convention of July 6th, 1906, takes the place of the Geneva Convention of August 22nd, 1864, in wars between Powers that are signatory to it. But should either of the belligerent Powers have not yet ratified the former, then the latter remains in force ; it is, therefore, necessary at present to have a knowledge of both Conventions. Twenty-seven out of the thirty-five Powers, whose representatives signed the Convention in 1906, had ratified it by the end of March, 1911. Great Britain ratified it on 16th April, 1907.

362. The chief points to be noted in the new Convention are that the sick and wounded must be taken care of irrespective of nationality ; that medical personnel must, as far as military exigencies permit, be left in charge of sick and wounded, and that, when they are captured by the enemy, they are to continue their duty under his directions. They will be sent back to their own side only when the enemy can arrange to do so conveniently to himself and by the route which he shall determine. They cannot claim to be sent back at once, but they can claim the same rates of pay and allowances from the enemy which are given to the corresponding ranks in the enemy's medical service. The same kind of protection is given to personnel in charge of convoys, and none of the personnel, medical or otherwise, including sentries and piquets appointed to protect medical units and convoys, are to be regarded as prisoners of war, if they fall into the hands of the enemy.

Sick and wounded who fall into the enemy's hands are, however, prisoners of war, and under the Convention are not entitled to any privilege different from those of unwounded and healthy prisoners, beyond that of proper medical attendance.

The commander who remains in possession of the field must cause a search to be made for wounded, and as far as possible prevent any acts of pillage to dead or wounded. Nominal rolls of all the enemy's wounded who have been received into any medical formation must be forwarded to the Bureau of Prisoners together with any identification marks or papers taken from the dead.

As regimental stretcher bearers are not exclusively engaged in the care of the wounded, they are not entitled, as such, to protection under the Convention or to wear the Red Cross brassard.

363 The protection afforded to the personnel of medical units is not forfeited by the fact that they carry weapons for self-defence, or hold the arms and ammunition of the wounded who are under their care.

In the Convention of 1864, these points were not clearly expressed, and the protection was only given when sick or wounded were actually found with the medical unit. In the new Convention the protection is granted in all circumstances.

364. The new Convention has somewhat complicated provisions regarding the method of dealing with the material of medical units and convoys. Briefly they are as follows :—

1. Material of mobile units of the Army Medical Service is not prize of war, and must be restored whenever this can be done. It can, however, be used by the enemy for the treatment of sick and wounded, pending restoration.

2. Material of fixed medical units is prize of war, but must not be diverted from its purpose, so long as there are cases to succour. In the case of a building, however, which the enemy want to use for purposes other than as a hospital, the Convention permits of this being done, if the sick and wounded in it are properly provided for elsewhere.

3. The medical material of convoys, including special ambulance and medical wagons along with their teams, ambulance trains, and river or lake ambulance boats, are to be restored, but not the general service or other military vehicles of convoys.

4. Material belonging to Voluntary Aid Societies is private property, in all circumstances where it is found, and can only be retained on requisition ; that is to say, a receipt must be given to the owner or representative of the owner, if it is necessary to make use of it, so that the cost may be recovered subsequently.

5. Similarly, civilian vehicles, belonging to convoys, can only be retained by the enemy on requisition.

365. The distinctive emblem of the Red Cross on a white ground is the emblem and distinctive sign of the medical services of armies and not, as is popularly supposed, of Voluntary Aid Societies. The latter are entitled to the use of the sign and the words " Red Cross " only when they are authorized by the State to render assistance to the regular medical service of its army and are employed with medical units and establishments of armies. That point is clearly defined in the Convention, although the previous Convention does not recognize Red Cross Societies in any way.

The national flag of the belligerent must always be hoisted along with the Red Cross flag (see para. 165, Chap. XV), except when a medical unit is captured by the enemy, in which case the Red Cross only is flown.

The other points in the Convention have no special bearing on the medical service, as such, but rather on the commanders of Armies and States.

GENEVA CONVENTION OF AUGUST 22nd, 1864.

(TRANSLATION.)

Article I.

Ambulances and military hospitals shall be acknowledged to be neutral, and, as such, shall be protected and respected by belligerents so long as any sick or wounded may be therein.

Such neutrality shall cease if the ambulances or hospitals should be held by a military force.

Article II.

Persons employed in hospitals and ambulances, comprising the staff for superintendence, medical service, administration, transport of wounded, as well as chaplains, shall participate in the benefit of neutrality whilst so employed, and so long as there remain any wounded to bring in or to succour.

Article III.

The persons designated in the preceding Article may, even after occupation by the enemy, continue to fulfil their duties in the hospital or ambulance which they serve, or may withdraw in order to rejoin the corps to which they belong.

Under such circumstances, when those persons shall cease from their functions, they shall be delivered by the occupying army to the outposts of the enemy.

Article IV.

As the equipment of military hospitals remains subject to the laws of war, persons attached to such hospitals cannot, in withdrawing, carry away any articles but such as are their private property.

Under the same circumstances an ambulance shall, on the contrary, retain its equipment.

Article V.

Inhabitants of the country who may bring help to the wounded shall be respected, and shall remain free. The Generals of the belligerent Powers shall make it their care to inform the inhabitants of the appeal addressed to their humanity, and of the neutrality which will be the consequence of it.

Any wounded man entertained and taken care of in a house shall be considered as a protection thereto. Any inhabitant who shall have entertained wounded men in his house shall be exempted from the quartering of troops, as well as from a part of the contributions of war which may be imposed.

Article VI.

Wounded or sick soldiers shall be entertained and taken care of, to whatever nation they may belong.

Commanders-in-chief shall have the power to deliver immediately to the outposts of the enemy soldiers who have been wounded in an engagement when circumstances permit this to be done, and with the consent of both parties.

Those who are recognized, after their wounds are healed, as incapable of serving, shall be sent back to their country.

The others may also be sent back, on condition of not again bearing arms during the continuance of the war.

Evacuations, together with the persons under whose directions they take place, shall be protected by an absolute neutrality.

Article VII.

A distinctive and uniform flag shall be adopted for hospitals, ambulances and evacuations. It must, on every occasion, be accompanied by the national flag. An arm-badge (*brassard*) shall also be allowed for individuals neutralized, but the delivery thereof shall be left to military authority.

The flag and the arm-badge shall bear a red cross on a white ground.

Article VIII.

The details of execution of the present Convention shall be regulated by the Commanders-in-Chief of belligerent armies, according to the instructions of their respective Governments, and in conformity with the general principles laid down in this Convention.

Article IX.

The High Contracting Powers have agreed to communicate the present Convention to those Governments which have not found it convenient to send Plenipotentiaries to the International Conference at Geneva, with an invitation to accede thereto; the Protocol is for that purpose left open.

Article X.

The present Convention shall be ratified, and the ratifications shall be exchanged at Berne in four months, or sooner if possible.

GENEVA CONVENTION OF JULY 6th, 1906.

(TRANSLATION.)

CHAPTER I.—THE WOUNDED AND SICK.

Article 1.

Officers and soldiers, and other persons officially attached to armies, shall be respected and taken care of when wounded or sick, by the belligerent in whose power they may be, without distinction of nationality.

Nevertheless, a belligerent who is compelled to abandon sick or wounded to the enemy shall, as far as military exigencies permit, leave with them a portion of his medical personnel and material to contribute to the care of them.

Article 2.

Except as regards the treatment to be provided for them in virtue of the preceding Article, the wounded and sick of an army who fall into the hands of the enemy are prisoners of war, and the general provisions of international law concerning prisoners are applicable to them.

Belligerents are, however, free to arrange with one another such exceptions and mitigations with reference to sick and wounded prisoners as they may judge expedient ; in particular they will be at liberty to agree—

To restore to one another the wounded left on the field after a battle ;

To repatriate any wounded and sick whom they do not wish to retain as prisoners, after rendering them fit for removal or after recovery ;

To hand over to a neutral State, with the latter's consent, the enemy's wounded and sick to be interned by the neutral State until the end of hostilities.

Article 3.

After each engagement the Commander in possession of the field shall take measures to search for the wounded, and to ensure protection against pillage and maltreatment both for the wounded and for the dead.

He shall arrange that a careful examination of the bodies is made before the dead are buried or cremated.

Article 4.

As early as possible each belligerent shall send to the authorities of the country or army to which they belong the military identification marks or tokens found on the dead, and a nominal roll of the wounded or sick who have been collected by him.

The belligerents shall keep each other mutually informed of any internments and changes, as well as of admissions into hospital and deaths among the wounded and sick in their hands. They shall collect all the articles of personal use, valuables, letters, etc., which are found on the field of battle or left by the wounded or sick who have died in the medical establishments or units, in order that such objects may be transmitted to the persons interested by the authorities of their own country.

Article 5.

The competent military authority may appeal to the charitable zeal of the inhabitants to collect and take care of, under his direction, the wounded or sick of armies, granting to those who respond to the appeal special protection and certain immunities.

Chapter II.—Medical Units and Establishments.

Article 6.

Mobile medical units (that is to say, those which are intended to accompany armies into the field) and the fixed establishments of the medical service shall be respected and protected by the belligerents.

Article 7.

The protection to which medical units and establishments are entitled ceases if they are made use of to commit acts harmful to the enemy.

Article 8.

The following facts are not considered to be of a nature to deprive a medical unit or establishment of the protection guaranteed by Article 6 :—

1. That the personnel of the unit or of the establishment is armed, and that it uses its arms for its own defence or for that of the sick and wounded under its charge.

2. That in default of armed orderlies the unit or establishment is guarded by a piquet or by sentinels furnished with an authority in due form.

3. That weapons and cartridges taken from the wounded and not yet handed over to the proper department are found in the unit or establishment.

Chapter III.—Personnel.

Article 9.

The personnel engaged exclusively in the collection, transport, and treatment of the wounded and the sick, as well as in the administration of medical units and establishments, and the Chaplains attached to armies, shall be respected and protected under all circumstances. If they fall into the hands of the enemy they shall not be treated as prisoners of war.

These provisions apply to the guard of medical units and establishments under the circumstances indicated in Article 8 (2).

Article 10.

The personnel of Voluntary Aid Societies, duly recognized and authorized by their Government, who may be employed in the medical units and establishments of armies, is placed on the same footing as the personnel referred to in the preceding Article, provided always that the first-mentioned personnel shall be subject to military law and regulations.

Each state shall notify to the other, either in time of peace or at the commencement of or during the course of hostilities, but in every case before actually employing them, the names of the Societies which it has authorized, under its responsibility, to render assistance to the regular medical service of its armies.

Article 11.

A recognized Society of a neutral country can only afford the assistance of its medical personnel and units to a belligerent with the previous consent of its own Government and the authorization of the belligerent concerned.

A belligerent who accepts such assistance is bound to notify the fact to his adversary before making any use of it.

Article 12.

The persons designated in Articles 9, 10, and 11, after they have fallen into the hands of the enemy, shall continue to carry on their duties under his direction.

When their assistance is no longer indispensable, they shall be sent back to their army or to their country at such time and by such route as may be compatible with military exigencies.

They shall then take with them such effects, instruments, arms, and horses as are their private property.

Article 13.

The enemy shall secure to the persons mentioned in Article 9, while in his hands, the same allowances and the same pay as are granted to the persons holding the same rank in his own army.

Chapter IV.—Material.

Article 14.

If mobile medical units fall into the hands of the enemy they shall retain their material, including their teams, irrespectively of the means of transport and the drivers employed.

Nevertheless, the competent military authority shall be free to use the material for the treatment of the wounded and sick. It shall be restored under the conditions laid down for the medical personnel, and so far as possible at the same time.

Article 15.

The buildings and material of fixed establishments remain subject to the laws of war, but may not be diverted from their purpose so long as they are necessary for the wounded and the sick.

Nevertheless, the Commanders of troops in the field may dispose of them, in case of urgent military necessity, provided they make previous arrangements for the welfare of the wounded and sick who are found there.

Article 16.

The material of Voluntary Aid Societies which are admitted to the privileges of the Convention under the conditions laid down therein is considered private property, and as such to be respected under all circumstances, saving only the right of requisition recognized for belligerents in accordance with the laws and customs of war.

CHAPTER V.—CONVOYS OF EVACUATION.

Article 17.

Convoys of evacuation shall be treated like mobile medical units subject to the following special provisions :—

1. A belligerent intercepting a convoy may break it up if military exigencies demand, provided he takes charge of the sick and wounded who are in it.

2. In this case, the obligation to send back the medical personnel, provided for in Article 12, shall be extended to the whole of the military personnel detailed for the transport or the protection of the convoy and furnished with an authority in due form to that effect.

The obligation to restore the medical material, provided for in Article 14, shall apply to railway trains, and boats used in internal navigation, which are specially arranged for evacuations, as well as to the material belonging to the medical service for fitting up ordinary vehicles, trains, and boats.

Military vehicles other than those of the medical service may be captured with their teams.

The civilian personnel and the various means of transport obtained by requisition, including railway material and boats used for convoys, shall be subject to the general rules of international law.

CHAPTER VI.—THE DISTINCTIVE EMBLEM.

Article 18.

As a compliment to Switzerland, the heraldic emblem of the red cross on a white ground, formed by reversing the Federal colours, is retained as the emblem and distinctive sign of the medical service of armies.

Article 19.

With the permission of the competent military authority this emblem shall be shown on the flags and armlets (*brassards*) as well as on all the material belonging to the medical service.

Article 20.

The personnel protected in pursuance of Articles 9 (paragraph 1), 10, and 11 shall wear, fixed to the left arm, an armlet (*brassard*) with a red cross on a white ground, delivered and stamped by the competent military authority, and accompanied by a certificate of identity in the case of persons who are attached to the medical service of armies, but who have not a military uniform.

Article 21.

The distinctive flag of the Convention shall only be hoisted over those medical units and establishments which are entitled to be respected under the Convention, and with the consent of the military authorities. It must be accompanied by the national flag of the belligerent to whom the unit or establishment belongs.

Nevertheless, medical units which have fallen into the hands of the enemy, so long as they are in that situation, shall not fly any other flag than that of the Red Cross.

Article 22.

The medical units belonging to neutral countries which may be authorized to afford their services under the conditions laid down in Article 11 shall fly, along with the flag of the Convention, the national flag of the belligerent to whose army they are attached.

The provisions of the second paragraph of the preceding Article are applicable to them.

Article 23.

The emblem of the red cross on a white ground and the words "Red Cross" or "Geneva Cross" shall not be used either in time of peace or in time of war, except to protect or to indicate the medical units and establishments and the personnel and material protected by the Convention.

CHAPTER VII.—APPLICATION AND CARRYING OUT OF THE CONVENTION.

Article 24.

The provisions of the present Convention are only binding upon the Contracting Powers in the case of war between two or more of them. These provisions shall cease to be binding from the moment when one of the belligerent Powers is not a party to the Convention.

Article 25.

The Commanders-in-chief of belligerent armies shall arrange the details for carrying out the preceding Articles, as well as for cases not provided for, in accordance with the instructions of their respective Governments and in conformity with the general principles of the present Convention.

Article 26.

The Signatory Governments will take the necessary measures to instruct their troops, especially the personnel protected, in the provisions of the present Convention, and to bring them to the notice of the civil population.

CHAPTER VIII.—PREVENTION OF ABUSES AND INFRACTIONS.
Article 27.

The Signatory Governments, in countries the legislation of which is not at present adequate for the purpose, undertake to adopt or to propose to their legislative bodies such measures as may be necessary to prevent at all times the employment of the emblem or the name of Red Cross or Geneva Cross by private individuals or by Societies other than those which are entitled to do so under the present Convention and in particular for commercial purposes as a trade mark or trading mark.

The prohibition of the employment of the emblem or the names in question shall come into operation from the date fixed by each legislature, and at the latest five years after the present Convention comes into force. From that date it shall no longer be lawful to adopt a trade-mark or trading mark contrary to this prohibition.

Article 28.

The Signatory Governments also undertake to adopt, or to propose to their legislative bodies, should their military law be insufficient for the purpose, the measures necessary for the repression in time of war of individual acts of pillage and maltreatment of the wounded and sick of armies, as well as for the punishment, as an unlawful employment of military insignia, of the improper use of the Red Cross flag and armlet (*brassard*) by officers and soldiers or private individuals not protected by the present Convention.

They shall communicate to one another, through the Swiss Federal Council, the provisions relative to these measures of repression at the latest within five years from the ratification of the present Convention.

GENERAL PROVISIONS.
Article 29.

The present Convention shall be ratified as soon as possible. The ratification shall be deposited at Berne.

When each ratification is deposited a *procès verbal* shall be drawn up, and a copy thereof certified as correct shall be forwarded through the diplomatic channel to all the Contracting Powers.

Article 30.

The present Convention shall come into force for each Power six months after the date of the deposit of its ratification.

Article 31.

The present Convention, duly ratified, shall replace the Convention of the 22nd August, 1864, in relations between the Contracting States. The Convention of 1864 remains in force between such of the parties who signed it who may not likewise ratify the present Convention.

Article 32.

The present Convention may be signed until the 31st December next by the Powers represented at the Conference which was opened at Geneva on the 11th June, 1906, as also by the Powers, not represented at that Conference, which signed the Convention of 1864.

Such of the aforesaid Powers as shall have not signed the present Convention by the 31st December, 1906, shall remain free to accede to it subsequently. They shall notify their accession by means of a written communication addressed to the Swiss Federal Council, and communicated by the latter to all the Contracting Powers.

Other Powers may apply to accede in the same manner, but their request shall only take effect if within a period of one year from the notification of it to the Federal Council no objection to it reaches the Council from any of the Contracting Powers.

Article 33.

Each of the Contracting Powers shall be at liberty to denounce the present Convention. The denunciation shall not take effect until one year after the written notification of it has reached the Swiss Federal Council. The Council shall immediately communicate the notification to all the other Contracting Powers.

The denunciation shall only affect the Power which has notified it.

PART IV.—ROYAL ARMY MEDICAL CORPS DRILLS AND EXERCISES.

CHAPTER XX.

GENERAL INSTRUCTIONS.

366. Portions of Infantry Training in use in R.A.M.C.— The portions of Infantry Training in use in the Royal Army Medical Corps are those dealing with :—Definitions ; Squad Drill (without arms*) ; Company Drill (without arms*).

367. Ceremonial.—The ceremonial drill for the R.A.M.C. is contained in " Ceremonial."

The official March of the Corps is " Her bright smile haunts me still." Published by Hawkes and Son, London.

368. R.A.M.C. Call.—The calls for the Royal Army Medical Corps are given in The Trumpet and Bugle Sounds for the Army.

The following is the Corps Call :—

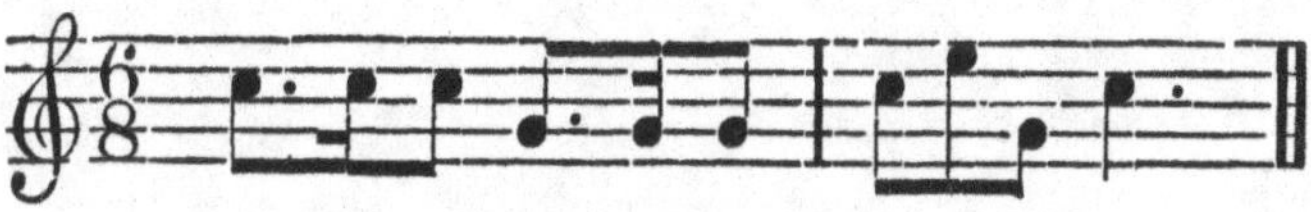

FIG. 65.—R.A.M.C. CALL.

369. Parties Marching.—The following rules are given for the guidance of officers marching parties from place to place :—

(1) Except for very short distances all movements should be in column of fours. When marching in fours, not more than four men should march abreast, including commanders and supernumeraries. Columns of fours will march on the left side of the road unless direct orders to the contrary are issued. Exact distances and covering are to be maintained at all times ; the fact of marching at ease is not to affect the relative position of men in the ranks, or that of supernumeraries or commanders, unless orders to the contrary are issued.

(2) If, on arrival at the destination, the party is to form up on a marker, it is better to advance from that flank on which it is intended to form up : *i.e.*, if to form up on a left marker, advance with the left leading ; if on a right marker, with the right leading.

(3) In other cases advance from whichever flank is the more convenient.

---

* Except for musketry instruction.

(4) An O.C. a party places himself three paces in advance of the leading section of fours, and leads the party to its destination : *i.e.*, on the march he does not require to give any words of command to wheel, etc., on coming to an angle in the road, he makes the wheel and his men follow him.

(5) The compliments to be paid on the march are laid down in the King's Regulations.

In addition, it is customary for officers' parties to pay the compliment of " EYES-RIGHT (OR LEFT)" to the following officers, the officer in command saluting with the right hand :—(i) G.Os.C. the command or division to which the party belongs ; (ii) Os.C. the R.A.M.C. in the command or division to which the party belongs ; (iii) The O.C. the company or group of companies to which the party belongs. To the C.O. this compliment is only paid once a day.

(6) Individual officers meeting a party salute the officer in command, if senior to them.

CHAPTER XXI.

FORMATIONS AND MOVEMENTS OF AMBULANCES.

The Field Ambulance.

370. On parade, and usually on the line of march, the bearer and tent sub-division of each section will parade together. To facilitate disengaging* when the bearer division is ordered forward the bearer sub-divisions (except wagon orderlies) will fall in on the right, the tent sub-divisions on the left of each section respectively. Field ambulances parade by the right in all formations.

371. Field Ambulance in Line.—(1) *Formation.*—The bearer and tent divisions will be drawn up as a company of three sections in line; A section on the right, B section in the centre, and C section on the left (Fig. 66).

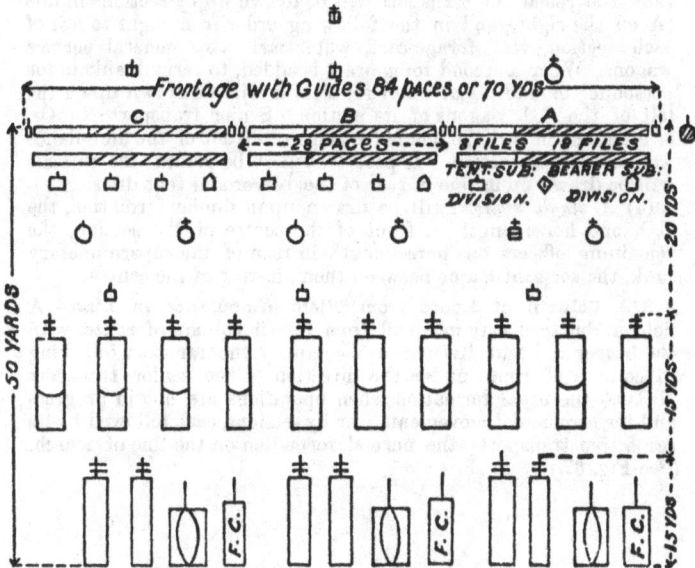

FIG. 66.—FIELD AMBULANCE IN LINE BY THE RIGHT.
(For key, see page ix.)

* *Note.*—A bearer sub-division may be disengaged and formed up in any convenient manner, *e.g.*, by being marched clear of the remainder, and ordered to fall in by squads (each man having been told off to his squad before taking the field). Nos. 3 supply stretchers. Nos. 4 provide themselves with surgical haversacks and water-bottles

(2) *Position of Officers.*—When the whole field ambulance is on parade together the senior captain of A section will act as a section commander. Section commanders will be one horse-length in front of the centre of their sections, the O.C. the field ambulance two horse-lengths in front of the centre of the line of section commanders. The other officers and the serjeant-major will be one horse-length behind the supernumerary rank of their respective sections, and the quartermaster, if on parade, four paces to the right of, and in line with, the front rank.

(3) *Transport.*—The transport will be drawn up in rear in two ranks at close (or half) interval, the first rank 20 yards in rear of the front rank of the bearer and tent divisions, the second rank 4 yards from the first, measured from tail boards to heads of leaders ; the directing flanks of the whole covering correctly. The ambulance wagons (with wagon orderlies on the near side of the box-seat) compose the first rank ; the wagons of A section on the right, those of B in the centre, and C on the left. In the second rank the remaining transport will be drawn up by sections in line (A on the right), and in the following order from right to left of each section, viz., forage-cart, water-cart, two general service wagons. When a second forage-cart is added, to carry blankets for personnel or additional tents for sick, it will be drawn up on the left of the G.S. wagons of its section. Senior transport N.C.Os. of each section will be one horse-length in front of the ambulance wagons of their section. If pack-transport be present the animals will be drawn up in line in rear of the bearer and tent divisions.

(4) *A single section* will be drawn up in similar formation, the C.O. one horse-length in front of the centre of the section, the remaining officers one horse-length in rear of the supernumerary rank, the serjeant-major between them, in rear of the centre.

372. Column of Route from Field Ambulance in Line.—A field ambulance may move off from line in column of route, with the bearer and tent divisions as a company, the transport following in column of route under the direction of the senior transport N C.O.—the usual formation when operations are not in progress and for ceremonial movements ; or by sections, each followed by its respective transport—the normal formation on the line of march. (See Fig. 67.)

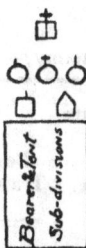

A. Section.

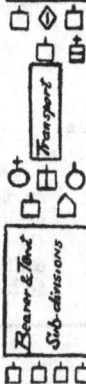

B Section.

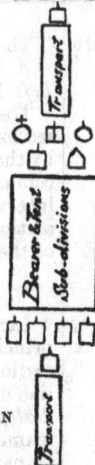

C. Section.

FIG. 67.—FIELD AMBULANCE IN
COLUMN OF ROUTE.
(For key, see page ix.)

Notes.—The normal position of commanders and supernumeraries is shown in the above diagram, but C.Os. and section commanders are authorized to march in the most suitable position to supervise their commands.

All vehicles should march on the left side of the road, and when a halt is ordered each vehicle should be drawn up at once on that side of the road, Cross-roads should be left clear,

(1) *As a Company :—*

Column of Route from Line.* **Move to the Right in Fours, Form—Fours. Right. Left Wheel, Quick—March.**	Bearer and tent divisions as in Infantry Training.
	Note.—This applies also to a single section.
Line, or Column, from Column of Route. (*See* detail.)	The field ambulance will form into line again on the command *On the Left, Form—Company,* or into column (*see* para. 373) on the command *On the Left, Form—Sections.* In both cases the caution *At the Halt* will be given if it is intended to halt in line or column.

(2) *By Sections :—*

Column of Route from Line. By Sections Column of—Route.	The section commanders give the orders :— *A (B or C) Section, Form—Fours. Right. Left Wheel, Quick—March.* The bearer and tent sub-divisions of each section, as it moves off in succession, are followed by the transport of the section in column of route, commanders of sections in rear, allowing an interval of 10 yards between the transport of the sections in front and the leading section of fours of their command.
Line, or Column, from Column of Route. (*See* Detail.)	Line, or Column, may be reformed on the principles mentioned in (1) of this paragraph, section commanders forming their sections into line or column on the order of the O.C., (*At the Halt*), *Form—Line,* or *Form—Column* ; commanders of sections in rear allowing for the transport of the preceding section.

* *Note.*—In this and following paragraphs the name of the movement is shewn in **thick type** in the left-hand column, and is followed by the caution or executive word of command, given by the O.C. or instructor, in SMALL CAPITALS. The right-hand column contains the detail.

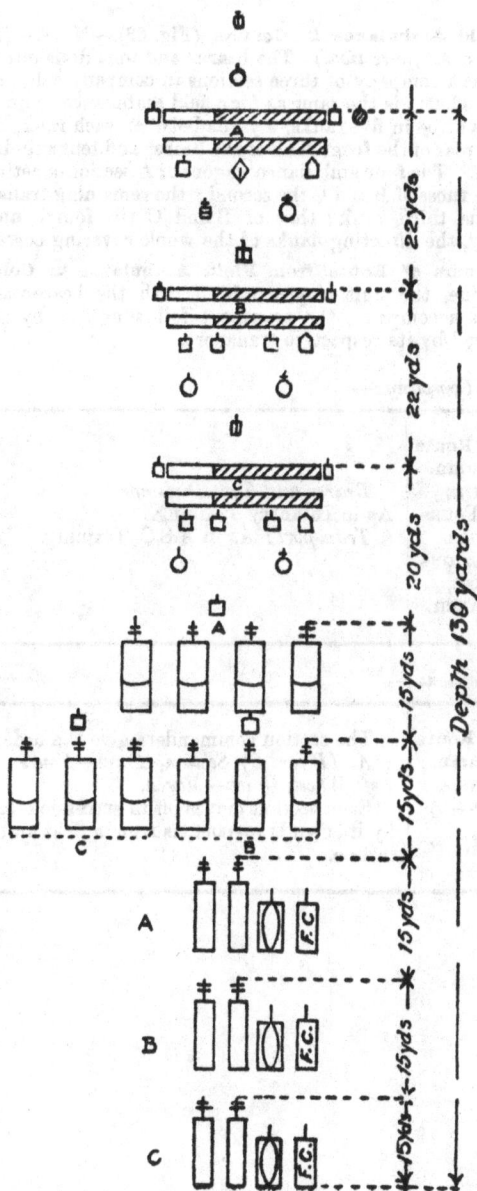

Fig. 68.—Field Ambulance in Column by the Right.

(For key, see page ix.)

373. Field Ambulance in Column (Fig. 68).—Note.—(*Not applicable to a single section.*) The bearer and tent divisions will be drawn up as a company of three sections in company column. The position of officers is the same as for a field ambulance in line. The transport will be in five ranks, 4 yards between each rank, the first 20 yards in rear of the front rank of the bearer and tent sub-divisions of C section. The four ambulance wagons of A section constitute the first rank; those of B and C the second; the remaining transport of A forms the third rank; that of B and C the fourth and fifth respectively, the directing flanks of the whole covering correctly.

374. Column of Route from Field Ambulance in Column.—As from line, the unit may march off with the bearer and tent divisions as a company, the transport following; or by sections, each followed by its respective transport.

(1) *As a Company :*—

Column of Route from Column. MOVE TO THE RIGHT IN FOURS, FORM—FOURS. RIGHT. SECTIONS, LEFT WHEEL, QUICK—MARCH.	*Bearer and Tent Divisions :* As in Infantry Training. *Transport :* As in A.S.C. Training.

(2) *By Sections :*—

Column of Route from Column. BY SECTIONS, COLUMN OF— ROUTE.	The section commanders give the orders :— *A, (B or C) Section, Form—Fours. Right. Left Wheel, Quick—March.* Each section moves off in succession, followed by its own transport, as from a field ambulance in line.

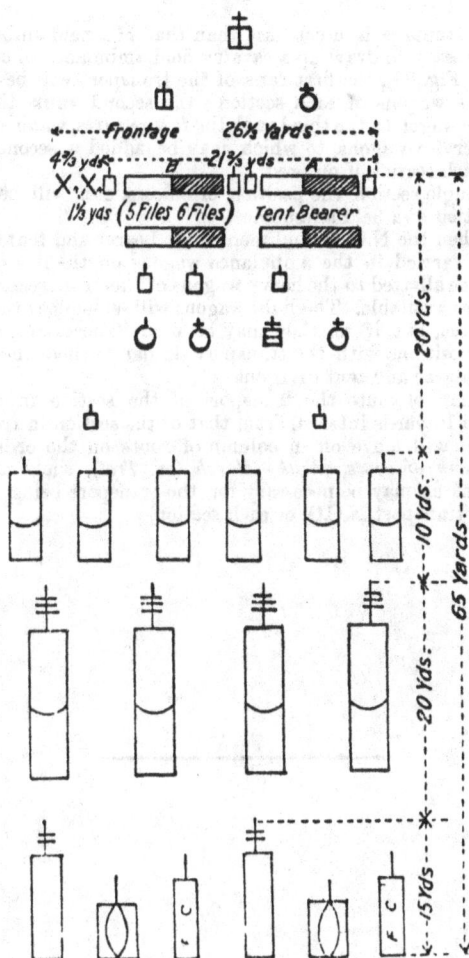

Fig. 69.—CAVALRY FIELD AMBULANCE IN LINE BY THE RIGHT.

(For key, see page ix.)

THE CAVALRY FIELD AMBULANCE.

375. The formations and movements (bearer and tent divisions on foot) are similar to those for a field ambulance in line, except that the transport will be drawn up in three ranks. The positions of the officers are as for a field ambulance in line, and the same distances will be preserved between the ranks of transport.

As the frontage is much less than that of a field ambulance, it is not necessary to draw up a cavalry field ambulance in column.

In line (Fig. 69), the first rank of the transport will be the light ambulance wagons of each section ; the second rank the heavy ambulance wagons ; the third rank the forage-carts, water-carts, and general service wagons, to which may be added a second forage-cart for each section if ordered.

For a single section the position of officers, etc., will be as for a single section of a field ambulance.

376. When the N.C.Os. and men of the bearer and tent divisions are to be carried in the ambulance wagons on the line of march, they will be allotted to the heavy wagons of their own sections as far as these are available. The light wagons will seldom be available for this purpose, but, if so, they may be used if necessary. Officers will take positions with the transport similar to those they occupy with the bearer and tent divisions.

In column of route the transport of the section in rear will close up to 10 yards interval from that of the section in front.

The unit will move off in column of route on the order of the C.O., *Column of route, Walk—March* (or *Trot*), such subsidiary instructions as may be necessary for the transport being given by the senior transport N.C.O. of each section

CHAPTER XXII.

STRETCHER EXERCISES.

377. General Remarks.—The following exercises have been framed for the instruction of bodies of men, with a view to the careful handling of the wounded, and their transport on stretchers and in wagons. When the bearers have become thoroughly proficient in these exercises on the parade ground, the instructor will take every opportunity of regularly practising them under conditions approaching as far as possible to those of field service. The squads should be exercised over rough ground, and each man taught the various means for the transport and carriage of wounded. The important point to impress on every man is that in the field he may form the No. 4 of the stretcher squad and so be responsible for the wounded man, until he is brought directly under the notice of the medical officer. A syllabus of exercises suitable for the practical training of trained soldiers in field work is given at the end of Chapter III.

378. Men detailed for stretcher exercises must be well grounded in squad and company drill. Knee-caps will be worn on the left knee at all exercises in which the men require to kneel, except when otherwise ordered. Soldiers to act as " patients " will be provided with ground-sheets to protect their clothing.

Regimental stretcher bearers should be especially practised in stretcher exercises with reduced numbers, and a regimental stretcher squad should normally consist of 4 bearers.

379. For instructional work the men will be taught the exercises "by numbers" (where so indicated); when sufficiently advanced, the various movements will be done " judging the time," or " working by the right."

FORMATION.*

---

380. Sizing the Bearers.† TALLEST ON THE RIGHT, SHORTEST ON THE LEFT, IN SINGLE RANK,— SIZE.	The whole will break off and arrange themselves according to their size in single rank, the tallest on the right and shortest on the left, and take up their dressing by the right.

---

* *Note.*—Previous to the parade the stretchers will be laid in a heap on the ground.

† *Note.*—In this and following paragraphs the name of the movement is shewn in **thick type** in the left-hand column, and is followed by the caution or executive word of command, given by the O.C. or instructor, in SMALL CAPITALS. The right-hand column contains the detail.

When, however, the words of command are given by the No. 4 of the stretcher squad, these are shewn in an additional (second) column, and the detail given in the third column.

NUMBER.	From right to left of the whole company.
ODD NUMBERS ONE PACE FORWARD, EVEN NUMBERS ONE PACE STEP BACK, —MARCH.	The odd numbers will take one pace forward, and the even numbers will step back one pace.
NUMBER ONE STAND FAST, RANKS, RIGHT AND LEFT—TURN.	The odd numbers, with the exception of Number One will turn to the right, the even numbers to the left.
FORM COMPANY, QUICK—MARCH.	The whole will step off, the even numbers wheeling round to the right and following the left-hand man of the odd numbers. No. 3 will form up two paces in rear of No. 1, No. 5 on the left of No. 1, No. 7 in rear of No. 5, No. 9 on the left of No. 5 ; and so on. The leading men of the even numbers will always form in the rear rank and the next man in the front rank. As the men arrive in their places they will turn to the left and take up their dressing.
381. Forming the Squads. BY FOURS (FIVES, OR SIXES)— NUMBER.	The front rank will number from right to left in order.
SQUADS AT THE HALT, LEFT—FORM. QUICK—MARCH. RIGHT—TURN.	As in Infantry Training.
RIGHT—DRESS.	The No. 1 of the squad on the right remains steady ; the remaining Nos. 1 will each take up positions one pace from the bearer on his right ; the other bearers will place themselves one pace in rear of and covering the bearer in front of them.

Notes.—If necessary, the bearers will be proved
as follows :—
   First Rank, No. 1 bearers, Stand-at-Ease.
   Second Rank, No. 2 bearers, Stand-at-Ease.
And so on. But this should be unnecessary as
bearers retain the same numbers in the squad as
when numbered for forming squads. When proved
in this manner, the squads will be called to ATTEN-
TION before proceeding with the next movement.
   Squads are composed of 4, 5, or 6 bearers.
   When the bearers are constantly employed in
the same positions, the squads will be formed up
on the command *By Squads, Fall—In*, when
each bearer will take up his proper position on
the No. 1 of the squad on the right.

NUMBER THE— SQUADS.	No. 1 bearers number from right to left.

382. Supplying Stretchers.

No. 3 BEARERS, RIGHT (OR LEFT)— TURN. SUPPLY STRETCHERS, QUICK—MARCH.	The No. 3 bearers will march by the shortest route to the pile of stretchers ; each bearer in turn will lay hold of the near handle of a stretcher, raise it to a perpendicular position in front of him, runners to the front ; stoop, grasp the lower runners with his right hand and place the stretcher on his right shoulder at the slope ; rise to the erect position and lead on, stepping short. As soon as the last bearer has provided himself with a stretcher he will give the command *About—Turn.* The whole will turn about, and rejoin their squads in quick time, halting without further word of command as they arrive in their places. Taking the time from the leading bearer they turn to the right (or left).
(TWO)	The lower handles will be rested on the ground, the stretchers held perpendicularly.
(THREE)	The bearers will place the stretchers on the ground to the right of the squad by passing the lower handles forward, runners to the right, front-ends of the poles in line with the toes of No. 1 ; and rise together working by the right.

STAND TO—
STRETCHERS.

The Nos. 1 place themselves with their toes in line with the front-end of the poles, Nos. 3 with their heels in line with the rear-end of the poles, allowing sufficient room for turning. The remaining bearers will take up positions one pace in rear of and covering the bearers in front of them.

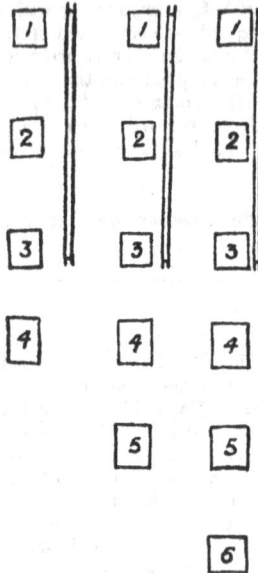

FIG. 70. "STAND TO STRETCHERS."

383. Lifting and lowering Stretchers.
LIFT—
STRETCHERS.

Nos. 1 and 3 stoop, grasp both handles of the poles firmly with the right hand, rise together holding the stretcher at the full extent of the arm, runners to the right.

LOWER—
STRETCHERS.

Nos. 1 and 3 stoop and place the stretcher quietly on the ground, runners to the right, and rise smartly together.

384. Storing or Piling Stretchers. LIFT— STRETCHERS.	As before detailed.
NOS. 1 AND 3, IN SUCCESSION FROM THE RIGHT (OR LEFT), DIS- ENGAGE, QUICK— MARCH.	The Nos. 1 and 3 on the flank named will dis-engage by taking a side-pace to the right, and move off in quick time followed by the remaining Nos. 1 and 3 in succession, dispose of their stretchers, and rejoin their squads.
SQUADS, STAND— EASY.	As in Infantry Training.
REMOVE—KNEE- CAPS.	Knee-caps are removed and collected (if necessary).
SQUADS, ATTEN— TION. DIS—MISS.	As in Infantry Training.

EXERCISES WITH CLOSED STRETCHERS.

385. Advancing and Retiring. LIFT— STRETCHERS.	As before detailed.
BY THE RIGHT (OR LEFT), QUICK— MARCH.	The squads will advance, the rules for marching as in Infantry Training being maintained, except that the hand holding the stretcher will be kept steady by the side.
SQUADS, ABOUT— TURN.	The whole turn about, the stretcher being passed from one hand to the other by the Nos. 1 and 3.

CHANGE—STRETCHERS.	If the squads are advancing, the Nos. 1 will pass the stretcher from one hard to the other behind them; the Nos. 3, seeing this done, will pass the stretcher from one hand to the other in front of them, the Nos. 2 moving diagonally to their places. If the squads are retiring the Nos. 1 act as for Nos. 3, and the Nos. 3 as for Nos. 1. The remaining bearers in each case continue in their respective positions.
	Note.—The stretcher must be held in the right hand when the command *About—Turn* is given. The runner must be to the left when the stretcher is in the left hand.
386. Moving to a Flank. (*See* Detail.)	When it is necessary to make a quick movement to either flank for a short distance only, the command *Right* (*or Left*)—*Turn* will be given. When a squad is marching to the right and the command *About—Turn* is given, the Nos. 1 and 3 will seize the handles of the stretcher with the left hand and cut away the right while turning about, resuming the grasp with the right hand —back of the hand to the rear—after the turn has been completed.
387. Changing Direction. AT THE HALT, RIGHT (OR LEFT)—FORM.	The No. 1 of the squad on the flank named will make a full turn to the right (or left), the remainder of the Nos. 1 a partial turn in the required direction, the other bearers a partial turn in the opposite direction.
QUICK—MARCH.	The No. 1 of the squad on the flank named will stand fast, the remainder step off by the shortest route to their places on the new alignment, halt, and take up their dressing independently.
	Note.—When it is intended to move off in the new direction after forming, the words *At the Halt* will be omitted, the bearers will mark time when formed and the word *Forward* will be given.

388. Extending.
FROM THE
RIGHT
(LEFT, OR
ANY NAMED
SQUAD), TO
FOUR PACES
—EXTEND.

On the March.—On the word *Extend*, the named squad will continue to move on in quick time, the remainder will make a partial turn outwards, double to their places and turn to their front, breaking into quick time as they arrive there and taking up their dressing by the directing flank or squad. On the commencement of the movement the Nos. 4, 5, and 6 bearers will place themselves on the right of the stretcher. (*See* Fig. 71.)

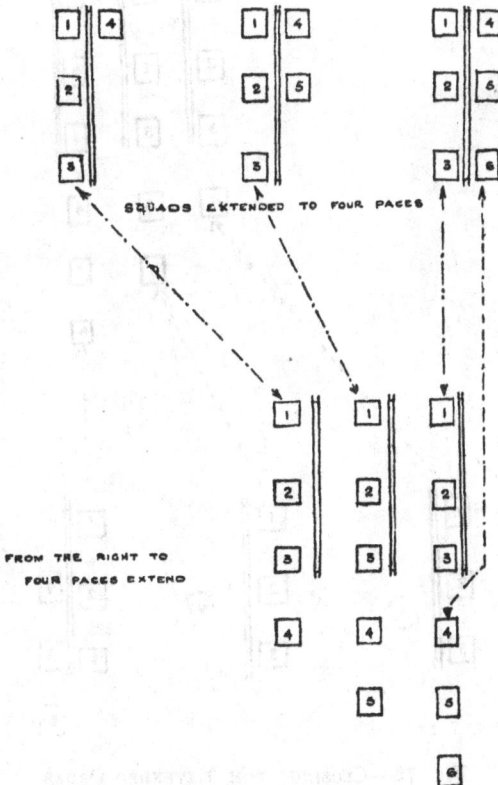

FIG. 71.—POSITION IN EXTENDED ORDER WITH CLOSED STRETCHERS.

P 2

389. Closing.	The named squad will continue to move on in quick time, the remainder will make a partial turn in the direction named, double to their places and turn to their front, breaking into quick time as they arrive there. The bearers on the right of the stretcher will drop back into their original places.
ON THE RIGHT (LEFT OR ANY NAMED SQUAD),— CLOSE.	

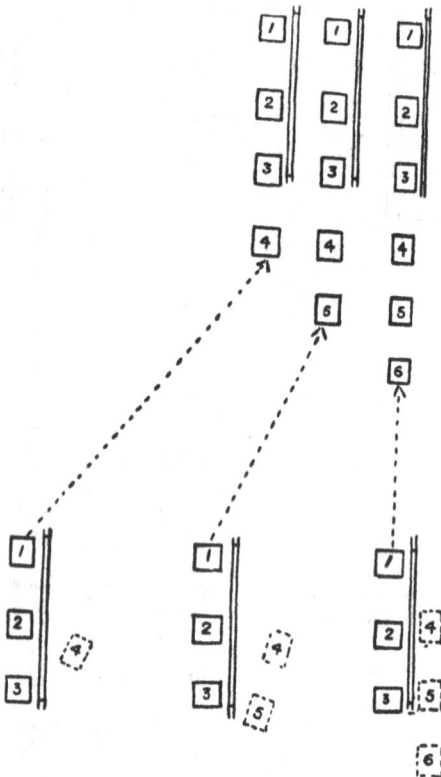

FIG. 72.—CLOSING FROM EXTENDED ORDER.

(Bearers on the right of stretchers dropping back into their original places.)

390. Preparing Stretchers. PREPARE— STRETCHERS.	The bearers on the right of the stretcher will take a side-pace to the right ; Nos. 1 and 3 then turn to the right, kneel on the left knee, unbuckle the transverse straps and place the slings on the ground beside them, separate the poles and straighten the traverses ; then, each takes up a sling, doubles it on itself, slips the loop thus formed on the near handle, and places the free ends over the opposite handle, grip-plate uppermost.
(TWO.)	On the word *Two*, they rise and turn to the left together, working by the right.
391. Closing Stretchers. CLOSE— STRETCHERS.	Nos. 1 and 3 turn to the right, kneel on the left knee, remove the slings and place them on the ground beside them, push in the traverses, raise the canvas, and approximate the poles.
(TWO.)	On the word *Two*, they rise, lifting the stretcher, and face one another ; place the handles of the poles between their thighs, runners to the right, and roll the canvas tightly over the poles to the right.
(THREE.)	On the word *Three*, each takes up a sling and passes the grip-plate† end to the other, and, holding the grip-plate end in the left hand, threads the transverse strap through the loop of the other sling and buckles it tightly close to the runner, keeping the sling on top. Then, grasping both handles in the right hand, back of the hand to the right, they turn to the right in a slightly stooping position, rise, and turn to the left together. The bearers on the right of the stretcher then take a side-pace to the left.

* *Note.*—The preparation of stretchers, and all movements with prepared stretchers, will be performed in extended order.

Note.—The older pattern sling has a buckle instead of a grip-plate.

392. Lifting and Lowering Stretchers. LIFT— STRETCHERS.	On the word *Stretchers*, Nos. 1 and 3 stoop, grasp the doubled sling midway between the poles with the right hand and sweep it off the handles, rise, holding it at the full extent of the arm, grip-plate to the front.
(TWO.)	On the word *Two*, they take a side-pace between the handles and place the sling over the shoulders, dividing it equally, grip-plate to the right. The sling should lie well below the collar of the frock behind and in the hollow of the shoulders in front.
(THREE.)	On the word *Three*, stoop, slip the loops over the handles, commencing with the left, and grasp both handles firmly.
(FOUR.)	On the word *Four*, rise slowly together lifting the stretcher, No. 3 conforming closely to the movements of No. 1.
ADJUST—SLINGS.	Nos. 2 turn about and step forward one pace ; Nos. 4 turn to the left ; they adjust the slings, taking care that they are well below the collar of the frock behind and in the hollow of the shoulders in front. The length of slings may be adjusted by means of the grip-plates if necessary.
(TWO.)	Nos. 2 turn about and step forward one pace ; Nos. 4 turn to the right.
	Note.—This movement is required only when the Nos. 1 and 3 have not adjusted the slings correctly when lifting stretchers.
LOWER— STRETCHERS.	Nos. 1 and 3 slowly stoop and place the stretchers gently on the ground, No. 3 conforming closely to the movements of No. 1 ; slip the loops from the handles, and stand up.

(Two.)	On the word *Two*, they remove the slings from the shoulders, hold them as before described, take a side-pace to the left, and stand to stretchers.
(Three.)	On the word *Three*, they stoop, place the slings on the handles as in "prepared stretchers," and rise together.
393. Changing Numbers. CHANGE— NUMBERS.	The bearers on the right of the stretcher will turn about; the whole will step off together, No. 1 wheeling round by the front of the stretcher and taking up the position of No. 4. Each man halts in the position of the bearer whose place he has taken. The new numbers on the right of the stretcher will turn about.

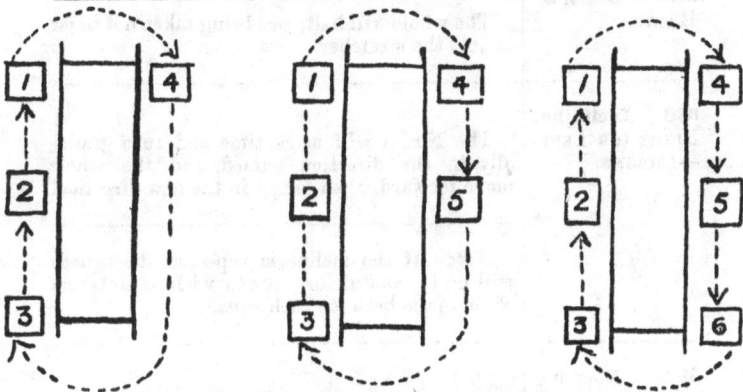

FIG. 73.—CHANGING NUMBERS.
(Bearers on the right of stretchers turn about.)

394. Advancing and Retiring. ADVANCE.*	The whole move off together, stepping short, No. 3 stepping off with the right foot, the remainder with the left, the Nos. 1 and 3 keeping their knees bent and raising the feet as little as possible. Special attention must be paid to the carriage of the stretcher so as to keep it level and avoid jolting or unnecessary swaying.

* *Note.*—When squads are ordered to advance, the directing squad or flank will be named.

Note.—The Instructor will see that the directing squad marches on a given point, taking the correct pace as regards length, and that the remainder preserve their interval.

RETIRE.

Each squad will move round by the right on the circumference of a circle of which No. 3 is the centre ; Nos. 3 will mark time, turning gradually in the direction named, and the whole will move forward when square.

ADVANCE.

Each squad will resume the original direction to the front by a movement similar to that detailed for retiring.

---

395.   Halting.
HALT.

The whole will halt, care being taken not to jar or jolt the stretcher.

---

396.   Inclining.
RIGHT (OR LEFT) —INCLINE.

The Nos. 3 will mark time and turn gradually in the direction named, and the whole move forward when facing in the new direction.

Note.—If the incline is repeated the squads will be in COLUMN OF SQUADS with an interval of one pace between each squad.

---

397.   Forming into line.
(*See* Detail.)

To form into line, the command will be given :
— *On the Right (or Left), Form—Line.* (*See* Detail for CHANGING DIRECTION, para. 387.)

---

398.   Unloading and   Loading Stretchers.

Notes.—Men provided with ground sheets, to act as patients, will be placed in front of the squads, extended to four paces, and directed to lie down with their heads towards the squads.

When the bearers have sufficiently advanced in these exercises, the Nos. 4 will take charge of their respective squads.

(1) *Loading.*
COLLECT—
WOUNDED.*

Each squad doubles by the shortest route to the corresponding patient, and halts without further word of command when one pace from the head of and in line with the patient.

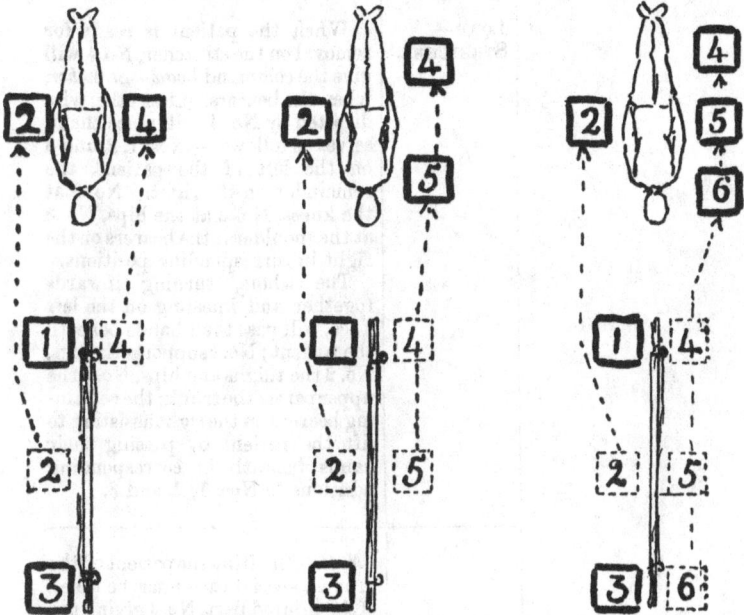

FIG. 74.—"COLLECT WOUNDED."

(The squads have advanced, halted, and lowered stretchers. While the stretchers are being prepared by Nos. 1 and 3, the disengaged bearers are rendering assistance to the patient.)

The No. 4 will proceed to the patient, examine and attend to his injury, and, if his carriage on the stretcher be necessary, he will give the following words of command :—

* *Note.*—The command *Collect Wounded* may be given when the squads are STANDING EASY, in which case they will come to ATTENTION, lift stretchers, and double out as above described.

LOWER—STRETCHER. PREPARE—STRETCHER.	While the stretcher is being prepared by Nos. 1 and 3, the disengaged bearers will proceed to the patient to render such assistance as may be required, No. 2 going to the left, the remainder to the right, unless otherwise directed by No. 4.
LOAD—STRETCHER.	When the patient is ready for removal on the stretcher, No. 4 will give the command *Load—Stretcher*, when the bearers, unless otherwise directed by No. 4, will place themselves as follows :—Nos. 1, 2, and 3 on the left of the patient, the remainder on the right. No. 1 at the knees, No. 2 at the hips, No. 3 at the shoulders ; the bearers on the right in corresponding positions. The whole, turning inwards together and kneeling on the left knee, will pass their hands beneath the patient ; No. 1 supports the legs, No. 2 the thighs and hips, No. 3 the upper part of the trunk; the remaining bearers on the right assisting to lift the patient by passing their hands beneath in corresponding positions to Nos. 1, 2, and 3.
	Note.—In lifting the patient off the ground, special care must be taken of the injured part, No. 4 giving the necessary instructions. In the case of a severe injury No. 4 will himself attend to the injured part in lifting, directing another bearer to replace him if necessary.
LIFT.	The patient will be carefully lifted on to the knees of Nos. 1, 2, and 3. The bearers on the right of the patient then disengage, rise, and step back one pace ; the bearer nearest the stretcher will turn to his left, double to the stretcher, take hold of it, left hand across, and rise

resting the near pole on the left hip, return to the patient and place the stretcher directly beneath him; then stand up and return to his former position. The bearers on the right of the patient will now step forward one pace, kneel on their left knees, and assist in lowering the patient when ordered by No. 4. (*See* Fig. 76.)

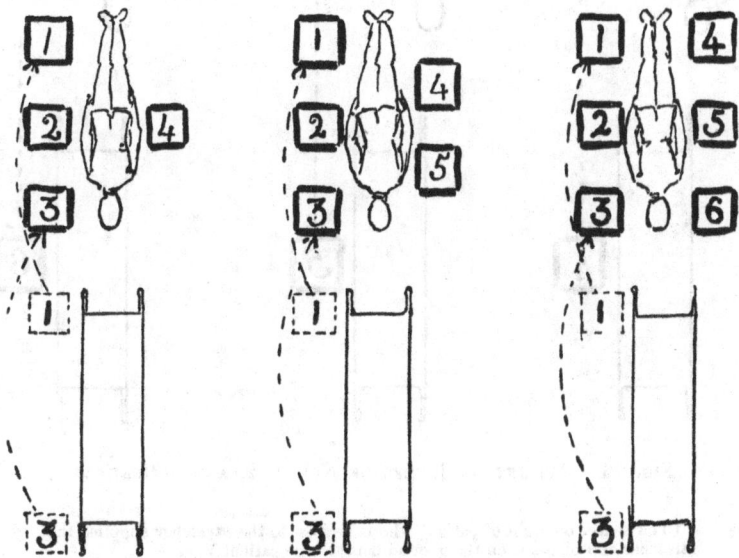

FIG. 75.—" LOAD STRETCHERS."

(The bearers in position ready to lift patient.)

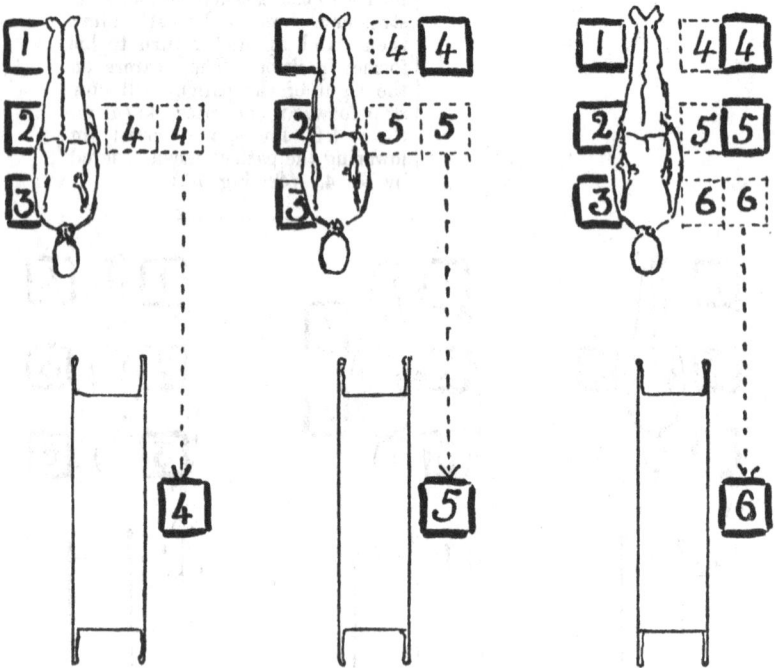

FIG. 76.— PATIENT ON KNEES OF NOS. 1, 2, AND 3 BEARERS.

(The bearer on right of patient who is nearest to the stretcher supplies the stretcher and places it on the ground beneath the patient.)

| LOWER. | The patient is lowered slowly and gently on to the centre of the canvas, special care being taken of the injured part. |
| | The bearers then disengage, rise, Nos. 1, 2, and 3 turn to the left, the bearers on the right of the patient to the right, and stand to stretchers as in " prepared stretchers." |

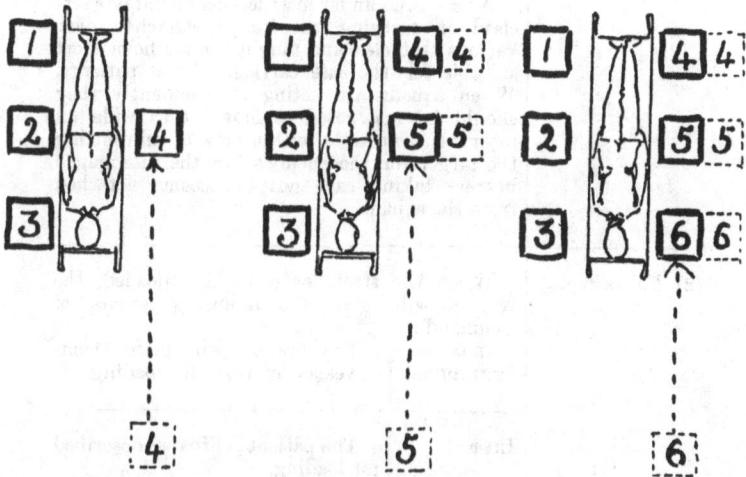

FIG. 77.—LOWERING PATIENT ON TO STRETCHER.

(The bearers on the right of patient step forward one pace to assist in lowering the patient on to the stretcher.)

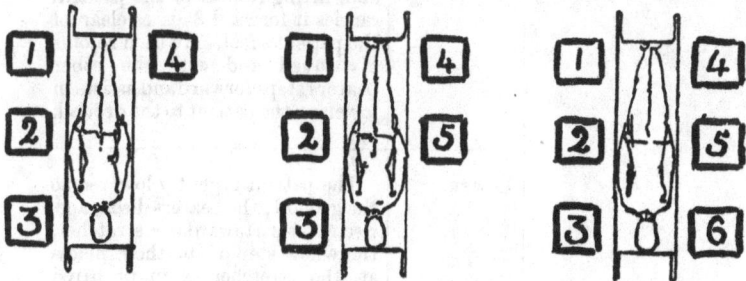

FIG. 78.—PATIENT ON STRETCHER.

(Patient on stretcher and bearers ready to move off.)

The No. 2, 5, or 6 will collect the arms and equipment of the patient. The rifle should be examined by pointing it in the air, opening the breech, and detaching the magazine to ensure that it is unloaded.

Note.—Men under instructions should be exercised in carrying the loaded stretcher over various obstacles, and taught the methods most suitable for the safe carriage of the patients. When squads are acting independently they should be instructed to move at as wide an interval as possible with a view of minimizing the target for the enemy's fire, the disengaged bearers taking care not to become detached from the squad.

(2) *Unloading.*	When the stretcher is to be unloaded, the No. 4 will give the following words of command :—
UNLOAD—STRETCHER.	The bearers will place themselves as described for loading.
LIFT.	The patient is lifted as described for loading. The bearers on the right of patient then disengage, rise, step back one pace ; No. 4 grasps the stretcher as described for loading, and, lifting it clear of the patient, carries it forward 3 paces clear of the patient's feet. He then rejoins his squad and with the other bearers steps forward and assists in lowering the patient to the ground.
LOWER.	The patient is gently lowered to the ground ; the bearers disengage, rise, and turn towards the stretcher, the whole step off to their places at the stretcher as in prepared stretchers. (*See* Fig. 80.)

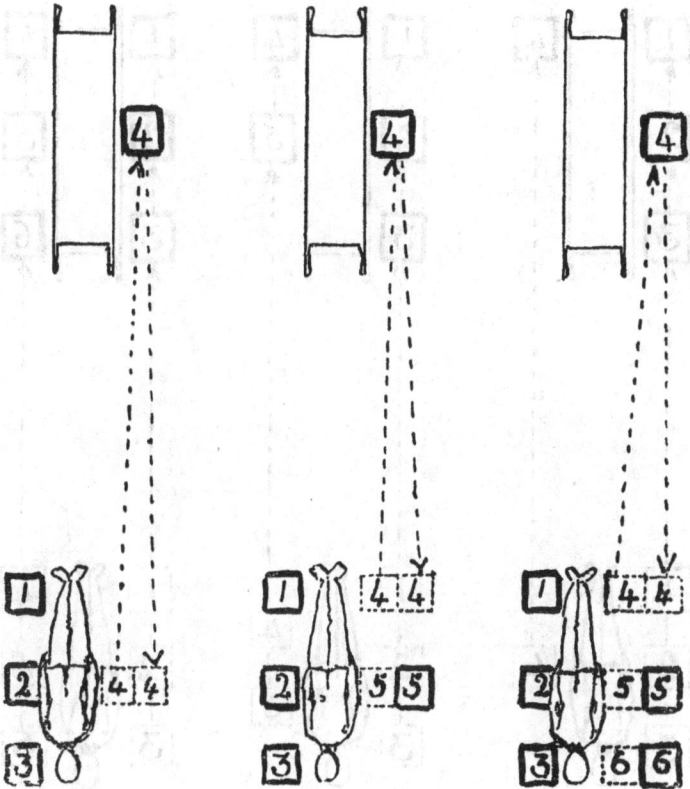

FIG. 79.--UNLOADING.

(No. 4 carrying the stretcher 3 paces clear of the patient's feet and returning.)

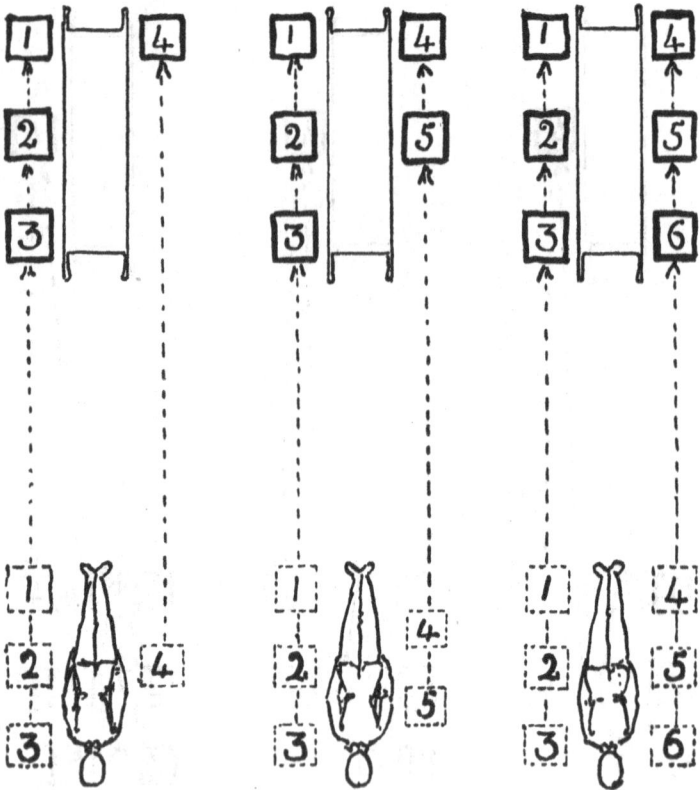

Fig. 80.—Unloading.

(Patient lowered to the ground and bearers taking up position at the stretcher as in prepared stretchers.)

Loading and Unloading Stretchers with reduced Numbers.

399. With Three Bearers.—In the event of there being only three bearers available, the stretcher will be placed at the patient's head, in the same line as his body. The bearers will then lift the patient, rise to the erect position, carry him head-foremost over the foot of the stretcher, the horizontal position of his body being maintained throughout the movement, and lay him in a suitable position on the canvas. When unloading, the patient will be lifted and carried head-foremost over the head of the stretcher. To lift the patient, one bearer, placing himself on the injured side in a line with the patient's knees, raises and supports the lower limbs, while the other two, kneeling on opposite sides of the patient, near his hips, facing each other, each pass an arm under his back and thighs, lock their fingers so as to secure a firm grip and raise and support the trunk.

400. With Two Bearers.—When only two bearers are available, the stretcher will similarly be placed at the patient's head, and in the same line as his body. The bearers will then lift the patient, rise to an erect position, carry him, in loading, head-foremost over the foot of the stretcher, and, in unloading, head-foremost over the head-end.

The method of lifting will vary according to whether the lower limbs are severely injured or not :—

(a) With a severe injury of one of the lower limbs, both bearers place themselves on the injured side; the one in a line with the patient's knees must raise and support the lower limbs, the one near the patient's hips, the body, assisted by the patient himself as far as possible, the horizontal position of the patient's body being maintained throughout the movement.

(b) With the lower limbs intact or only slightly injured, the patient may be lifted by the improvised seat described in the next chapter, provided there are no symptoms of shock present; in the latter case, method (a) must be resorted to.

EXERCISES FOR STRETCHER, MARK I, SPECIAL.

401. With Six Bearers.—When supplying stretchers, care should be taken that the stretchers are placed on the ground with the hooded or head-ends of the stretchers towards the Nos. 3.

(i) *Loading.*—The patient having been placed on the stretcher, Nos. 2 and 5 raise the hood, adjust the front pair of lines, passing them through the leather loops fixed on the stretcher, and fastening off. Nos. 3 and 6 at the same time pass the rear lines through the eyes in the rear of the canvas and secure them. Bearers then rise together, Nos. 1, 2, and 3 turn to the left, Nos. 4, 5, and 6 turn to the right.

(ii) *Lifting.*—On the command *Lift—Stretchers*, the Nos. 1 and 3 lift the stretcher as before described. As soon as this is carried out, Nos. 4 and 5 step back and place themselves by the side-handles on the right of the stretcher. Nos. 2 step up and place themselves by the side-handles on the left, in line with Nos. 4. The Nos. 6, turning outwards and passing round by the head of the stretcher, place themselves on the left of the stretcher in line with Nos. 5.

(iii) *Advancing.*—On the command *Advance*, the whole move off. Nos. 1, 2, and 6 with the left foot, Nos. 3, 4, and 5 with the right; Nos. 2, 4, 5, and 6, laying hold of the side-handles, will assist in carrying the stretcher,

(B 10977)

Q

(iv) *Lowering.*—On the command *Lower—Stretchers* the stretcher will be lowered to the ground, and the bearers will place themselves at the stretcher as for unloading (Nos. 1, 2, and 3 on the left, Nos. 4, 5, and 6 on the right).

(v) *Unloading.*—On the command *Unload*, Nos. 2 and 5 unfasten the front lines, Nos. 3 and 6 the rear lines, and lower the hood. As soon as this is done the patient is lifted as before.

(vi) *Loading wagons.*—Previous to the stretchers being placed in the wagons, the side-handles will be pushed under the stretcher.

AMBULANCE WAGON EXERCISES.

402. For instructional purposes the squads will be numbered by fours.

The ambulance wagons will be drawn up in single rank on the drill ground. A corporal or private will be told off as wagon orderly to each wagon. They will lower the seats and rails of the upper compartments and prepare the wagons for the reception of the wounded.

403. Loading Wagons. ON WAGONS— RETIRE.	The stretcher squads retire towards the line of wagons ; the four squads on the left, as the line is retiring, proceeding to the wagon on the extreme left, the next four squads to the next wagon, and so on to the right of the line, closing in to two paces interval between the squads, and halting without further word of command when four paces from the tail-board of the wagon.
LOWER— STRETCHERS.	As before detailed.
FIX—SLINGS.	Slings will be fixed as follows :—Nos. 1 and 3 turn to the right, kneel on the left knee, pass the loop of the grip-plate end over the near handle, grip-plate downwards, carry the sling under and round the opposite handle close up to the canvas, back to the near handle, round which two or three turns are made, pass the transverse strap round the pole between the runners and traverse, and fasten the buckle outside the sling between the poles ; the bearers then rise and stand to stretchers.

While this is being done, the patient's rifle and kit will be stored in the wagon, and the bearers will take up position as follows :—Nos. 1 and 3 on the left, 2 and 4 on the right of the stretcher, No. 2 placing himself opposite No. 3 ; the remaining bearers taking a side-pace of 30 inches to the right. (*See* Figure 81.)

Note.—When the bearers have learned to fix slings, the order *Lower Stretchers and Fix Slings* will be given as one order by No. 4, and carried out accordingly.

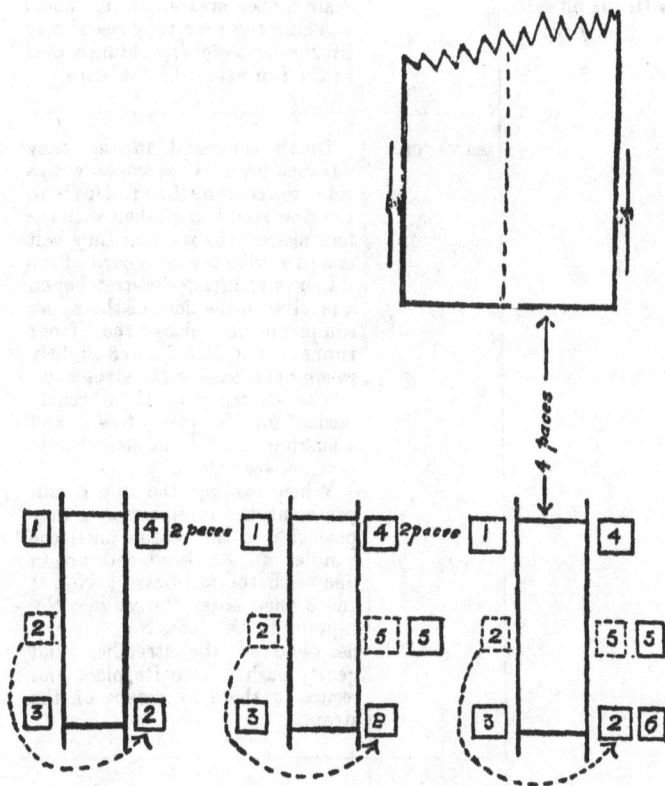

FIG. 81.—" ON WAGONS—RETIRE."
(Three squads of four, five, and six bearers in position ready for loading wagon.)

Q 2

STAND—EASY.	As in Infantry Training.

SQUADS, IN SUC-CESSION FROM THE RIGHT,—LOAD.		When the squads are sufficiently advanced in these exercises, the Nos. 4 will take charge of their respective squads and give the following words of command :—
Note.—The upper compartments will be loaded first, commencing with the off-side.	No.—SQUAD, ATTEN— TION. LOAD —WAGONS.	The Nos. 1, 2, 3, and 4 bearers turn inwards, stoop, grasp the poles of the stretcher, hands wide apart, palms uppermost ; the remaining bearers stand fast. Then, working together, they rise slowly lifting the stretcher, holding it level at the full extent of the arms.
	ADVANCE.	On the command *Advance*, they advance towards the wagon with a side-step crossing their feet in front, the first step being taken with the foot nearest the wagon ; they halt one pace from the tail-board of the wagon, and, lifting the stretcher on a level with the floor of the upper compartment, place the front runners on it, Nos. 2 and 3 slightly raising the head of the stretcher. The stretcher is then gently pushed into its place, Nos. 1 and 4 making way for the stretcher to pass between them. When loading the upper compartment the stretcher is gently pushed into the wagon until the handles at the head end are in line with the tail-board ; Nos. 1 and 3 then enter the wagon, No. 1 going to the foot, No. 3 to the head-end of the stretcher, and gently push it into its place and secure it there by means of the strap.
	FALL—IN.	As soon as the stretcher is in its place, the No. 4 will give the command *Fall—in*, when the bearers will fall in, as in file, facing the wagon.

RE-FORM SQUAD QUICK— MARCH.	The bearers will wheel round to the right and re-form squad, as in file, facing the field, four paces behind and to the right of the remaining squads. (*See* Fig. 83.)
HALT, STAND— EASY.	As in Infantry Training.

Notes.—When loading the upper compartment, it may be necessary for the No. 1 to enter the wagon as soon as disengaged, and guide the front runners over the rubber blocks which retain the stretcher in position in the wagon. As soon as the off upper compartment is loaded, the next squad will be ordered to load the near upper compartment. As soon as this is completed the lower compartments will be loaded in the same way. When loading the lower compartment it will not be necessary for Nos. 1 and 3 to enter the wagon.

When the wagon is fully loaded the upper seats will be securely strapped to the side of the wagon by the wagon orderly, and the tail-board lifted and secured in its place.

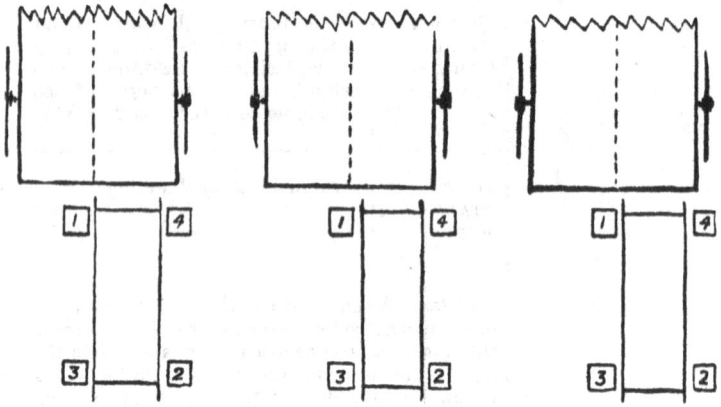

FIG. 82.—" LOAD WAGONS."
(Squads advanced towards the wagons to load.)

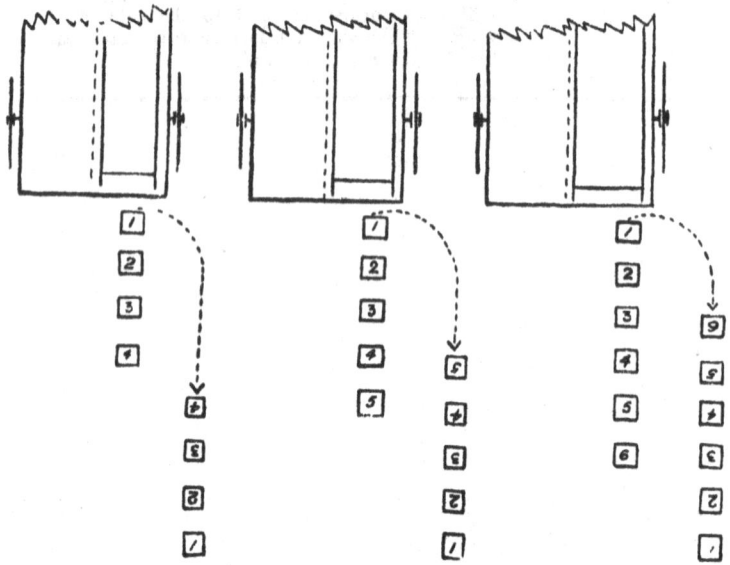

FIG. 83.—RE-FORMING SQUAD.
(Facing the field.)

404. Unloading Wagons.	*Notes.*—The requisite number of squads will be drawn up ten paces from and facing the tail-boards of the wagons. The squads will be numbered by fours.
SQUADS, STAND—EASY.	As in Infantry Training. The wagon orderlies will prepare the wagons as for loading. The lower compartments will be unloaded first, commencing with the off compartment.

SQUADS, IN SUCCESSION FROM THE RIGHT,— UNLOAD.

When the squads are sufficiently advanced in these exercises, Nos. 4 will take charge of their respective squads and give the following words of command:—

No.—SQUAD, ATTEN— TION. FOR UNLOADING, TAKE— POST.	The squad moves off towards the wagon, Nos. 1, 2, and 3 stepping short to allow the remaining bearers to come up on their right; the whole will then move forward in quick time, halting without further word of command one pace from the tail-board of the wagon. (*See* Fig. 84.)
UNLOAD— WAGONS.	The bearers on the right will take a side-pace of 30 inches to their right ; Nos. 2 and 3 pass up between Nos. 1 and 4 (No. 2 going to the right), lay hold of the handles, and, raising the head of the stretcher about 6 inches, gently withdraw it. As the stretcher is withdrawn, Nos. 1 and 4 take hold of the handles at the foot-end, and, taking the weight, lower it to the full extent of the arms; great care being taken to keep the stretcher level and to avoid jarring the patient as the stretcher leaves the compartment.

Retire.	The squad will retire and place the stretcher on the ground selected for the purpose ; then stand to stretchers, being joined by Nos. 5 and 6 with the patient's rifle and kit. If there are only four bearers to the squad, No. 2 will return to the wagon for the patient's kit, etc.
Stand— Easy.	As in Infantry Training.

Note.—In unloading the upper compartment Nos. 1 and 3 enter the wagon as in Loading, withdraw the stretcher until the handles at the head-end are in line with the tail-board of the wagon, then rejoin their squad : the stretcher is withdrawn as in previous detail.

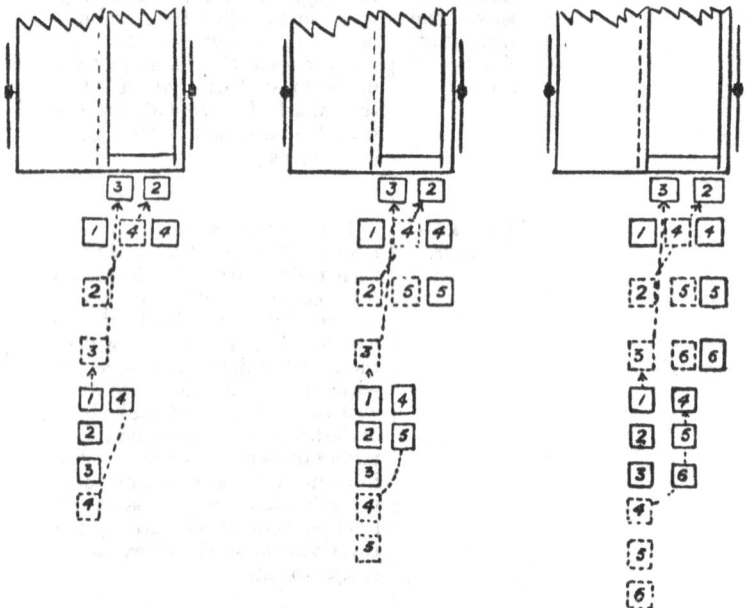

Fig. 84.—Unloading Wagons.
(Squads taking posts and unloading.)

HAND-SEAT EXERCISE.

The "Hook-Grip" Seat.

405. The bearers will be formed up in double-rank and numbered:—

> Odd Numbers : Right Files.
> Even Numbers : Left Files.

FORM TWO-HANDED—SEATS.	The right files turn to the left, the left files to the right.
TWO.	The right files bend the fingers of the right hand at the second joint, back of the hand uppermost. The left files bend the fingers of the left hand at the second joint, back of the hand downwards. The right and left files hook the hands together, each placing the disengaged hand upon the other's hip. (*See* Figs. 85 and 86.)
FILES, RIGHT AND LEFT—TURN.	The files resume the position of ATTENTION, and turn in the original direction.

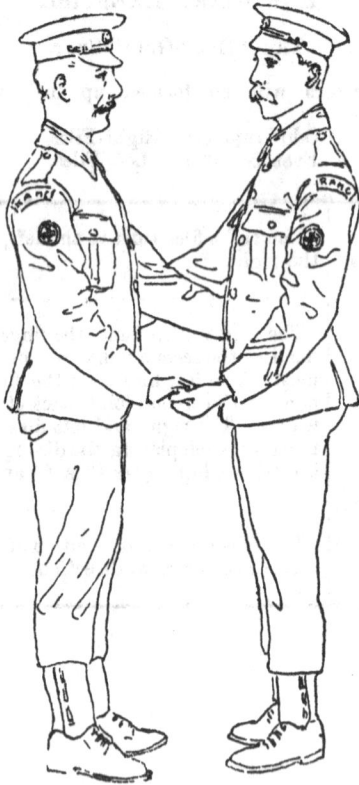

FIG. 85.—THE "HOOK-GRIP" SEAT.

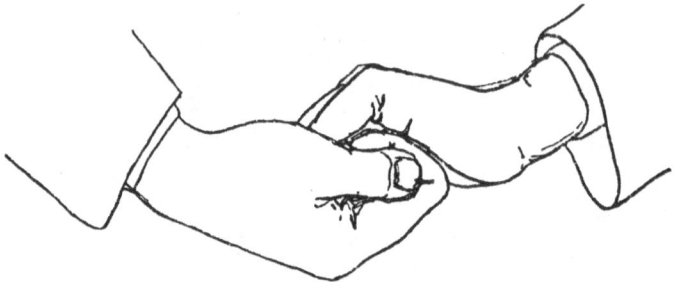

FIG. 86.—METHOD OF FORMING "HOOK-GRIP."

CHAPTER XXIII

EXERCISES WITH RAILWAY WAGONS.

406. No special instructions are necessary for loading and unloading wounded men who are able to walk and assume the sitting posture; recumbent patients alone are alluded to in the text. Various methods of adapting railway wagons for the carriage of wounded have been mentioned in paras. 352 to 356, Chapter XVIII. Zavodovski's plan for adapting wagons and the method of loading and unloading patients in wagons so arranged is herein described.

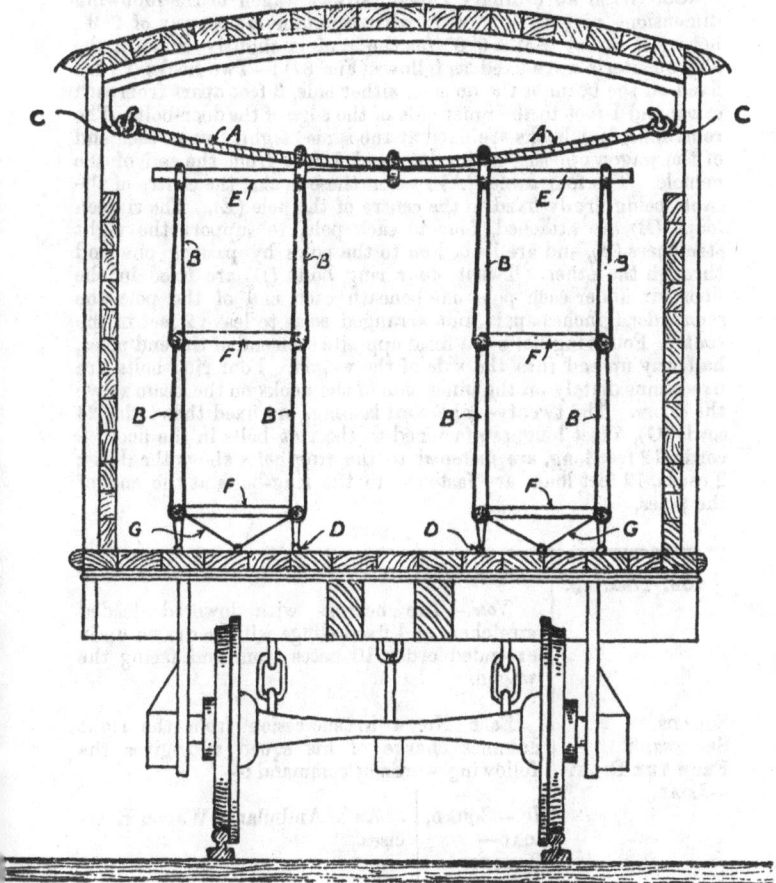

Fig. 87.—Transverse Section of a Railway Goods Wagon Fitted on Zavodovski's Method.

407. Zavodovski's Method.—To prepare a wagon according to Zavodovski's method the following stores are required :—(1) 4 cables 9′ long and over 1″ thick, ringed at each end, the inner portion of the ring strengthened by a metal collar-shaped band. (2) 16 stout looped ropes (the thickness of a drag rope) tied in the centre so as to support the upper tier of stretchers. (3) 8 large iron hooks. (4) 32 small ring-bolts. (5) 4 solid circular poles, 6′ long and 2″ thick. (6) 8 stretchers (army pattern). (7) 28 stout cords for lashings.

408. Given an ordinary closed railway wagon of the following dimensions, viz., 18′ × 7′ × 6′, with a minimum doorway of 4′ 9″, height of van at centre 6′ 6″ (as the roof is slightly curved), the above materials are fixed as follows (Fig. 87) :—Two hooks (C) are fixed on the beam of the door on either side, 3 feet apart from each other and 1 foot to the inner side of the edge of the door-bolts. The remaining four hooks are fixed at the same height, two at each end of the wagon opposite each other, and 1 foot from the end of the vehicle. The four cables (A) rest on these hooks, the centre of the cable being firmly fixed to the centre of the pole (E). The sixteen loops (B) are attached, four to each pole, to support the eight stretchers (F), and are looped on to the poles by passing one end through the other. Twenty-four ring bolts (D) are fixed in the floor, six under each pole, one beneath each end of the pole, the remainder 9 inches apart, but arranged so as to leave 2 feet in the centre. Four ring-bolts are fixed opposite each end of the end poles, half-way up and into the side of the wagon. Four ring-bolts are fixed immediately on the inner side of the hooks on the beam above the doors. The twenty-eight cord lashings are fixed thus : the 24 cords (G), 5 feet long, are fastened to the ring-bolts in the floor ; 2 cords, 12 feet long, are fastened to the ring-bolts above the door ; 2 cords, 12 feet long, are fastened to the ring-bolts at the end of the poles.

---

409. Loading.

Note.—The bearers with lowered loaded stretchers and fixed slings will be drawn up in extended order 10 paces from and facing the wagon.

SQUADS, IN SUCCESSION FROM THE RIGHT, —LOAD.

Each No. 4 in succession from the right assumes charge of his squad and gives the following words of command :—

| No.—SQUAD, LOAD—WAGONS. | As in Ambulance Wagon Exercises. |

ADVANCE.	The squads advance by the nearest way to the wagon, wheeling when opposite to, and one pace from, the doorway, and the stretcher is carried into the wagon head-first. The stretcher is carried to the far right-hand corner, where it is raised, and the handles of the poles are placed in the upper loops of the ropes.
FALL-IN.	The bearers fall in outside the wagon, as in file, facing the wagon, one pace from the doorway.
ABOUT TURN. REJOIN SQUADS, QUICK— MARCH. HALT. ABOUT— TURN. STAND AT— EASE.	As in Infantry Training.

410. Similar words of command are given by the Nos. 4 of the successive squads when they see the squad on their right falling in outside the wagon. No. 2 squad loads the upper, near, right-hand corner; No. 3 the lower, near, right-hand corner. The lashings are fixed by No. 4 squad as follows :—The lashing attached to the ring in the floor of the wagon immediately beneath the handles of the stretcher is carried up round the handle, back through the ring, and fastened off. The lashing attached to the ring lying between the handles is passed up round the left handle, back through the ring, round the right handle, and back to the ring, thus forming a V, where it is fastened. The upper tier is steadied by a lashing starting from a ring-bolt in the side of the wagon which is carried across and secured to the opposite side, a firm hitch being taken round each handle. The lashings must be drawn tight to prevent the swaying of the stretchers. The left half of the wagon is loaded in a similar manner.

411. Unloading. SQUADS, IN SUCCESSION FROM THE LEFT, —UNLOAD.	The Nos. 4 will take charge of their respective squads, and give the following words of command :—
No.—SQUAD, ATTEN—TION. FOR UN-LOADING, TAKE—POST	As in Ambulance Wagon Exercises, but halting one pace from the doorway.
UNLOAD—WAGONS.	The bearers on the right take a side-pace of 30 inches to the right, Nos. 2 and 3 then enter the wagon and proceed to the head of the stretcher, Nos. 1 and 4 to the foot, lift and remove it from the loops, and carry it clear of the wagon. As it is brought through the doorway, the remaining bearers take up their positions at the stretcher, and the whole, working together, retire and place the stretcher gently on the ground selected for this purpose. The bearers then rise and take up their positions as in " prepared stretchers."

CHAPTER XXIV.

CAMPS, BIVOUACS, AND BILLETS.

412. Camps.—Field and cavalry field ambulance camps are shown in Figs. 88 and 89. These plans are drawn up for guidance, but need not always be rigidly adhered to. The unallotted spaces are to permit of expansion. It may be left to the discretion of the O.C. the unit as to whether he will have bivouacs for the bearer and tent personnel in front or in rear of the tents for the sick, or he may elect to place the horse-lines in rear of the transport ; the transport personnel, however, should always be in proximity to the horse-lines. The point to be aimed at, taking into consideration the nature of the ground, is to arrange a compact camp, so that the space allotted for the accommodation of the sick is not too cramped, and that the whole can be effectively guarded in the case of attack. In pitching such a camp the instructions laid down in Field Service Regulations, Part I, will be followed.

413. The site having been chosen, and the line decided upon, the camp will be marked out as follows :—Mark the base-point with a tent-peg or flag ; measure off the distance required for the front of the camp, viz. (if sections are pitched together), for a field ambulance 120 yards, for a cavalry field ambulance 80 yards ; mark this with a second tent-peg or flag.

The front of the camp being thus laid down, the rear of the ground will now be determined. Place a tent-peg or flag on the front alignment 6 feet from the base-point, another tent-peg or flag 8 feet from the base-point towards the rear, and 10 feet diagonally from the other tent-peg or flag ; the angle thus formed will be a right angle. Place a third tent-peg or flag in the same straight line as the 8-feet side of the triangle, and distant from the base point 200 yards for a field ambulance and 180 yards for a cavalry field ambulance. The rear line of the camp will be equal in length and parallel to the base-line, and will be marked with a fourth flag.

If it is considered that a mobilized force on taking the field requires blankets for personnel, or additional tents for the accommodation of sick, or both, twelve extra tents per section for a field ambulance and seven extra tents per section for a cavalry field ambulance are carried, for the transport of which an extra forage cart per section is allowed.

For sanitation, watering arrangements, picketing of animals, and parking of vehicles, the instructions contained in Field Service Regulations, Part I, and Field Service Pocket Book, will be followed.

Methods of field sanitation are described in Part II of this manual.

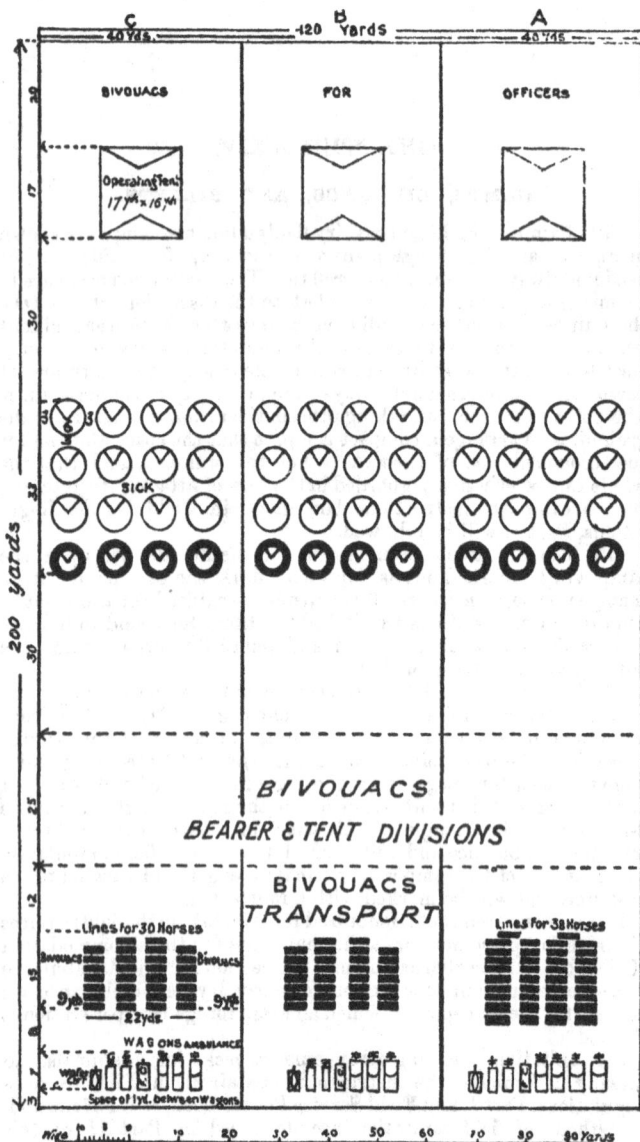

Kitchens & Conservancy arrangements according to circumstances and requirements.

This diagram is drawn up as a guide only (see Para. 412).

Fig. 88.—Field Ambulance Camp, Showing Full Tentage
for Sick.

Note.—When a blanket for each man is specially ordered to be carried,
an extra forage-cart per section will be required, in addition to those shown
in the foregoing diagram. Also 3 extra drivers and 6 extra draught-horses
for these vehicles.

This extra transport is sufficient for the carriage of tents in addition, if
these are ordered to be taken. Additional number of tents are shown above
in thin outline.

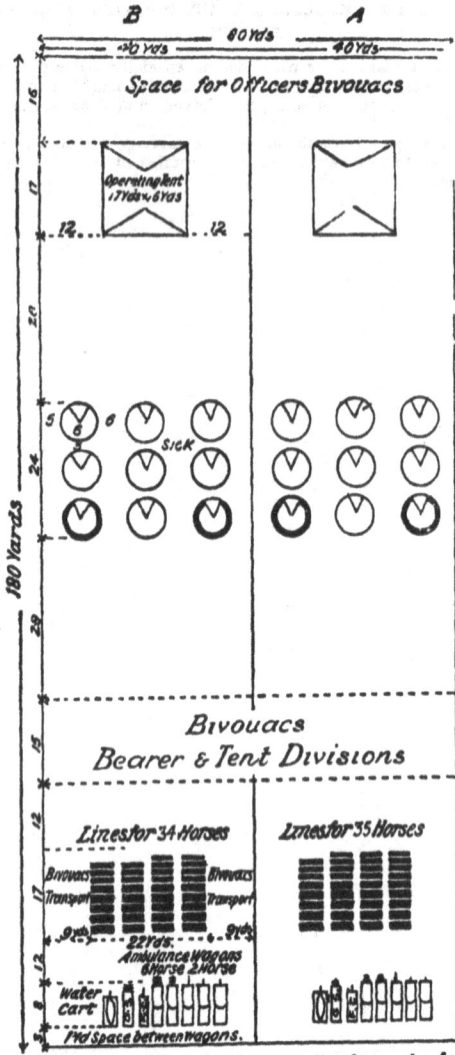

Kitchens & Conservancy arrangements according to Circumstances & requirements This diagram is drawn up as a guide only

Fig. 89.—Cavalry Field Ambulance Camp, Showing Full
Tentage For Sick.

Note.—When a blanket for each man is specially ordered to be carried,
an extra forage-cart per section will be required, in addition to those shown
in the foregoing diagram. Also 2 extra drivers and 4 extra draught horses
for these vehicles.

This extra transport is sufficient for the carriage of tents in addition, if
these are ordered to be taken. Additional tents are shown above in thin
outline.

414. Bivouacs.—As the personnel of field medical units will
normally not be provided with tents, and billets may not be available,
it is essential that officers and men should know how to construct
simple shelters for themselves and the wounded who may be in their
charge. Information regarding the construction of bivouacs and
shelters will be found in the Manual of Field Engineering.

415. Billets.—The use of buildings as billets for personnel and
for hospital purposes is the normal method of accommodation on
field service in countries where suitable conditions exist. The
general rules regarding billets are contained in Field Service Regulations, Part I, and instructions regarding the utilization of buildings
for the accommodation of sick and wounded are given in para. 210,
Chap. XV, and para. 256, Chap. XVI, of this manual.

CHAPTER XXV.

TENT-PITCHING EXERCISES.*

Bell Tent.

416. Description.—In field medical units the single-circular or bell tent is used for the accommodation of the sick. This tent weighs 83 lb. It is fitted with 3 ventilators, 20 tying-up lines, and from 22 to 24 ropes or bracing lines according to the particular pattern of tent, *e.g.*, Mark II, 22 bracing lines, Mark III, 23 bracing lines, Mark IV and Mark V, 24 bracing lines. A valise and a pin-bag containing 47 pins and 2 mallets with handles are supplied with each tent.

417. Pitching a Bell Tent by Two Men.—No. 1 is told off as pole-man; No. 2 as tent-man. No. 1 falls in with the pole in his left hand, and mallet and five pegs in his right; No. 2 covers him, carrying tent and pin-bag. When No. 1 is moved to the position his tent is to occupy, No. 2 will follow with the tent, and fall in five paces in rear of him. No. 1 having put the pole together takes up his dressing.

No. 2 drives a peg upright between the feet of No. 1 at the foot and in front of the pole ; he then shakes the tent out of its valise, and spreads it on the ground with the door uppermost. No. 1, when the peg is driven, lays the pole on the ground. He then takes three and a half paces from the centre peg to his front, *i.e.*, the way the door is to face, and drives in the front peg. He then turns about, goes to the centre peg, takes three and a half paces to the rear from it, drives in another (the rear peg), returning to the centre, and following a like course to the right and left.

Both men now proceed to the tent; one to the right, the other to the left of the door. Each takes the second rope on either side, commencing to count from the lower corner rope of the door-flaps, and draws the tent on to the ground it is to occupy. Both these ropes are then attached to the front peg. The men then count the ropes until they come to the seventh (sixth in Mark II pattern), and attach them to the right and left pegs. No. 2 counts five more ropes on either side and fastens them (one rope only in Mark III pattern) to the rear peg at full length. No. 1, in the meantime, takes up the pole and fits the smaller end of it into the cap of the tent (in the case of a double-circular tent passing it through the hole in the inner lining), keeping the bottom of the pole to the front. No. 2 assists in fitting the pole into the top of the tent. No. 1 gets inside the tent, and No. 2 then hooks the fly of the tent over the pole and under the ropes. No. 1 then raises the pole about 3 feet from the ground, keeping the bottom of it on the ground.

---

* Various useful knots are illustrated in the Field Service Pocket Book.

On the command being given to raise the tent, No. 1 works the bottom of the pole inwards until it comes against and immediately behind the centre peg, lifting the upper end of the pole at the same time. No. 2, when the tent is raised, tightens the ropes already fixed to the four pegs. No. 1 continues to support the pole upright until this is done.

When the tent is secure, No. 1 comes out and assists No. 2 in driving pegs and fastening ropes in the following manner :—The two second ropes, which were first fixed to the front peg, are now separated. The runner of each rope is slid half-way up. The loop thus formed is drawn out in a line with the seam of the tent. It is then brought down to the ground, and at the spot where it touches the ground a peg is driven. This is continued until all the ropes have been made fast.

The curtain of the tent should now be pegged down. The door of the tent should be opened, the ropes attached to its lower corners being fastened to the second peg on the right and left of the doorway.

The mallets, spare pegs, and pin-bag are put into the valise which is placed inside the right-hand side of the door of the tent.

When the tent is correctly pitched the pegs should form a perfect circle.

418. Trenching a Bell Tent.—If it is necessary to trench a tent, it is done in the following manner :—Before the curtain of the tent is pegged down, a cut is made with a spade all round where the edge of the curtain touches the ground. This cut is made about 6 inches deep with the spade held upright. A second cut is made leading into it, about 6 inches from it all round. The turf so cut out is laid with the grass downwards round the outer edge of the trench. The curtain is then pegged down into the inner side of the trench.

419. Precautions in wet weather.—When rain comes on, the ropes, as they become wet, get tight and, if not attended to, will pull the pegs out of the ground or break the poles. They will also get tight with a heavy dew. Thus it will be necessary to slacken them when rain is expected, and also at night if the dew is heavy. Again, if the ropes have become wet, they will slacken as they dry, and will require to be braced up, otherwise the tent may flap and draw the pegs.

Note.—The foregoing instruction applies to all canvas tents.

420. Striking a Bell Tent.—To strike a tent, both men will take off and coil down all the ropes except those attached to the two front, right, left, and rear pegs. The fly is unhooked ; No. 1 goes inside and takes hold of the pole ; No. 2, in the meantime, draws out all the pegs to which the ropes are not fixed.

Note.—The pegs holding the curtain will have been drawn out already.

On the command to strike being given, No. 1 runs out of the door of the tent with the pole. The five remaining ropes are now cast off and coiled down. No. 2 now takes hold of the point of the tent and draws it to the rear, door upwards. Keeping the door upwards, in the centre the tent is spread out flat on its side.

No. 1 places his foot on the point of the tent; No. 2, taking the edges, folds them over so that they meet at the door. This is again done, and then the right half of the tent is folded over the left. No. 1 now takes the point and brings it half-way down the tent. Nos. 1 and 2 then roll the tent as tightly as possible, from the smaller to the larger end, and put it into its valise.

Mallets are taken apart, and their heads put into the peg-bag with the pegs. Their handles are put into the tent-valise. The pin-bag is then put into the valise on top of the tent, and the valise laced up. No. 1 takes the pole to pieces and holds it in his left hand. No. 2 falls in in rear of him with the valise.

HOSPITAL MARQUEE.

421. Description.—A hospital marquee, inside dimensions 29 feet long and 14 feet wide, weighing 512 lb. complete, consists of :—One inside linen roof, 1 outside ditto, 8 walls (4 inside and 4 outside), 82 bracing-lines (40 inside and 42 outside), with wooden runner and button to each, 2 wooden vases painted red, and 2 weather lines (90 feet each) with large runners, all packed in a canvas valise, laced up in the centre, and marked on the outside "Hospital Marquee"; 180 small tent pegs, 4 large ditto (for weather-lines), and 2 mallets, all contained in one peg-bag, marked on the outside with contents and marquee to which it belongs; 1 set of poles, consisting of 8 pieces, viz., 1 ridge in two pieces, and 3 standards or uprights in two pieces, and lashed together in one bundle by two box-cords; 1 waterproof bottom, made of painted canvas, in four pieces, each piece measuring 15 feet by 8 feet, rolled in a bundle round a thin pole, and tied by three box-cords.

422. Pitching a Marquee.—Undo and empty the peg-bag (keeping the four large pegs for the weather-lines by themselves), fit the handles in the mallets, and fix the two pieces of the ridge-pole together. This done, proceed to lay out the ground for pitching the marquee as follows :—Lay the ridge-pole on the ground selected, and drive in a peg at its centre and at each of its two end holes. These pegs will mark the positions of the standard or upright poles, and will be 7 feet apart. With each end peg as a centre, in a semi-circle with a radius of 6 yards, lay thirteen pegs with their points inwards where they are to be driven. This will be easiest done as follows: Step 6 yards from one of the end pegs, and, in a straight line with the three standard pegs, lay the centre peg of the semi-circle; next step 6 yards to each side of the end peg, and, on a line at right angles to the three standard pegs, lay a peg for each end of the semi-circle; then lay at each side, between the centre peg of the semi-circle and its two end pegs, equal distances apart, five pegs, and the semi-circle of thirteen pegs is complete. The other end will be done in the same way.

For the sides of the marquee, on a straight line parallel to the three standard pegs, and 5 yards distant, lay six pegs, the first and the last of which will be 18 inches distant from the lines formed

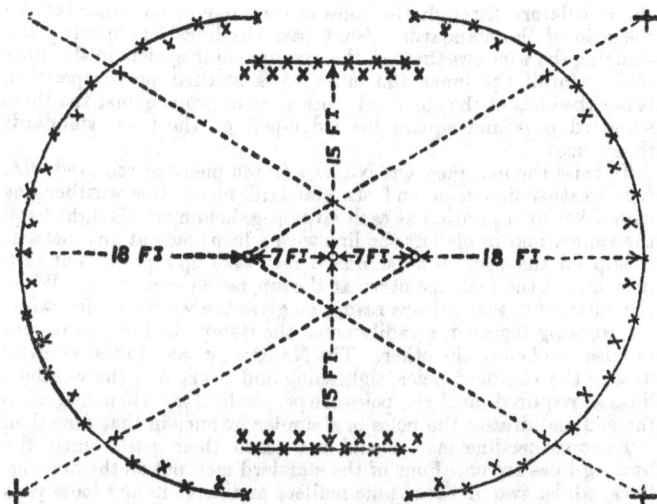

FIG. 90.—GROUND PLAN OF THE PEGS OF THE MARQUEE.
(Showing direction of weather-lines.)

by each end standard peg and the two end pegs of each semi-circle. Now the pegs for the outer roof are all laid, and should be driven in before proceeding further.

For the inner roof, lay a peg between each two pegs of the outer roof, but on a line 1 foot further in. The space, however, between the third and fourth pegs on each of the straight lines of pegs is to be left blank for the doorway. These driven, the pegs are complete for the marquee, except the four weather-line pegs. These are each driven at a corner where lines, drawn from each end and centre peg of the semi-circle, would meet to form a right angle.

The ground being laid out, carry the marquee within the line of pegs, unlace the valise, and arrange and spread out the marquee, the roofs one inside the other, in such a manner that the base and ridge will be parallel with the line of the standard pegs and the base will be touching them. Roll up the upper side of the outer roof as far as the ridge, so as to expose the web slings of the inner roof, insert the ridge-pole, and roll up the upper side of the inner roof in a similar manner.

Fix the two pieces of each standard pole together according to their numbers. This done, pass the standards through the openings in the inner roof; then pass their pins through the holes in the ridge-pole, through the eyelets in the two end web slings, and also through the eyelet holes in the ridge of the outer roof. Now fit the vases on the pins of the end standards, and pass the opening lines of the ventilators through the holes in the ridge of the inner roof by the side of the standards. Next pass the lines for opening and shutting the windows through the corresponding eyelets in the inner roof. Unroll the inner and outer roofs to their proper position, bring the ends of the standard poles so as to prop against the three standard pegs, and square the ridge-pole on the three standards thus placed.

To raise the marquee, one N.C.O. and ten men are required, viz., four weather-line men and six standard men. One weather-line man takes up a position at each large peg, holding in his right hand the runner and in his left the line with a loop ready at any moment to slip on the peg. Two standard men take up a position at each pole, one at the foot, the other at the top, facing each other. When the instructor sees all are ready, he gives the word to raise, when all, working together, steadily erect the standards, taking care not to raise one before the other. The N.C.O. now goes to the side and dresses the standard poles, tightening and slackening the weather-lines as required until the poles are perpendicular. He next goes to the end and dresses the poles in a similar manner in that direction.

The weather-line men should not leave their posts until the bracing-lines are on. Four of the standard men put on the bracing-lines, whilst two of them take mallets and drive in any loose pegs there may be. To put on the bracing-lines, two men go to each side of the marquee, commencing with the outer roof ; one takes the line at one side of the window, and the other the line at the other side, which should be put respectively on the third and fourth pegs of the outer straight line, thus working towards the ends until meeting the men from the other side. In tightening the bracing-lines the marquee should be pulled towards the pegs so as to slacken the line, otherwise the pegs will be pulled out of the ground. The lines of the inner roof should be put on in a similar manner, beginning at each side of the window, and working round to the ends. When two lines are together, they should for the present go on the same pegs, but afterwards be shifted.

The curtains are in eight pieces, four for the inner wall and four for the outer wall. The outer curtain should be so put on that the ground-flap is inside, and that it can be pegged on the outside. The inner curtain should be put on with the flap out, so that it can be pegged on the inside. Commence with the outer curtain at each side of the doorway and work round towards the ends, taking care to leave enough to overlap and close the doorway. When the curtains are on, they should be pegged down inside and outside.

The doorway of the marquee should be on the sheltered side. The curtains should be taken off the pegs and raised daily for ventilation. They can be fastened to the bracing-lines by the buttons of the peg loops.

423. Trenching a Marquee.—A trench, 9 inches broad and 4 to 6 inches deep, should be dug round the curtain, especially on the upper side if the ground be sloping. The trench should be cut well under the curtain, so as not to leave a ledge, otherwise the water will drip on the ledge and run under.

424. Striking a Marquee.—Unfasten the curtains at the bottom, and unhook them from the roof, beginning with the inner one. Fold each piece into eight parts. The four weather-line men now stand by the weather-lines while four men unfasten and do up into a skein the bracing-lines, beginning with the inner roof at each side of the doorways and working round to the ends. The two mallet men take up the pegs as the lines are taken off them, and put them away in the peg-bag.

To lower the marquee, the men take up positions as in pitching, one to each weather-line and two to each pole. When all are ready, the N.C.O. gives the word to lower. The weather-line men take the lines off the pegs but keeping a firm hold, the standard men having hold of the poles. All together they steadily lower the poles against the wind, the men at the feet of the poles keeping them from slipping, and the other men lowering them by walking backwards towards the ridge, in the same way as men lowering a ladder.

To repack the marquee, roll up the four weather-lines and take the vases off the pins, leaving them attached by the ventilating-cords. Spread out the roofs and roll up the upper flap, so as to expose the ridge-pole. Next pull away the standard poles, and remove the ridge-pole from the slings.

This done, unroll the upper fold of the roof. Bring over each end to the centre, across the middle of the window, and fold the square thus made from side to side into three equal parts. Place the eight pieces of curtain on the roofs lengthwise, overlapping in the centre, the flaps towards the thick end. Roll up the whole thus placed, evenly, commencing with the thick end, taking care not to have the roll too wide or too narrow for the valise.

Spread out the valise, and pushing one of the side-flaps under the marquee, roll it in. Having arranged the flaps, lace them, commencing with the ends.

OPERATING TENT.

425. Description.—The tent is rectangular in shape, and has a doorway at each end. It is fitted with six ventilators of the ordinary type, and also with a large ventilator on each side, to give extra light and air. The wall is permanently attached to the tent. The poles used with it consist of two upright poles and one ridge-pole, each made in two pieces.

It is 20 feet in length, 14 feet in width, and 9 feet 4 inches in height, the wall being 3 feet high. The tent itself weighs 116 lb., or, with poles and appurtenances complete, 181 lb.

The duck used in making this tent is of the same quality as for Mark V circular tents (S. 7359). For the main part of the tent the duck is 27 inches in width, and $10\frac{1}{4}$ oz. per yard in weight. For the wall, 36-inch duck is used, of about $13\frac{3}{4}$ oz. per yard in weight.

The valise and the pin-bag are the same as used for the laboratory tent. The pins and mallets are of the ordinary Service pattern. The complement is 2 mallets, 1 pin-bag, 60 small pins, and 8 large pins; this allows 2 spare small pins.

Note.—On account of the rods in the large ventilators, this tent must be folded and rolled up lengthwise, and the weather-lines must not cross the ventilators when the tent is pitched.

426. Pitching an Operating Tent.—One N.C.O. and six men are required, two as pole-men, four as tent-men. The pole-men take the ridge-pole and uprights; the tent-men the pegs and mallets (a maul is required to drive large pegs).

The tent-men unpack the tent and spread it flat on the ground, the lower edge about two paces from the ridge-pole, and top to windward.

The pole-men put the ridge-pole together, and lay it on the ground on the site of the tent, and a peg is driven in at each end of it. The pole-men stand back to back with these pegs between their feet.

Two tent-men take post at the pegs, their backs to the faces of the two pole-men; take five paces to their front, dress themselves on the pole-men, and turn to windward. Two other tent-men join them, and stand back to back with them; the four now take six paces to their front and halt.

The pole-men take a maul and four large pegs, and drive them at points marked by the feet of the tent-men.

The four tent-men return to the pegs marking the ends of the ridge-pole, and, after taking two paces in continuation of the line marked by it, turn back-to-back at right angles to the line, take six paces to the front, and halt. Four large pegs for weather-lines are driven at their feet by the pole-men; the pole-men return to the poles and lay the frame with the feet of the uprights against the pegs first driven, ridge to windward.

The tent-men roll up the upper side of the tent until the top is exposed, and, the pole-men raising the poles, the underside of the tent is drawn beneath them, and the poles adjusted, taking care that each ventilating-cord is on its own side of the ridge-pole. The vases with weather-lines are now fitted on, the lines uncoiled, and the four tent-men, each taking one, move towards the weather-line pegs. The pole-men working with them, the tent is raised and the lines fastened to the pegs. The lines must not be crossed. The four tent-men each take an upper corner rope (distinguished by its being fastened to a ring through which another line passes), and adjust it to the large pegs first driven in. The doors are now laced and hooked.

The tent-men take the four lower corner ropes, and fasten them to the small pegs driven in a line with but two paces nearer the tent than, the upper corner pegs. The pole-men adjust the windows, the tent-men drive pegs and adjust the front and side lines of the roof, drawing them square with the tent, and fasten down the curtain.

Note.—In fixing the upper corner bracing line, it may be necessary to apply a bowline or sheepshank to shorten it.

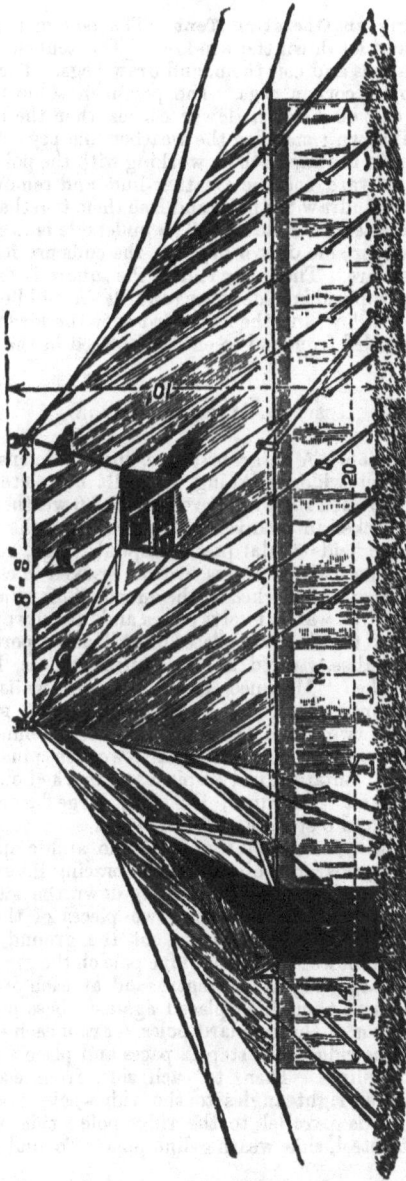

FIG. 91.—OPERATING TENT (MARK I).

427. Striking an Operating Tent.—The pole-men pull up the curtain-pegs and let down the windows. The tent-men cast off all ends and side-lines and coil them, and draw pegs. They then take post at the lower corner pegs. The pole-men stand to the poles : the tent-men cast off first the lower corner, then the upper corner ropes, and coil down ; stand to the weather-line pegs, cast them off and hold them in the hand ; then, working with the pole-men, lower the tent to windward, coil the weather-lines and remove the vases. The pole-men withdraw the poles and lash them together. The tent-men fold up the tent as follows :—The underside is first spread out flat, and the upper side drawn over it ; the ends are folded over so as to form a square. The lower end of the square is folded over to the middle ; the top end is folded over towards the middle as far as the ventilator-irons allow, and then refolded over the lower half. The whole is then rolled from end to end and placed in the valise.

Hospital Marquee (Large).

428. Description.—A large marquee, inside dimensions 35 feet long and 17 feet wide, weighing 1,149 lb. complete ; consisting of :—One outside linen roof, with two vases and 6 weather-lines (each 45 feet long), packed in a canvas valise, laced up the centre, and marked on the outside " Marquee, Hospital, large, roof, outer " ; 1 inside cotton roof, 4 porchways, cotton, packed in canvas valise, laced up the centre, and marked on the outside " Marquee, Hospital, large, roof, inner" ; 1 wall in twelve pieces, and 8 porchway-poles, viz., 2 side, 2 end, and two doorway-pieces of wall, and 4 porchway-poles packed in each valise, packed in two canvas valises, laced up the centre, and marked " Marquee, Hospital, large, walls " ; 1 set of poles consisting of 8 pieces, viz., 1 ridge-pole and 3 standards or uprights, each in two pieces, lashed together in two bundles by four cords ; 94 large wooden pins, 116 small wooden pins, 3 mallets, 3 vases for poles, contained in two pin-bags, marked on the outside with contents and " Marquee, Hospital, large " ; and a sledge-hammer, 14 lb., and 6 steel pins, 3 feet, loose.

429. Pitching a Large Marquee.—Undo and empty the two pin-bags (keeping separate the large pins for bracing-lines of inner and outer roofs and the small pins for pegging down the walls) ; fit the handles in the mallets and fix the two pieces of the ridge-pole together. This done, proceed to lay out the ground for pitching the marquee as follows :—Lay the ridge pole on the ground selected and drive in a large peg at its centre and at each of its two end holes ; the " bases " should be placed against these pegs, and will mark the positions of the standard poles. From each end peg, and in a line with the ridge-pole, step 12 paces and place a steel pin for the end weather-lines. Then, to each side, from each end peg, and on a line at right angles to the ridge-pole, take 11 paces and a pace inwards parallel to the ridge-pole ; this will give the positions of the steel, side weather-line pins. To find the position

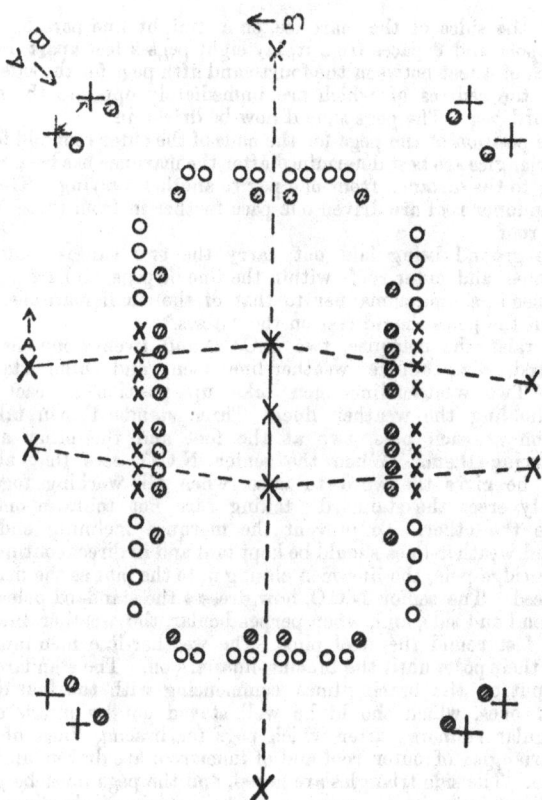

FIG. 92.—GROUND PLAN OF PEGS OF MARQUEE (LARGE).
(Showing direction of weather lines.)

  ✕ Pegs driven in before marquee is raised.
  ○ Pegs driven in after marquee is raised.
  ● Pegs for inner roof
  A and B showing manner in which positions of pegs for corner bracing-lines are found.
  Pitching space, 80 feet by 55 feet.

of pegs for the double corner bracing-lines, one man, "A," places himself one pace from the side of the side weather-line pin and parallel to the ridge-pole, and another man, "B," at the side of the end weather-line pin and at right angles to the ridge-pole; they will then march straight to their front, halting where they meet; they then face the end standard peg, take three paces towards it, halt, turn outwards, take a pace forward, and lay down a peg.

For the sides of the marquee, on a straight line parallel to the ridge-pole and 6 paces from it, lay eight pegs 2 feet apart, leaving a space of 4 feet between the fourth and fifth pegs for the side door-ways, the centres of which are immediately opposite the centre standard peg. The pegs should now be driven in.

The position of the pegs for the ends of the outer roof and for the side triangles are best determined after the marquee has been raised, owing to the distance from one peg to another varying. The pegs for the inner roof are driven one pace further in from those for the outer roof.

The ground being laid out, carry the two valises containing the inner and outer roofs within the line of pegs, and arrange the marquee in a similar manner to that of the small marquee. The ends of the poles should rest on the "bases."

To raise the marquee, two N.C.Os. and twenty-one men are required, viz., twelve weather-line men, and nine standard men. Two weather-line men take up position at each steel pin, holding the weather lines. Three standard men take up position at each pole, two at the foot and the other at the top facing them. When the senior N.C.O. sees that all are ready he gives the word to raise, when all, working together, steadily erect the standards, taking care not to raise one end before the other. To prevent the marquee inclining endways, the end weather-lines should be kept taut and in direct continuation of the ridge-pole, the linesmen closing in to the pins as the marquee is raised. The senior N.C.O. now dresses the standard poles from both end and side, and, when perpendicular, the weather lines are made fast round the steel pins. The weather-line men must not leave their posts until the bracing-lines are on. The standard men now put on the bracing-lines, commencing with the four double corner ones, which should be well stayed out by means of the triangular runners ; after which pegs for bracing lines, of ends, and triangles of outer roof and of inner roof are driven, and lines put on. The side triangles are gored, and the pegs must be placed in a direct line with the seams, so that the strain will be direct from the top of the end poles. The porchway-poles should now be fixed.

The wall is in twelve pieces, fitted with brass eyelets, through which the loops of the inner roof are reeved. Four of the pieces of wall are marked "side" ; four, "end" ; and four, "doorway" ; and the four flaps that form the roof of the four porchways are marked "centre" on the inside lining. It is most important to note that the centre of each of the four doorway-pieces of wall where marked "centre of porchway," must be exactly under that point of the roof-flap of each of the four porchways where marked "centre" before commencing to lace on the side-wall, which is done in continuation of the doorway-piece. The end-wall is laced to the side-wall. The loops on the walls are so placed as to permit of the walls being interchangeable. The wall when laced on should be securely pegged down. The marquee can be ventilated as required by disconnecting and unlacing the wall.

430. Striking a Large Marquee.—Unlace the wall from the inner roof, freeing the loop-lines from the pegs ; detach the wall ;

unfasten and roll up the bracing-lines, commencing with the inner roof. The pegs should be taken up as the lines are removed from them and put away in the peg-bags.

To lower the marquee, the men take up positions as in pitching, two to each weather-line and three to each pole. The marquee should then be lowered in the same manner as the small marquee. The end weather-lines must be kept taut in lowering.

To repack the marquee, roll up the six weather-lines, and take the vases off the pole-spikes. Spread out the roofs and roll back the upper portion of the outer roof so as to expose the ridge-pole; next pull away the standard poles and remove the ridge-pole from the slings.

The roofs are folded thus: For the inner roof, the ends are folded over to the centre, and three folds are then made from side to side; the porchways should be folded up with the inner roof, and should not be unlaced from it when the tent is struck. The inner roof is then rolled up.

For the outer roof, the under side is spread out flat and the upper side drawn over it; next fold the roof in two equal parts by bringing over one end and laying it on top of the other; see that the ventilating-irons are together. Turn back the ends in a line with and as far as the ventilating irons; now make two folds about the width of the valise from the opposite direction and then fold over the remaining portions of the ends; the corner containing the irons is turned back, thus bringing them on top and in a proper position for rolling. Roll up the outer roof from the thick end.

To put a roof into its valise spread out the valise, and pushing one of the side-flaps under the roof, roll it in. Having arranged the flaps, lace them, commencing with the ends.

The wall is rolled up the width of the bamboos inserted in the wall; two side, two end, two doorway-pieces of wall, and four bamboo porch-poles being packed in each valise. Two of the poles in each valise are turned the reverse way, *i.e.*, the bottoms are placed alongside the spikes: this prevents the spikes from piercing the canvas valise.

CHAPTER XXVI.

FIELD COOKING.

431. To cook rapidly and well is an art not difficult to acquire, and one which soldiers should be encouraged to learn. The means generally used for cooking in the field are camp-kettles and the mess-tin, the lid of which can be used as a frying-pan. Troops should, in all circumstances, have their dinners ready an hour and a half after the rations are issued.

Messes should be by kettles, that is, the number of men composing a mess should depend on the kettle used. Full instructions with regard to this, as well with regard to cooking in mess-tins, preserved meat tins, etc., and the improvisation of field ovens, are given in the Manual of Military Cooking, together with useful recipes for cooking in the field.

432. Camp Kettles.—Camp-kettles are as follows :—

Name.	Weight.	Contents.	Surface diameter.	Depth, outside measure.	Number of men will cook for.	
					With vegetables.	Without.
	lb.	gals.	inches.	inches.		
Oval, large	8	3	18½ × 9	11	8	15
,, small... ...	4¾	1¼	12½ × 8½	8	5	8

433. Field Kitchens.—On a unit's arrival in camp the cooks will at once proceed to make the kitchen. This can either be a trench-kitchen or one without a trench.

The Trench-kitchen.—If the encampment is only for one night, one or two trenches, according to the number to cook for, should be dug 7 feet 6 inches long, 9 inches wide, and 18 inches deep at the mouth, and continued for 18 inches into the trench, then sloping upwards to 4 inches at the back, with a splay mouth pointing towards the wind, and a rough chimney 2 feet high at the opposite end formed with the sods cut off from the top of the trench. If the upper 6 inches of the edge of the mouth are bevelled off, air is more freely admitted to the trench. It will be advantageous if these trenches are cut on a gentle slope. This trench will hold seven of the large oval kettles.

Iron cooking-bars are placed across the trench to support the kettles. The kettles are placed side-by-side with their bottoms resting on the ridges of the trench. The spaces between them are packed with wet earth or clay, which should reach as high as the

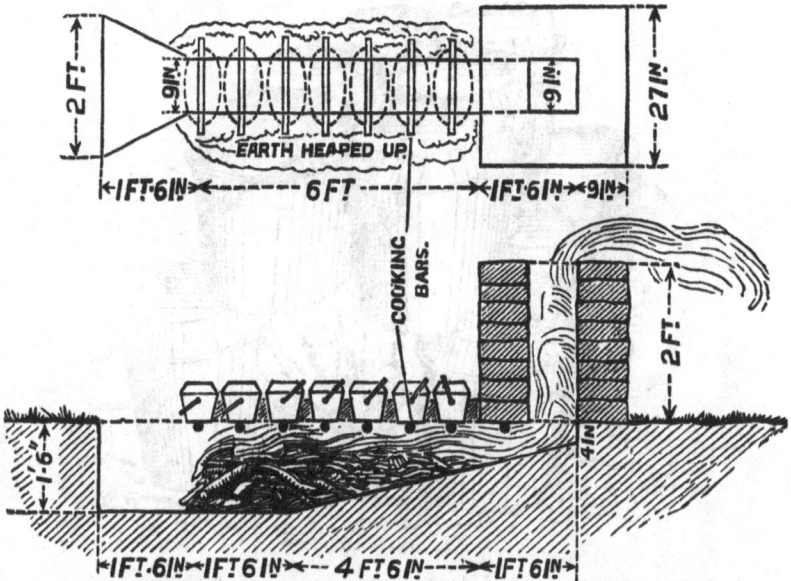

Fig. 93.—Plan and Sectional Elevation of Trench-kitchen with Camp-kettles, to show Dimensions and Detail.

loops of the handles. The fuel, generally wood, is fed into the trench from the splay mouth. (See Fig. 93.)

Without a Trench.—The simplest and best arrangements for cooking in the field for any party over twenty, if the stay in camp is for a night only, is to place a proportion of the kettles on the ground in two parallel rows about nine inches apart, handles outwards; block the leeward end of the channel so formed with another kettle, lay the fire, and place over it one or two rows of kettles resting on those already placed in position. (See Figs. 94 and 95.)

Mess-tins can be arranged similarly, but of these not more than eight should be used together.

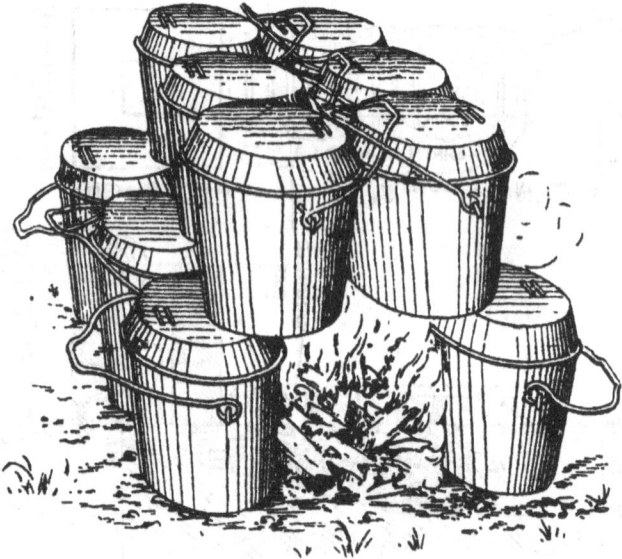

FIG. 94.—KITCHEN, WITHOUT A TRENCH, WITH CAMP-KETTLES.

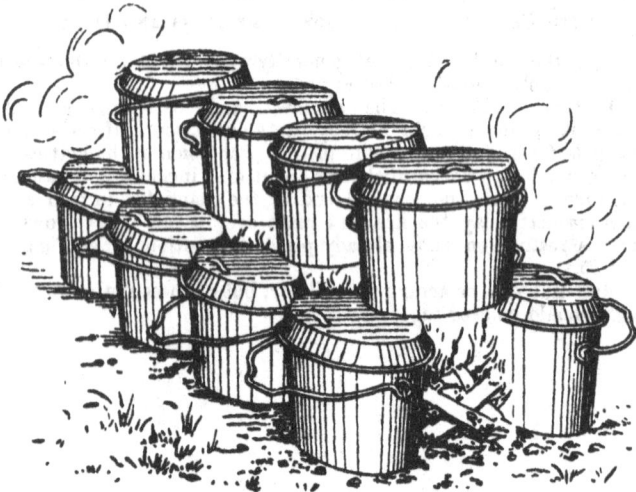

FIG. 95.—FIELD KITCHEN WITHOUT A TRENCH.

434. Improvised Field Oven.—Given an empty kerosene oil tin and a few bricks or stones, a very simple form of improvised oven for a small party can be made on the lines indicated below. The following materials are required to construct the oven :—An empty kerosene oil tin with the top removed, two pieces of iron (hoop-iron if obtainable) for the tin to rest upon, and some bricks or stones ; using mud or clay to cement the stones together. Build the base to form a cross as shown in Fig. 96 ; on this place the bars and the tin lying on its side, and proceed to build up the stones and mud round the tin, at the same time forming the side and back flues as shown in Figs. 97 and 98. The top is built, as in the Fig. 96, to form a cross-flue, the chimney being formed by means of an empty coffee tin or a piece of rolled tin. The opening to the oven can be closed with the top cut from the kerosene oil tin, and made tight with clay, or a stone may be used for the same purpose. The whole of the exterior should be covered with watery clay, or mud, as often as is necessary. The fire should be lighted under the tin, wood being used as fuel.

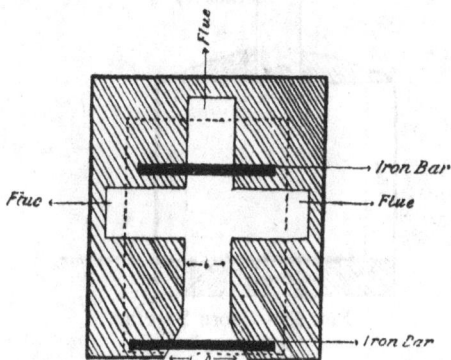

FIG. 96.—PLAN.

Dotted lines indicate tin in position.

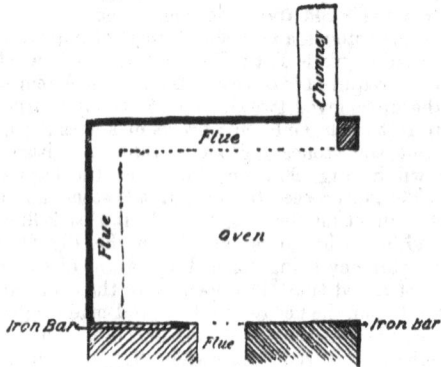

FIG. 97.—LONG SECTION.
(Shaded parts indicate brick or stone.)

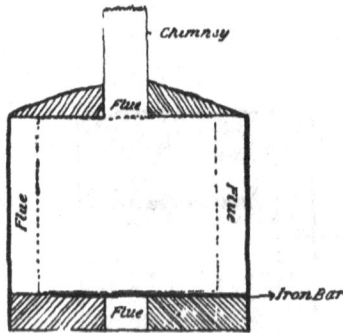

FIG. 98.—CROSS SECTION.

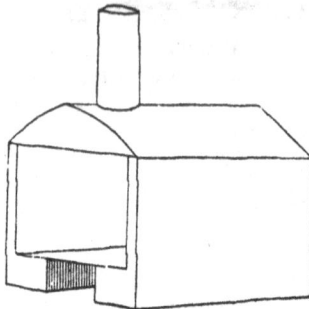

FIG. 99.—ELEVATION.
FIGS. 96–99.—IMPROVISED FIELD OVEN.

435. The Portable Stove.—This stove (Fig. 100) is for use in medical units in the field. It consists of two ovens, two boilers with lids, four baking-dishes, one grate, and two shelves. The ovens (one of which is smaller than the other) are made of steel-plate. The grate is made of wrought-iron, and the boilers and baking-dishes of tin-plate. Each apparatus is considered capable of cooking for 50 patients.

To put the stove together for use, place the ovens back-to-back, leaving space between them to receive the grate, which is provided with four hooks to engage in slots in angle pieces fixed to the bottoms of the ovens. Before the grate is set in its place, connect the ovens together by means of the plates pivoting on the sides of the smaller oven and furnished with hooks to fit into slots cut in the top of the larger oven. These plates, when in position, close in the fire-place. The doors of the oven have their hinges at the top, and open upwards. Each oven has a movable shelf of plate-iron to rest on a ledge and intended to receive one baking-dish, the second being placed on the bottom of the oven. The boilers rest on top of the ovens over the fire.

PACKED.

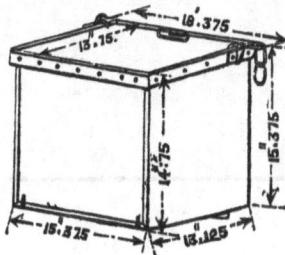

READY FOR USE.

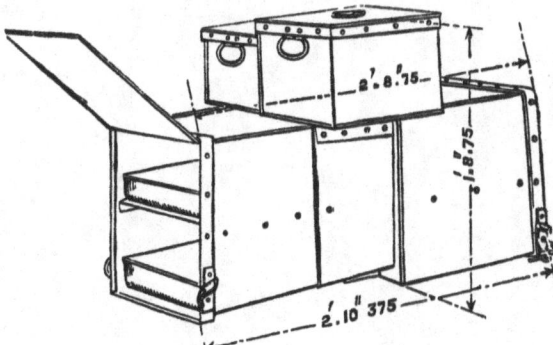

FIG. 100.—PORTABLE STOVE.

To pack the stove for transport, place the small oven inside the large one, with the large shelf on its top, and the small shelf at one side of it. Put the small boiler into the large one, and place the latter with the baking-dishes inside the small oven. Place the grate in last, resting on the boiler. In packing the grate, place the bottom bars, not the hooks, next the boiler, or the latter will be injured.

The large oven is fitted with links for pack-transport.

The portable stove weighs 90½ lbs., and, when packed for transport, is 14 inches in height, 18¾ inches in length, and 16¾ in depth.

PART V.—TRAINING OF THE MEN IN FIRST AID, NURSING, COOKING, &c.

CHAPTER XXVII.

PRELIMINARY REMARKS ON THE GENERAL SCOPE AND OBJECTS OF INSTRUCTION.

436. The Royal Army Medical Corps, both in peace and war, at home and abroad, is responsible not only for the nursing of the sick and the dispensing of medicines, but it is also called on to perform various duties connected with the charge of equipment, the requisitioning for fuel, light, provisions, and all necessary supplies and repairs, the cooking and expenditure of diets, the custody of patients' kits, the cleanliness of the hospital and its surroundings, and the preparation of the accounts, abstracts, and vouchers of expenditure. The detailed instructions relating to these duties are contained in the Standing Orders for the Corps.

In the field, the Corps is further charged with another duty. It supplies to the Army an organization designed expressly for the purpose of speedily collecting and succouring the wounded during and after an engagement, and removing them from the battlefield to a place of safety, and with attending to the sick and wounded in all sick-convoys, hospital trains and ships, and the various hospitals in connection with an army in the field. Instructions regarding this are contained in Part III.

To the above are added various duties in connection with sanitation and the purification of water, for which see Part II.

437. To enable men to undertake these duties efficiently they must of necessity undergo not only a course of preliminary technical training, but continuous training throughout their service, so that in war their duties may be performed with that thoroughness and efficiency which must be the aim and object of every soldier of the Corps.

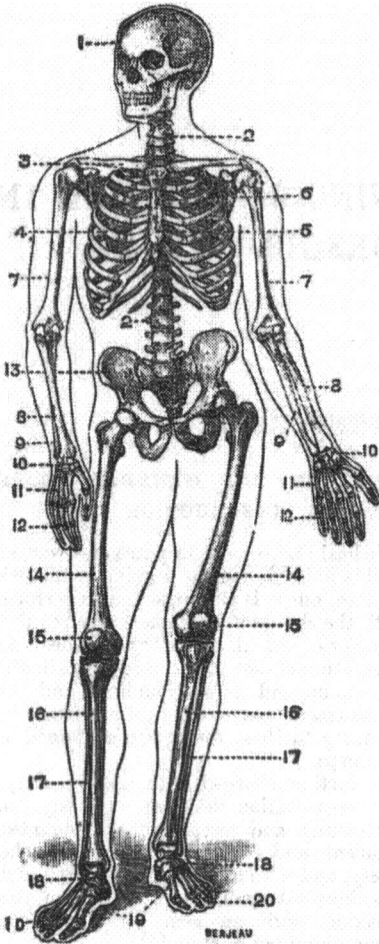

1. Cranium, or skull.
2. Spine formed of vertebræ.
3 Clavicle, or collar-bone.
4. Ribs.
5. Sternum, or breast-bone.
6. Scapula, or shoulder-blade
7. Humerus, or arm-bone.
8. Radius.
9. Ulna.
10. Carpus, or wrist-bones.
11. Metacarpal bones.
12. Phalanges, or finger-bones
13. Pelvis.
14. Femur, or thigh-bone.
15. Patella, or knee-cap.
16. Tibia, or shin-bone.
17. Fibula.
18. Tarsus, or ankle-bones.
19. Metatarsal bones.
20. Phalanges, or toe-bones.

Fig. 101.—The Skeleton.

CHAPTER XXVIII.

ANATOMICAL AND PHYSIOLOGICAL OUTLINES.

438. Construction of the human body.—The human body is made up of :—(1) The skeleton or bony framework with its joints ; (2) the Muscles, which make every movement ; and (3) the Nervous System, which receives impressions and governs all these movements. Further, as every movement of the body causes waste, some means are required for removing the products of waste and for supplying nourishment to make up for it. The following are concerned in supplying such needs, viz., (4) the Circulatory System— heart, blood, and blood-vessels—to carry to different parts of the body nourishment and oxygen ; (5) the Respiratory System—lungs and air-passages—to take in air and so give oxygen to the blood ; (6) the Digestive System—mouth, stomach and intestines, and certain glands—to take in and give to the system food and water ; (7) the Excretory System—kidneys, lungs, and skin—to extract from the blood the products of waste and to eliminate them and (8) the Skin, enclosing the whole, for the protection of the body and the regulation of its heat.

The Bones, Joints, and Muscles.

439. The Skeleton.—The skeleton consists of a number of bones, some long, some short and irregular, held together by bands or ligaments to form joints, which allow of greater or less movement between them. The bones determine the general shape and proportions of the body, give attachment to the muscles, and form levers on which the muscles act to move the body or limbs from one position to another. They also form cavities for the protection of important organs.

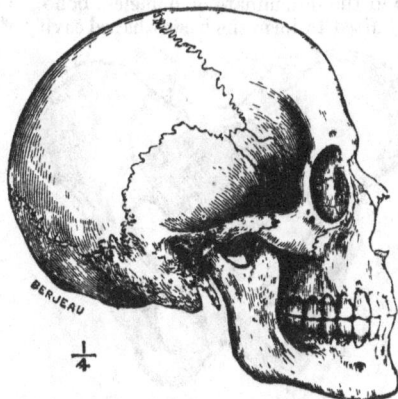

$\frac{1}{4}$

Fig. 102.—The Skull.

440. The Skull.—The bones of the head and face are together called the skull. The skull consists of two portions, namely, the cranium, a strong bony case for the protection of the brain, and the face, which consists of a number of bones, of which one only, the lower jaw, is movable.

441. Bones of the Trunk.—The bony parts of the trunk are the spinal or vertebral column, the chest or thorax, and the pelvis formed by the two large hip-bones and the sacrum.

The spinal column or backbone may be said to consist of thirty-three bones, but only twenty-four of these are movable. These are called vertebræ (see paras. 470 and 471). Through the centre of this column runs a canal or cavity, the spinal canal, which contains and protects the spinal cord. The spinal canal ends in the sacrum.

The chest or thorax is a large bony cavity formed by the union of the twelve dorsal vertebræ with the ribs, and the breast-bone or sternum in front, containing the heart, lungs, œsophagus or gullet, and the great blood-vessels.

The ribs or costæ are twenty-four in number, twelve on each side, connected in pairs with the dorsal vertebræ behind, and, with the exception of the last two pairs, with the sternum or breast-bone in front. Each of these pairs of ribs forms a circular arch called the costal arch.

The sternum is a long, flat, soft bone, the lower portion of which is composed of flexible cartilage.

The first seven pairs of ribs are called the true ribs, and have their own costal cartilage connecting them directly with the sternum. The next three pairs are each connected with the cartilage next above it, so that they are united to each other before they reach the sternum. The remaining two pairs are not connected in any way with the breast bone. The last five pairs are termed false ribs; and of these the last two pairs are called free or floating ribs.

The sacrum, and the innominate or nameless bones, one on either side, are firmly united to form the basin-shaped cavity of the pelvis,

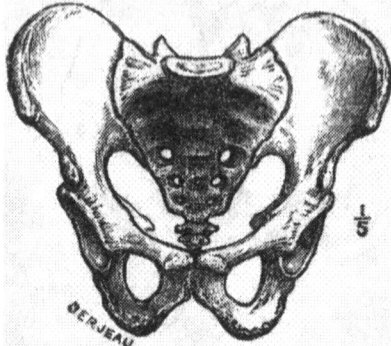

FIG. 103.—THE PELVIS.

which contains and protects the bladder and the lower end of the bowel or rectum, and to it the lower extremities or limbs are attached.

442. Bones of the Upper Limb.—The upper limb is divided into the shoulder, the arm, the forearm, and the hand.

The shoulder connects the arm to the trunk, and includes two bones : the collar-bone or clavicle, and the shoulder-blade or scapula. The former is a long, curved bone situated in front at the bottom of the neck and connecting the shoulder-blade to the breast-bone, whilst the latter is a large, flat, triangular bone lying upon the ribs behind.

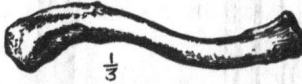

$\frac{1}{3}$

FIG. 104.—THE RIGHT COLLAR-BONE (seen from above).

The bone of the arm is called the humerus ; it is a long bone, having at its upper end a rounded head, which works in a socket in the scapula or shoulder-blade, and at its lower end a roller-shaped surface, which, with the bones of the forearm, forms the elbow-joint.

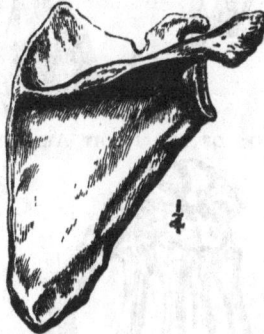

$\frac{1}{4}$

FIG. 105.—THE RIGHT SHOULDER-BLADE (seen from behind).

The bones of the forearm are the radius and the ulna. The radius extends from the outer side of the elbow to the thumb-side of the wrist. The ulna extends from the inner side of the elbow to the little finger side of the wrist. At its upper end is a projection, called the olecranon, which forms the point of the elbow. There is a space between the radius and ulna.

The bones of the hand are arranged in three rows : firstly, in the wrist or carpus are eight small bones, called the carpal bones ; secondly, a row of five long bones, called the metacarpus, forming the palm ; and lastly, small bones, named the phalanges, three for each finger and two for the thumb.

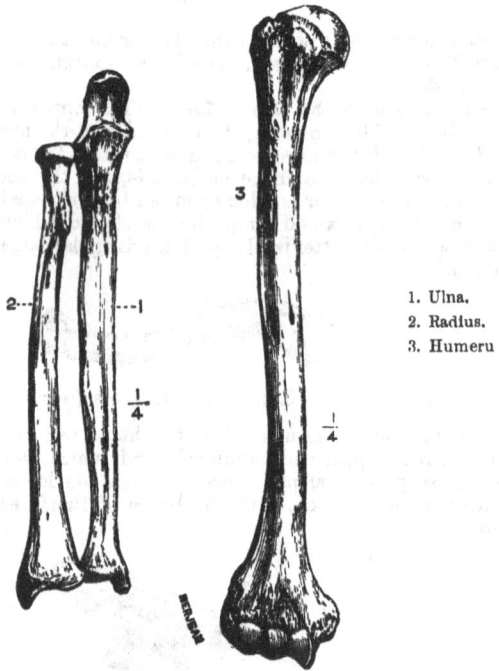

FIG. 106.—BONES OF THE RIGHT ARM AND FOREARM.

1. Ulna.
2. Radius.
3. Humeru

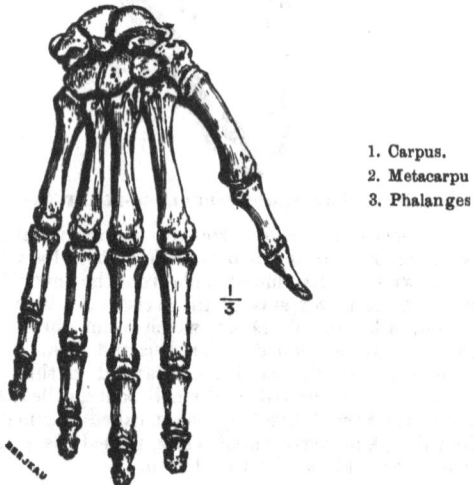

1. Carpus.
2. Metacarpu
3. Phalanges

FIG. 107.—THE BONES OF THE RIGHT HAND.

448. Bones of the Lower Limb.—The lower limb is divided into the thigh, the leg, and the foot.

The thigh is that portion which extends from the hip above to the knee below; its one bone is named the femur or thigh-bone, and is the largest and strongest in the body. At its upper end there is a rounded head, which fits into a deep, cup-shaped depression in the innominate bone forming the hip-joint; below, the expanded end of the bone enters into the formation of the knee-joint. Protecting the knee-joint in front there is a small bone called the patella or knee-cap.

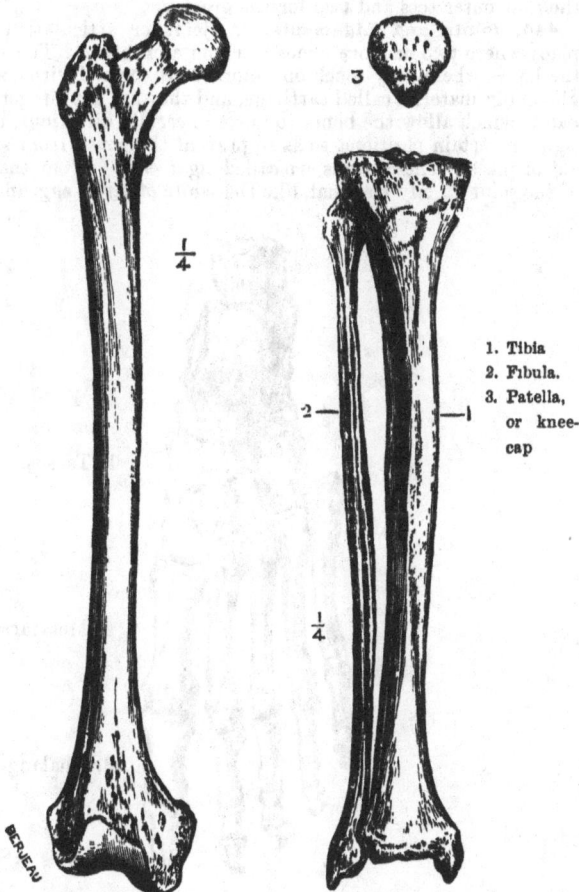

1. Tibia
2. Fibula.
3. Patella, or knee-cap

Fig. 108.—The Right Thigh-bone (right side).

Fig. 109.—The Bones of the Right Leg (right side).

The leg, extending from the knee to the ankle, has two bones, a larger one lying on the inner or great-toe side, called the tibia or shin-bone, upon the flat expanded head of which rests the lower end of the thigh bone, and a more slender one on the outer side, called the fibula.

The construction of the foot is like that of the hand; it has three rows of bones: the hinder part, or tarsus, is formed of seven short strong bones, called the tarsal bones; secondly, a row of five longer bones, the metatarsus, corresponding to the sole of the foot and instep; lastly, small bones, named the phalanges, three for each of the four outer toes and two for the great toe.

444. Joints and Ligaments.—A joint or articulation is the place where two or more bones work on each other. The ends of the bones where they touch one another are covered with a smooth, glistening material called cartilage, and they are kept together by bands which allow the bones to move in certain directions, but are tight in certain positions, so as to prevent the bones from slipping out of place. These bands are called ligaments. From the inside of the joint an oily material, like the white of a raw egg, and called

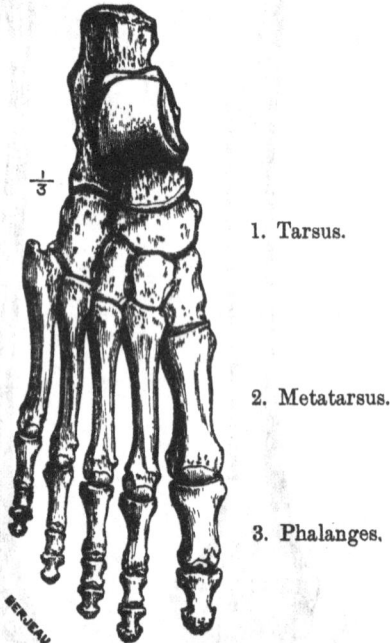

1. Tarsus.

2. Metatarsus.

3. Phalanges.

Fig. 110.—The Bones of the Right Foot.

synovia, is poured out, which allows the ends of the bones to glide smoothly over one another. The membrane which lines the joint and provides this material is called the synovial membrane.

The two principal kinds of joints are the ball-and-socket and the hinge-joint. The ball-and-socket joint allows one of the bones to move freely in all directions. The shoulder and hip are joints of this description, the scapula and the innominate bone each having a cup-like hollow, into which fit the rounded, ball-shaped ends of the long bones of the arm and thigh. The second kind of joint, working like the hinge of a door, allows of movement up and down, or backwards and forwards only, as seen in the elbow and knee.

445. Muscles.—The muscles form the red flesh of the body, and are arranged in bands. These bands pass from one bone to another and are attached to the bones, very commonly by means of leaders or tendons. These muscles have the power of contracting or shortening themselves under the influence of the will, and so of moving the bones to which they are attached. In this manner the limbs and different parts of the body are made to move.

THE ORGANS OF CIRCULATION.

446. The organs of circulation consist of the heart and blood-vessels, and contain the blood. They are the means by which the nourishment and oxygen are carried round the body, and waste matters conveyed to places where they are to be got rid of.

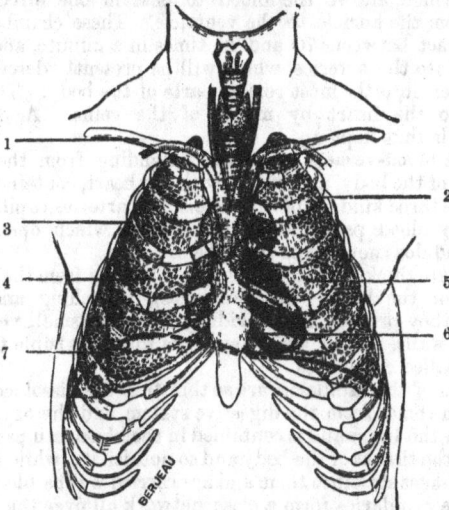

FIG. 111.—THE THORAX OR CHEST.
1. Collar-bone. 2. Second rib. 3. Third rib. 4. Right lung. 5. Left lung.
6. Heart. 7. Cut edge of diaphragm.

447. The blood is a fluid of a red colour, which coagulates or changes into a jelly-like mass or clot when it escapes from the blood-vessels. It is made up of two parts: a clear fluid called the liquor sanguinis, which is what is seen in a blister; and many millions of very minute, coin-shaped bodies which give to the blood its colour and substance, and which collect together in the blood-clot. These little discs are too small to be seen by the naked eye: over 3,000 placed in a line side-by-side would not make up 1 inch. They are called corpuscles. The blood in the right side of the heart and in the veins of the body is dark-coloured, and requires aeration, *i.e.*, to be supplied with oxygen from the air; that in the left side of the heart and the arteries of the body is bright-scarlet, and is aerated, *i.e.*, it has obtained oxygen from the air during its passage through the lungs. The dark-coloured blood is called venous blood, the bright-coloured blood is called arterial blood.

448. The heart is a hollow, muscular pump about the size of a closed fist, lying in the middle of the chest between the two lungs, with its point or apex toward the left side.

It is divided into a right and left half, separated by a partition, so that nothing can pass directly from the right to the left side of the heart. Each half is divided by another partition into an upper, thin-walled receiving-chamber and a lower, thick-walled pumping-chamber. The upper chamber is called an auricle, the lower a ventricle. There is a flap or valve between each auricle and ventricle, which allows the blood to pass in one direction only, namely, from the auricle to the ventricle. These chambers of the heart contract between 70 and 80 times in a minute, and so force the blood into the arteries, which will be presently described, and through them into the most remote parts of the body. The blood is returned to the heart by means of the veins. A continuous circulation is thus kept up.

449. The blood-vessels are tubes extending from the heart to every part of the body, and which, with the heart, contain the blood.

There are three kinds of blood-vessels, viz., arteries, capillaries, and veins. The blood passes along these tubes, which open into one another, and does not escape from them.

Arteries are thick-walled, strong tubes, leading from the pumping-chambers of the heart (the ventricles), branching and getting smaller as they proceed, and dividing into very small vessels with very thin walls, which are so small as to be invisible to the eye. These are called capillaries.

The walls of the capillaries are so thin that the dissolved nourishment which comes from the digestive system, and the oxygen which comes from the lungs and is contained in the blood, can pass through them into the tissues of the body and so nourish it; while impurities from the tissues soak into them and are carried by the blood into the veins. The capillaries form a close network all over the body, and gradually collecting together and getting larger, they become veins.

The veins, thin-walled tubes, commencing thus in the capillaries, become fewer in number and larger in size as they get nearer the heart, until they end in the large veins which open into its upper chambers (the auricles).

The arteries carry the blood from the heart to the capillaries, the veins from the capillaries to the heart. The blood travels rapidly in the arteries and veins, and very slowly in the capillaries, so as to allow the work above described to be done.

450. Circulation.—In the body there is a double circulation, owing to the fact that the oxygen required to aerate the blood cannot be taken into the blood at the same time as nourishment. Consequently, the blood has to make one round to take in nourishment and to distribute nourishment and oxygen, and a second round through the lungs to take in the oxygen from the air which is drawn into them. Of these two rounds or circulations, the first is called systemic, the second pulmonary. The systemic circulation is that of every part of the body except the lungs. The pulmonary circulation takes place in the lungs alone, and is for the sole purpose of aerating the blood. The pulmonary veins are the only veins in the body containing bright-coloured blood, and the pulmonary arteries the only arteries in the body containing dark-coloured blood. The blood, when it passes from the capillaries of the lungs, is aerated and bright-scarlet ; it remains so while it circulates through the veins of the lungs into the left auricle, from thence into the left ventricle, from thence into the systemic arteries, until it passes into the systemic capillaries, where it loses the oxygen with which it has been charged and becomes dark-coloured. It remains dark-coloured while flowing from the systemic capillaries into the systemic veins, from thence into the right auricle, right ventricle, thence into the arteries of the lungs, and from thence into the capillaries of the lungs, where aeration again takes place and the bright-red colour is restored. This is the course of the circulation. The blood in the systemic capillaries takes up nourishment from the stomach and bowels.

The pumping action of the heart produces a wave through the arteries, which can be felt where they come near the surface of the body, as at the wrist just above the root of the thumb. This wave or beat is called the pulse, each beat corresponding with the contraction or beat of the heart.

In the veins there is no beat or pulse, the force of the blood-current having been expended while passing through the wide network of capillaries lying between the ends of the arteries and the commencement of the veins, so that the blood flows in the latter in a steady, even stream.

THE ORGANS OF RESPIRATION.

451. The organs of respiration or breathing are the means by which air is taken into the lungs, and one of its gases, called oxygen, is given to the blood. While the oxygen is being taken into the blood, carbonic acid gas, certain other gases, and watery vapour pass from the blood into the air in the lungs, and are breathed out.

The organs of respiration consist of the trachea or windpipe and the lungs.

The trachea is a stout tube through which the air passes into and out of the lungs. Its upper part, called the larynx, is the organ of voice, and opens into the back of the mouth and nose. The windpipe can be felt in the throat under the skin where it lies immediately in front of the gullet. In the chest it divides into two tubes, the bronchi, one for each lung.

There is a flap, called the epiglottis, at the upper opening of the larynx, which covers it and prevents food from passing into the windpipe when swallowing.

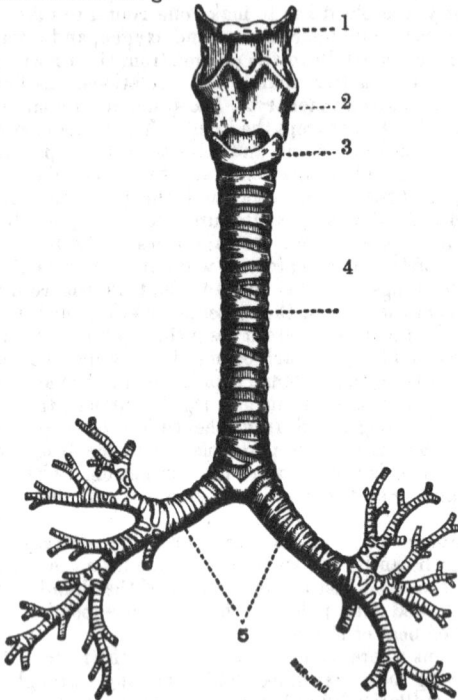

FIG. 112.—THE LARYNX, TRACHEA, AND BRONCHI.

1. Hyoid bone ; 2. thyroid cartilage ; and 3. cricoid cartilage, forming the Larynx. 4. Trachea or Windpipe. 5. Bronchi.

The bronchi are stout tubes leading from the windpipe to the lungs. In the lungs the bronchi branch out in all directions, becoming smaller and their walls thinner as they proceed to their closed endings, the air-cells.

The lungs, two in number, lie in the cavity of the chest, one on either side. Each consists of a mass of minute, extremely thin-walled cells, the air-cells, which are the blind endings of the bronchial tubes. In the extremely thin walls of the air-cells are spread networks of capillaries.

The air-cells thus communicate directly with the external air through the bronchi, windpipe, larynx, mouth, and nose.

Vessel bringing venous blood to the lung.

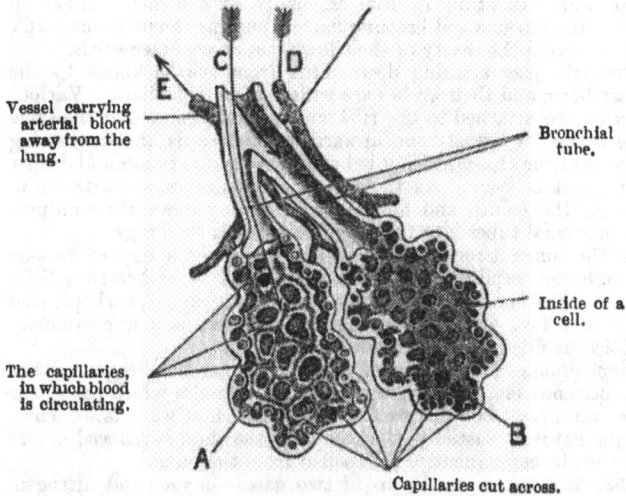

FIG. 113.—TWO AIR-CELLS OF THE LUNG CUT ACROSS (MAGNIFIED).

A, showing the arrangement of the capillaries around the air cells.
B, showing the appearance of the inside of an air-cell.
C, is a bronchial tube. The arrow in it shows the direction of the air in inspiration.
D, a blood-vessel taking the dark blood to be aerated in the cell.
E, a blood-vessel returning the bright aerated blood to the left auricle.

452. Description of Respiration.—Respiration or breathing is produced by the alternate enlargement and contraction of the chest-walls, by means of which air is drawn into and expelled from the lungs.

A complete respiration consists of :—Inspiration or drawing-in of air to the lungs, immediately followed by expiration or breathing-out, expulsion of air from the lungs. This is followed by a pause while one may slowly count two.*

A complete respiration occurs in health 15 to 18 times a minute. The rate is increased during exertion and also in many diseases. The act of respiration is carried out in the following way:—

Inspiration.—In inspiration the chest is enlarged by the action of various muscles.

---

* The importance of impressing the relation to one another of these three phases of respiration becomes manifest when the practice of artificial respiration is being taught.

One of these, the diaphragm or midriff is situated between the chest and the belly or abdomen. The diaphragm when not in action is arched upwards, being attached to the lower end of the breast-bone, the lower ribs, and the backbone, forming the floor of the chest and separating it from the belly or abdomen. When in action, it contracts and becomes flatter, pushing the belly outwards, and enlarging the cavity of the chest from above downwards.

The ribs pass slanting downwards from the backbone to the breast-bone, and their arches are wider below than above. Various muscles are attached to the ribs which raise them and at the same time carry the breast-bone upwards and forwards, thus increasing the size of the chest, making it broader from side to side and deeper from front to back. As the chest cavity enlarges, air is drawn in through the mouth and nostrils, and passing down the windpipe and bronchial tubes into the air-cells, expands the lungs.

In the lungs it remains long enough to allow the oxygen to pass through the capillaries into the blood. At every breath a little additional air is drawn in, and some watery vapour, carbonic acid and other foul gases passed out. The chest is not completely emptied or filled at each breath.

Expiration.—At the end of inspiration the diaphragm relaxes and becomes more arched upwards : the muscles which raised the ribs and breast-bone cease to act, and the chest-walls fall. Thus, by its natural elasticity, the cavity of the chest is reduced in size and the air, consequently, is expelled from the lungs.

453. The air is made up of two gases—oxygen and nitrogen. Oxygen is what is required in the blood : the nitrogen passes out just as it went in. Oxygen has the effect of making the corpuscles bright scarlet, as in the systemic arteries. As the oxygen passes out of the corpuscles the blood becomes darker in colour, as in the systemic veins.

The Nervous System.

454. The nervous system consists of (1) nerve-centres, (2) nerve-cords, or nerves, (3) nerve-endings.

The nerve-centres are the brain and spinal cord and receive all messages from the skin and organs of sense, sending out orders to the muscles to make them move in any desired way. All the thinking is done in the brain. It is contained in, and protected by, the skull.

The spinal cord proceeds from the brain down the spinal canal, and both brain and spinal cord give off all the nerve-cords which proceed to every part of the body.

The nerve-cords are the connecting threads between the nerve centres and nerve-endings. They are, therefore, attached at one end to the brain or spinal cord, and at the other end terminate in the nerve-endings, whether in the skin, organs of sense, or muscles.

Nerve-endings are to be found in every part of the body ; for instance, it is not possible to touch with the point of a needle any portion of the skin which does not contain a nerve ending. They are able to communicate to the brain information of what is taking place in the part to which they are distributed. For instance, with the end of the finger we can tell whether anything we touch is rough or smooth, hot or cold. Other nerve-endings in the ear, eye, tongue, or nose send to the brain information as to hearing, sight, taste, and smell. Acting on this information, the brain can send an order to any muscle, or set of muscles, instantaneously, by the nerves which pass into them, and so make them move.

THE DIGESTIVE SYSTEM.

455. The digestive system consists of two portions, viz., (1) a long tube called the alimentary canal, and (2) glands which prepare juices to be mixed with the food and digest it.

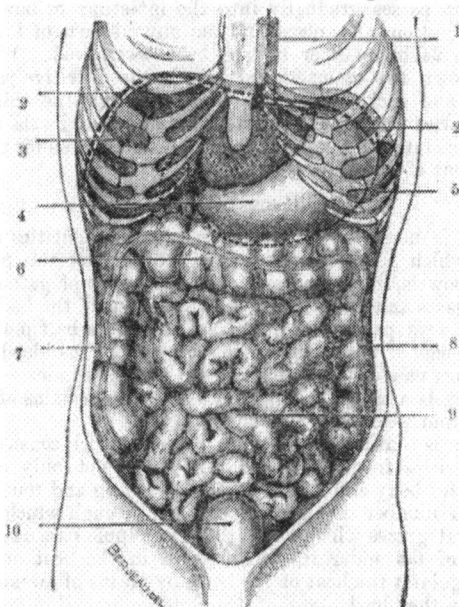

FIG. 114—THE ABDOMEN.

1. Gullet. 2, 2. Cut edge of diaphragm. 3. Liver. 4. Stomach. 5. Spleen.
6. Transverse colon. 7. Ascending colon. 8 Descending colon.
9. Small intestines. 10. Bladder.

The alimentary canal begins at the mouth and ends at the anus or lower opening of the bowel. It is altogether about 30 feet long.

The different parts of the alimentary canal are the mouth, gullet or œsophagus, stomach, small and large intestines.

The glands, or organs which pour juices into this canal or tube, are the salivary glands in the mouth, the gastric glands in the stomach, the liver which makes bile (two pints a day), the pancreas which makes a juice similar to the saliva, and other glands in the walls of the small intestine.

The position of the digestive organs is referred to in para. 461.

456. It is necessary for proper digestion that the teeth should be in good order and kept from decay. One great means of preventing decay is to brush the teeth regularly every day. This removes the remains of food, which when left among the teeth helps to cause their decay.

457. The food passes through the gullet from the mouth, after being chewed or masticated and mixed with the saliva, into the stomach. As it become sufficiently liquefied by the action of the stomach, it passes gradually into the intestines or bowels, where further digestion takes place, and the unused parts of it are passed out about 24 hours after having been swallowed. While it is passing down the stomach and bowels the nutritive part of it is dissolved and sucked into the blood, through the thin walls of the capillaries on the inside of the stomach and bowels, and passes from thence into the veins, and so into the circulation for the general nourishment of the body.

THE EXCRETORY SYSTEM.

458. It is necessary to life to get rid of impurities and waste matters which accumulate in the blood, and for this purpose the kidneys, bowels, lungs, and skin have the power of gathering these matters, gases and fluid, and passing them out of the body.

The kidneys pass out daily about two and a half pints of urine which consists of water and waste matter from the blood.

The lungs pass out impure gases in the expired air.

The bowels assist in casting out, with the remains of the food certain impurities.

The skin is continually passing off sweat, which consists of water and impurities from the blood. The skin not only covers and protects the body and has the sense of feeling and touch, but also has in it a number of minute apertures, through which sweat and the natural grease which keeps the skin supple pass out. It has a quantity of fat under it, which keeps in the heat of the body. It also regulates the heat of the body by means of sweating, which cools down the blood.

In order to keep the skin healthy, great attention should be paid to cleanliness.

THE CHEST AND ABDOMEN.

459. There are two large cavities in the trunk, namely, the chest or thorax, and the belly or abdomen. The organs of respiration and circulation are contained in the chest; those of digestion and excretion in the belly.

460. The Chest.—The cavity of the chest occupies the upper third of the trunk and is a cone-shaped chamber the base of which is below. The walls are principally made of a frame-work of bone, namely, the backbone, the ribs, and the breast-bone or sternum ; the spaces between the ribs being filled in by muscles and fibrous tissue. (See Fig. 111.)

The chest contains the lungs, heart, the large blood-vessels, and part of the gullet. Above, it communicates with the neck by an opening through which pass the windpipe, gullet, and blood-vessels from the head and neck. Below, it is shut off from the abdomen by the diaphragm, through which pass, at the back of the chest, the gullet leading to the stomach, and the main artery and vein of the body.

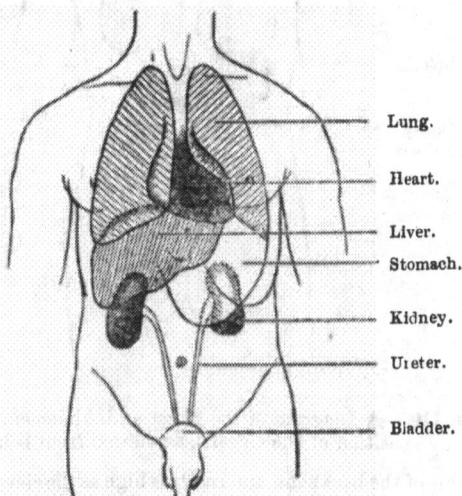

FIG. 115.—A Diagram of the Chest and Abdomen, to show the position of the Organs, as Viewed from the Front.

461. The Abdomen.—This cavity lies immediately below the chest, being roofed in by the diaphragm. The walls in front and of the sides are formed by layers of muscles, and behind by the back-bone. The floor is formed by the pelvis (see Fig. 103).

The belly contains the stomach, bowels (small and large intestines), the liver, spleen, pancreas, kidneys, and bladder. The liver is a very large organ. It is placed below the diaphragm, under the ribs, on the right side, and fills nearly a sixth part of the belly. The stomach is under the ribs on the left side, and varies in size according as it is empty or full. The pancreas or sweetbread lies across the front of the spine just above the level of the navel. The spleen is a large, soft organ about the size of the fist. It is concerned in the formation of the blood, and is placed deeply under the left ribs, behind the stomach, and close under the diaphragm. It is apt to be enlarged in certain tropical diseases. The kidneys are deeply placed in the loins, one on

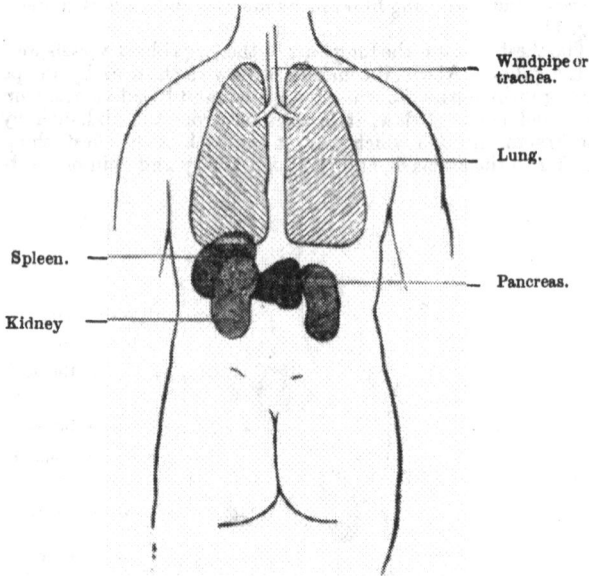

Fig. 116.—A Diagram of the Chest and Abdomen, to show the
position of the Organs, as viewed from behind.

each side of the backbone, and reach as high as the eleventh rib. They
are placed at the back of the abdomen. The bladder is quite low down,
in the middle of the front of the belly, and only rises above the pelvis
when it is very full. The bowels fill up the whole of the rest of the
space in the belly. The urine reaches the bladder from the kidneys
by two tubes, called the ureters, one to each kidney. It remains in
the bladder until such time as it is convenient to pass it. The tube
by which it is passed is called the urethra.

CHAPTER XXIX.

FURTHER INSTRUCTION IN ANATOMY AND PHYSIOLOGY.

The Bones.

462. Bones are composed of animal matter and lime, and are surrounded by a membrane, called the periosteum, from which blood-vessels pass into the bone to nourish it, and which is essential to its proper union in case of fracture. The longer bones have a cavity in their shaft called the medullary or marrow cavity, containing yellow marrow : in this, as well as in the periosteum, are found blood-vessels for the supply of the bone. The outer layers of the bones are hard and compact, but the inner portions are made of a kind of network of interlacing laths of bone, with spaces between them containing many blood-vessels and red marrow which plays an important part in the formation of the blood. This porous bone is called cancellous tissue.

The Skull.

463. The skull (para. 440), as has been said, has many bones entering into its structure, and it is really made up of a number of cavities for the protection of the brain and the delicate organs of special sense (as the eye, the ear, and the nose), and of other air-cavities which add lightness to its structure and give resonance to the voice. Many bones go to form the brain-case or cranium, and the face with its air-cells and cavities.

464. Cranium.—The cavity of the cranium contains the brain ; is continuous with the spinal canal (para. 441), and opens into it by means of a large hole at its base, called the foramen magnum. The bone which has this hole in it is called the occipital bone. On either side of the foramen are the condyles, which are rounded pieces of bone which rest and move upon the topmost vertebra of the spinal column. The whole weight of the skull is thus borne through the condyles upon the top vertebræ of the spinal column.

The occipital bone is permanently united by its fore-end to the sphenoid bone, which forms a sort of keystone to the base of the cranium, and which has wing-like extensions passing upwards and outwards, supporting a great part of the base of the brain. It has other extensions passing downwards which form the back part of the hinder nostrils and give attachment to some of the muscles of the lower jaw.

The great blood-vessels for the brain enter through holes in the base of the skull near the sphenoid bone.

The eye-socket or orbit is partly formed by the wing of the sphenoid, which also appears on the outside of the skull.

Attached to the fore-end of the sphenoid at the base of the skull is the frontal bone ; it has a horizontal part forming the front portion of the floor of the cranium and the roof of both orbits, and a rounded ascending plate which forms the whole of the forehead and the front of the skull.

A small bone called the ethmoid is placed in the front part of the base of the cranium, between the frontal and sphenoid bones, and forms part of the roof of the nasal cavity.

The lateral parts of the base of the cranium are formed by the occipital bone, the temporal bones (which are wedged in between the occipital and sphenoid, but which do not meet in the central portion of the skull's base), the wings of the sphenoid, and the frontal bone ; the dome and sides of the skull by the occipital bone behind, the two parietal and two temporal bones, a small portion of the sphenoid, and the frontal bone.

The base of the skull is very thin in certain spots, such as the roof of the orbit and the roof of the nasal cavity ; these are, however, generally protected by their position. The central portions of the base are very strong, as must be the case to withstand the shock of the weight of the head in jumping from a height.

The cranium contains the brain, from which the nerves of special sense pass through the holes in its base, and is lined by a strong membrane called the dura mater, which supports nerves and vessels, and forms partitions to hold the brain in its place, and which also contains blood-vessels to nourish the inner layers of the skull's bones, as the periosteum does in the case of other bones.

The muscles which move the head and form the flesh of the neck are attached to the base of the skull.

465. Bones of the Face.—The face is formed of a good many bones which, as said, form cavities for the protection of the organs of special sense, and give lightness to the structure of the head and resonance to the voice. These bones, with the exception of the lower jaw, are fixed together immovably. (Para. 440.)

The fixed bones are the superior maxillæ, the malar bones, the nasal bones, the palate bones, the vomer, and the turbinate bones.

The upper jaws (superior maxillæ), one on each side, underlie the greater part of the cheeks, carry the upper teeth, and form most of the bony palate, the opening of the nostrils, and the inner side of the eye-socket.

The cheek-bones (malar bones) are small and strong and are joined to the upper jaw-bones by their inner ends, and to the prong (or zygomatic process) of the temporal bone by their outer ends, and form the lower and outer part of the rim of the eye-socket or orbit. They are joined by their upper ends to the frontal bone, which last completes the eye-socket above, and joins with the upper jaw-bone to its inner side.

The two small nasal bones are joined to the frontal bone above, to one another by their inner edges, and to the upper jaw-bone by their outer edges to form the bridge of the nose.

The bony palate is completed by two bones called the palate-bones, which unite together in the centre, and join the upper jaw in front and form much of the hinder opening of the nostrils into the throat or pharynx.

A thin bone, called the vomer, forms the division between the nostrils, passing from the base of the skull and ethmoid bone above, to the junction of the palate and palate portions of the upper jaw-bones below.

There are some very thin, curled bones called the turbinate bones, fixed to the outer walls of the nasal passages, projecting into the passage, and which are covered with mucous membrane which has many large blood-vessels in it, in order to warm the air as it passes through the nostrils to reach the lungs. These bones also serve for the spreading out of the nerves of smell in the upper part of the nostrils.

466. There are numerous air-chambers opening into the nasal passages, a very large one being situated in the back part of the upper jaw above the back teeth, and there is one in the forehead behind the brow in the thickness of the frontal bones ; others exist between the two eye sockets and above the back part of the nasal passages.

467. The lower jaw-bone is strong and heavy and carries the lower teeth. It is flattish in section, and bent on the flat at its centre which forms the chin, and edgeways behind the rows of teeth to form two upward projections for attachment to the temporal bones of the cranium with which it is articulated. The upper ends of these two projections are rounded and smoothed to form a movable joint. They are called condyles.

Very powerful muscles are attached to the lower jaw. One, called the temporal muscle, covers much of the side of the skull, and passes beneath a bony arch, formed by the temporal prong or zygomatic process and the malar bone, to be attached to the upper projection of the lower jaw in front of its rounded articular head or condyle. Other very strong muscles are attached to both sides of it lower down, and by their other ends to the bones of the face and the downward-projecting plates of the sphenoid bone (see Cranium), which muscles give the side-to-side movement of the jaw (the temporal muscle simply moving it up and down).

468. Special sense organs located in face cavities.—It has been mentioned that most of the organs of special sense are located in the cavities of the face. The eyes are contained in the orbits or eye-sockets, formed as described ; the organ of smell is contained in the upper part of the nasal passages, the lower part of these passages being for breathing. The internal ear is in the thickness of the temporal bone, and the external meatus or earhole opens behind the joint of the lower jaw. The internal ear has a communication with the back of the throat through a tube called the Eustachian tube. The sense of taste is situated in the tongue and palate.

469. The Teeth.—There are two sets of teeth grown in a lifetime from the upper and lower jaw.

The first set, which is complete in childhood, is of twenty teeth only, and these in grown-up people give place to thirty-two.

The teeth in both halves of the upper and lower jaw and in the two jaws correspond in number and shape. The eight front, chisel-shaped teeth are called incisors or cutting teeth ; the four on each side of these are called canines or dog-teeth. In childhood there are eight grinding teeth behind these, called molars. Adult people have the same number of incisors and canines, but in place of the eight molars of childhood they have eight bicuspids or narrow grinders with two points or cusps each, and in addition twelve molars with three or four points each. Those four furthest back are called the wisdom teeth, and may not come through till the age of thirty.

The child teeth are called "temporary" and the adult teeth "permanent." The buds of both sets are contained in the thickness of the jaws at birth.

The Spinal Column.

470. Vertebræ.—The vertebræ (para. 441) are a number of bones which make up the spinal column. They form a jointed, elastic pillar for the support of the trunk and skull by means of their bodies, which are placed one on top of another with cushions between them (the intervertebral fibro-cartilages). The spinal column so formed gives attachment to the ribs and limbs.

The vertebræ have projections from the hinder part of their bodies forming rings, and these rings placed one above the other form the spinal canal, a bony canal which encloses and protects the spinal cord. Projecting from the sides of each ring are two lateral bars called transverse processes, which in the twelve dorsal vertebræ support the ribs ; and from the back of the ring project central pieces called spinous processes, which can be seen and felt under the skin of the back as knobs of bone.

471. Regions of Spine.—The different regions of the spine receive different names, each containing a certain number of vertebræ ; these are : —The neck or cervical region with seven vertebræ ; the back or dorsal region with twelve ; the loins or lumbar region with five ; the sacrum with one piece of bone consisting of five vertebræ welded together ; and the coccyx or tail with four joints which are incomplete vertebræ.

The Muscles.

472. Structure and Action.—Muscles (para. 445) are responsible for all movements of the body, whether under the control of the will or not, and all movements are caused by impulses travelling along the nerves to the muscles. Consequently all muscles have nerves passing into their substance, and branching so as to give a nerve-fibre to each muscle-fibre.

Muscles are made up of threads or fibres, which in a simple muscle lie side by side, enclosed in a sheath, and generally end in tendons at one or both ends attaching them to bones or other parts they are intended to move. The movement of these bones or parts is caused by the muscle contracting or shortening itself in response to the impulse sent along its nerve, and so bringing its points of attachment nearer together and moving the part, e.g., bending or straightening the limb.

The muscles moving the head, trunk, and limbs are under the command of the brain and are termed "voluntary" muscles. They are made up of fibres which are striated, *i.e.*, striped transversely, and are capable of most rapid movements, and movements of very complicated kinds. The muscles of the limbs are grouped to perform such habitual actions as walking, bringing the hand to the mouth in taking food, etc. There are, however, muscles, such as those of the heart and intestines, which are not under control of the will. Such muscles are said to be "involuntary." Involuntary muscles (with the exception of that of the heart) are not striped, and are of paler colour as a rule than the striped ones. They are slower in their movements and carry on the more mechanical functions of the body. They are under the control of the sympathetic system of nerves. Layers of involuntary muscles surround the blood-vessels and the alimentary canal, the calibre of which they control, and it is by their means that the contents of the intestines are pushed along.

473. Blood-supply.—Muscles are very freely supplied with blood as every movement causes the consumption of some of their substance, which must be removed and replaced, otherwise they would soon be clogged and so prevented from doing more work. The well-known feeling of stiffness after severe exercise is due to the accumulation of waste products in the muscles.

474. Muscular development.—Moderate exercise and good feeding enlarge the muscles: disuse and poor feeding cause them to dwindle. Great development of muscle is seen in persons who systematically exercise every muscle.

The effect of disuse in causing the dwindling or atrophy of the muscles is particularly striking in the case of a stiff joint, when the limb affected may decrease to half its proper size. When the nerves supplying muscles are destroyed, the condition of the muscle which becomes powerless and would otherwise atrophy can be preserved to a certain extent by massage and passive movement. Muscles can be made to contract by the electric current, which is often used to keep up their activity in cases of paralysis.

475. Internal work done.—There is always much muscular work going on in the body, even during sleep; and when one considers that the heart never ceases to beat, that the breathing-muscles never rest, and that the food in the alimentary canal is continually kept moving by muscular action, it is not surprising to find that enough energy is daily expended (without counting what is used in external and visible work) to raise a weight of 260 tons to a height of 1 foot in the twenty-four hours. The body-tissues, particularly the muscles, also produce by their slow combustion a great quantity of heat, enough in the twenty-four hours to boil sixty pints of water, previously at freezing point.

476. Necessity for oxygen.—The combustion or burning of the body-tissues, as in the case of every fire, requires oxygen to keep it up and produces carbonic acid gas. When, as in making great exertion, the rate of the breathing is much increased, it is because more oxygen is wanted to supply the muscles in action, as it is only by spending them that movement can take place.

The Nervous System.

477. The nervous system (para. 454) is the most delicate and complex of all the parts of the body. The great difference between human beings and other living creatures consists in the high development of their nervous system.

478. Cerebro-spinal.—The brain and spinal cord are the centres of the " cerebro-spinal system," which is the voluntary and will-controlled system.

479. Sympathetic.—There is a system of nerves called the sympathetic system, which consists of chains of ganglia or knots, connected together and to the spinal nerves, and which automatically regulate the movements of the vital parts and blood-vessels which are not controllable by the will. This system is to be found in the very lowest animals, which have no brain proper, and no spinal cord.

480. Brain.—The brain consists of countless numbers of nerve-cells and nerve-fibres ; the nerve-cells are in two great masses called the cerebrum or brain, and the cerebellum or small brain. The spinal cord also contains masses of nerve-cells. The cerebrum and cerebellum are contained in the cranium, the brain being uppermost.

The cerebrum consists of two halves or hemispheres, which are to all intents duplicates of one another. The halves are united together and to the cerebellum below, and are separated above by a deep furrow from front to back, into which a partition of the dura mater fits. The outer surface of the brain is covered with rounded ridges and furrows, and is plentifully supplied with blood-vessels which run into these furrows. The main blood-supply of the brain passes into its base.

From the base of the brain nerve-cords proceed, viz., the nerves of smell, sight, hearing, and taste, and for the movements of the eyes, tongue, jaw, and the muscles of the face.

481. Spinal Cord.—At the junction of the spinal cord with the brain, there is a piece of the cord called the medulla oblongata from which come very important nerves governing the movements of the heart, of breathing, and of the stomach ; and the spinal cord contains all the nerve-centres for the lower physical functions of the body.

The spinal cord proceeds from the base of the brain and is contained in the spinal canal. It extends as far as the upper lumbar vertebræ. From the spinal cord a pair of nerves passes between every two vertebræ for the sensations and movements of the trunk and limbs.

482. Functions of the Brain.—The cerebrum is the seat of thought, the higher voluntary originations, and is the seat also of most of the special senses ; while the cerebellum serves to " co-ordinate " or combine the various groups of muscles in movement which together carry out such habitual actions as walking and eating. It is possible for life to continue for a time without the higher brain, as the centres for the mere vital and non-intellectual functions are in its base and in the medulla and spinal cord. Breathing and swallowing can go on even when, as in concussion of the brain, sensibility is quite absent, but if the nerve-centres which govern the vital functions are in any way interfered with, instant death is the consequence.

To perform any voluntary movement an impulse must proceed from the brain to the nerve moving the muscles required, and there must always be some reason for the movement which, however, may be physical or mental.

There are, again, many acts which are not performed intentionally, though they are done by the voluntary muscles ; the acts, for instance, of coughing, sneezing, vomiting, yawning, and hiccupping are independent of the will, and are what are called *reflex* acts, that depend upon the state of the air-passages and digestive organs, and the impulse causing the muscular movement proceeds from centres in the medulla and spinal cord, short of the higher brain.

483. Sensory and Motor Nerves.—Nerves are either " afferent " or sensory nerves which convey sensations to the nerve-centres, or " efferent " or motor nerves which convey impulses from the nerve-centres to the muscles. All nerves are in connexion by their central ends with nerve-cells.

The sensory nerves are the nerves of the special senses, *e.g.*, sight, taste, smell, and hearing, and those of common sensation carrying impressions of heat, cold, and pain. The motor nerves cause the muscles to move, the glands to produce their secretions, and the blood-vessels to enlarge or contract.

The nerves are made up of many strands of fibres, which are insulated like wires intended to carry electric currents. The great sciatic nerve, which passes into the thigh, is the largest nerve in the body and is as thick as the little finger.

484. Injury to Nerves.—Injury to nerves causes paralysis of the parts they supply, *i.e.*, loss of sensation and of the power of movement, and the nourishment of the paralysed parts also suffers ; bed-sores are especially likely to occur in paralysis.

The spinal cord consists principally of nerve-fibres coming from the brain to supply the trunk and limbs, and when it is torn through or badly crushed paralysis of both sides of the body is the result, extending as high as the point of origin of the lowest uninjured nerves coming off from it.

When a nerve is completely severed it may be repaired in time, but it takes long, and sensation and power are only gradually recovered.

The Blood and Blood-vessels.

485. White Blood-corpuscles.—The blood and its circulation have already been described briefly (paras. 446 to 450). In this description no mention was made of the white blood-corpuscles. These bodies, though not so-numerous as the red corpuscles, have very important duties in the body. There are about 500 red to one white corpuscle.

The white corpuscles have the power of altering their shape, and of passing through the walls of the capillaries ; and they also seize and envelop and destroy germs of disease which gain access to the blood, thus protecting the body from invasion ; when an injury has been done to some part of the body and it has become inflamed, the white corpuscles flock there in great numbers to deal with the cause of the inflammation, and if they are successful in removing it, they return into the circulation ; if not, they become pus-corpuscles, which may be regarded as dead white blood-corpuscles, collections of which form abscesses.

The white blood-corpuscles are made in the spleen and lymphatic glands.

486. Red Blood-corpuscles.—The red corpuscles have been described in para. 447. They are coloured by a compound of iron, which is called *hæmoglobin*, and the red colour of the blood is entirely due to them. Their principal duty is to absorb oxygen from the air taken into the lungs (para. 552), and to carry carbonic acid gas from the system to the lungs, where it passes into the air in exchange for the oxygen, and is breathed out (see under The Muscles).

487. It must always be remembered that every movement causes the combustion or spending of some of the body tissues, and the result is transference of energy to some object, such as a cricket-ball when thrown, and secondly, the production of heat, and thirdly, the formation of carbonic acid gas or carbon dioxide, which is the gas produced by all burning or rapid oxidation of organic matter. To make combustion possible there must always be a supply of oxygen, and the necessity for the continuous supply of oxygen from the lungs and its carriage to every part of the body by means of the blood is apparent when the above-described conditions are understood.

488. Blood-plasma.—The fluid part of the blood in which the corpuscles float (para. 447) is called *plasma*, and its function is to carry nourishment to the tissues by passing or soaking through the walls of the capillaries, and to take up waste products from the tissues and carry them into the lymphatic system (see under Lymphatic System), returning to the blood-stream by way of the thoracic duct.

489. Blood-vessels.—All the blood-vessels are surrounded by muscle-fibres, which, however, are more numerous in the arteries than in the veins, and these fibres by their contraction regulate the calibre of the vessels and admit more or less blood to the parts they supply.

490. It must be borne in mind that all the work of the blood is done in the capillaries while it is moving slowly and that there is far more blood in the venous system than in the arterial. The vessel-muscles are under the control of the sympathetic system of nerves. Flushing and pallor are caused by the dilating and con-tracting, respectively, of the capillaries of the skin, and are caused by

"CIRCULATORY SYSTEM"

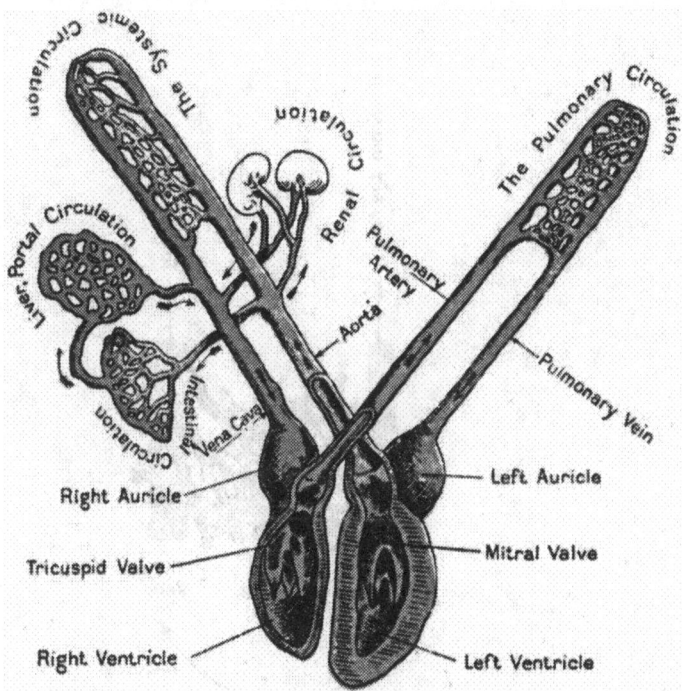

Fig.117.   *Diagram of the circulation of the blood*
The ventricles are seen in section to show the valves
The right & left side of the heart are shown separated

To face page 295

"BLOOD VESSELS"

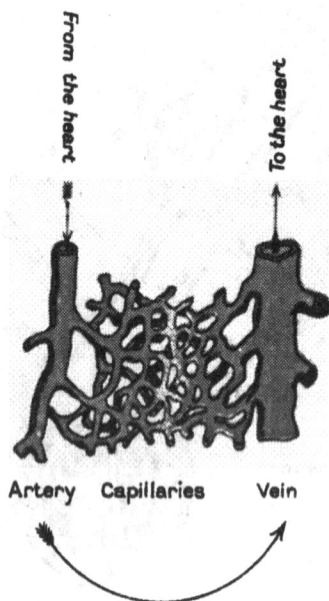

Fig. 118. *Diagrammatic sketch to show the three classes of blood vessels*

emotion, heat, cold, pressure, etc., acting on the local sympathetic ganglion, whether through the brain or reflexly.

491. The blood-supply of vital organs.—It is important that the supply of blood to all parts of the body should be uninterrupted, and that the vital organs should receive a copious supply. The vital organs, therefore, are placed in the chest and abdomen near the heart, which is the source of supply. The brain, which is a little further off, has a particularly free supply, being fed by four large arteries, into two of which (the carotids) the blood passes direct from the arch of the aorta ; the two others (the vertebrals) are branches of the subclavians which come from the arch of the aorta.

492. The arrangement of main vessels of the limbs.—The main arteries of the limbs are so placed that they are protected from pressure and stretching, which would arrest the flow of blood through them ; in the case of the limbs the most protected side is the flexor side, *i.e.*, that towards which the limb bends.

The artery of the upper limb, for instance, passes underneath the collar-bone, and thence deeply into the axilla or arm-pit ; then passing down the inner side of the humerus it goes in front of the bend of the elbow, where it divides into two branches which both pass down on the inner side of the forearm (when the arm hangs in a natural position), and pass over the wrist on the side towards which it bends ; the deep palmar arch formed by the junction of these two arteries is protected from pressure by being buried beneath the tendons deep in the palm of the hand.

In the lower limb, the main artery after passing out of the abdomen gains the centre of the groin (which is on the flexor side of the thigh), and then passes deeply down on the inner side of the thigh till it arrives at the middle of the back of the knee-joint. It divides into two branches a little distance below the knee, one branch keeping along the back of the tibia and going to the inner side of the back of the ankle, the other running down the front of the leg between its muscles to reach the front of the ankle, the two meeting in the sole of the foot where the plantar arch formed by them is placed in such a position under the arch of the instep that it cannot be compressed by the weight of the body in the standing position.

The Portal Circulation.

493. When describing the systemic circulation, it was stated that the blood in the systemic capillaries takes up nourishment from the stomach and bowels, but it was not mentioned that the whole of the veins which carry blood from the alimentary canal pass into a large vein called the portal vein, which splits up in the substance of the liver into which it enters. After passing through the interstices of the liver the blood is gathered into the hepatic or liver-veins and by them passed into the main vein which enters the heart.

In the kidneys, also, there is a secondary circulation of similar description.

(B 10977)   U

The Lymphatic System.

494. There is a circulatory system in the body which has not yet been alluded to, called the lymphatic system. It will be remembered (para. 449) that liquid nourishment is conveyed in the blood to every·part of the body by the blood-vessels, and oozes through the thin walls of the capillaries into the tissues, from which certain waste matters soak back into the capillaries and are conveyed into the veins. But the greater part of this necessary absorption is carried on by the lymphatic system, which receives the name of "absorbent system," also, on account of its important functions.

The lymphatic system is made up of :—(a) Lymphatic capillaries and lymph-spaces, into which fluids from the tissues soak, and which are to be found in every part of the body ; (b) lymphatic glands, to which all the lymphatic vessels converge and which are factories of white blood-corpuscles and in which filtration of the lymph takes place; (c) large lymph-vessels which collect lymph after it has passed through the glands, and empty it directly into the blood as it passes towards the heart in the veins; (d) the lymph itself, which is a clear, colourless, or faintly yellow fluid such as is seen in a blister. The lymph which passes from the intestine during digestion, however, becomes milky from being charged with fat.

495. Movements of the lymph.—The lymph is constantly moving from the extremities towards the centre. A large lymphatic vessel which returns it into the great vein in the chest is called the thoracic duct.

There is no outward going stream as in the case of the blood-circulation, and no heart to drive the lymph ; but all the vessels have many valves, and every movement of the body moves it forward and the valves prevent its return.

496. Lymph-capillaries.—Lymph-capillaries are larger and less regular in shape than blood capillaries, and commence in spaces in the tissues ; they are to be found in all parts of the body, as also are blood-vessels, and by their junction they form lymphatic vessels which join and branch to form networks of lymphatics, and pass into and out of the lymphatic glands.

497. Lymphatic glands.—The lymphatic glands are small bodies which are situated in various parts of the body, such as the bend of the knee and elbow, the groin and axilla, the back and sides of the neck, the mesentery, and the root of the lungs ; each set of glands receiving the lymph from the parts of the limbs and organs near which it is situated. If there is a "septic" or festering sore on the foot, the glands below the fold of the groin become inflamed from the poisoned lymph they have intercepted ; in case of such a sore occurring on the hand, the glands in the axilla are affected. In some general diseases the glands all over the body become enlarged. Medicines which are rubbed into the skin and those also which are hypodermically injected, become diffused by means of·the·lymphatic system.

THE DIGESTIVE SYSTEM.

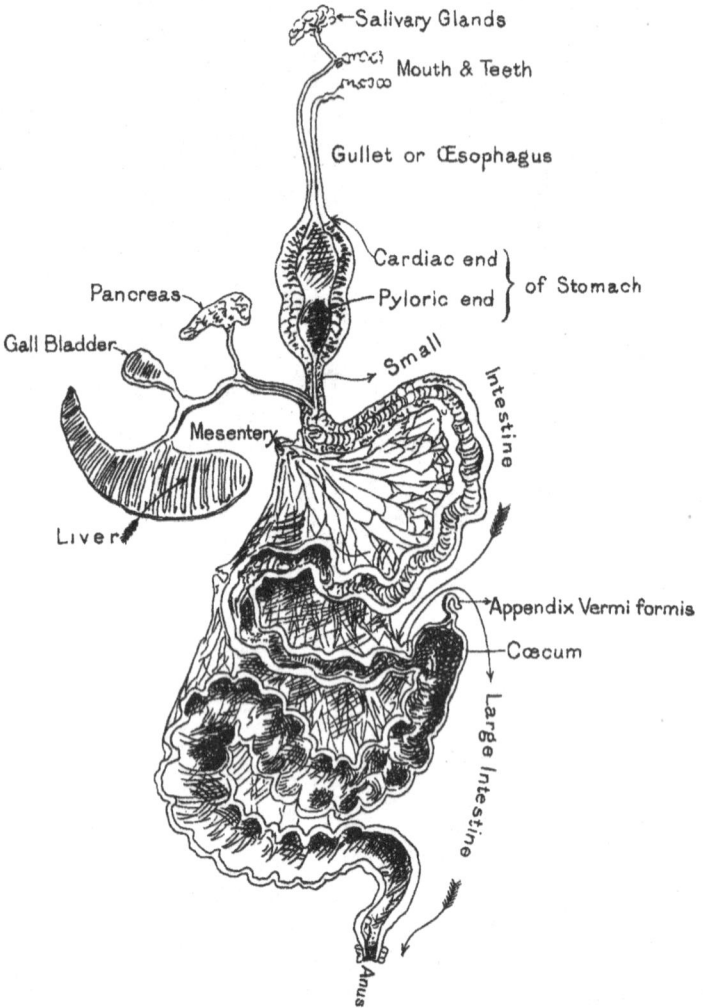

Fig.119 *Diagram to show Regions of Alimentary Canal.*
The Alimentary Canal is shown in section and
the mesentery is diagrammatic.

498. Lacteals.—The intestines are highly equipped with lymphatic vessels which take an active part in the absorption of fats into the system, and are called lacteals ; they are found in the *villi* (Fig. 120). These carry the digested fats into the mesenteric lymphatic vessels, which pass it into the thoracic duct which discharges into the great veins of the root of the neck.

499. Organs of a lymphatic nature.—The tonsils, Peyer's patches (see para. 505), and parts of the spleen are of the nature of lymphatic apparatus.

THE DIGESTIVE SYSTEM.

500. By digestion is understood the preparation of food to be received into the blood.

It is obvious that before it can be absorbed it must be dissolved.

501. Swallowing.—Food, which must consist of proper proportions of certain substances, viz., meats, fats, starches, salts, and water, is first placed in the mouth, where by the movements of the tongue and cheeks it is turned about and crushed between the teeth, the saliva running into it, until it is mixed up and can be swallowed ; this is done by the tongue pushing it into the upper part of the throat or pharynx, whose muscles seize it and pass it quickly down over the top of the larynx which is covered by the flap of the epiglottis until it has passed ; the muscles of the œsophagus now push it into the stomach.

The saliva begins the digestion of the starchy parts of the food.

502. Stomach.—The food remains in the stomach, which is represented in Fig. 119 as a very thick bag with a slight constriction in the middle. This constriction does not really exist, but is illustrated to show that the digestion in the stomach has two phases and that two different sorts of glands are at its opposite ends, producing two different sorts of gastric juice. The peptic glands are situated at the left end of the stomach (its first part), and the acid-forming glands towards the pyloric end, on the way to the intestine. The pyloric funnel-shaped end of the stomach itself has no acid forming glands, but has alkaline pepsine-glands.

Food remains about four hours in the stomach ; after which it is pressed out into the upper end of the small intestine or duodenum in an acid condition. The digestion of meat is done to a considerable extent in the stomach. A short distance down the intestine the duct carrying the bile and juice of the pancreas opens into it, and these juices are poured into the liquid food which is coloured yellow by the bile.

503. Small Intestine.—The small intestine is about 22 feet in length, and it and the greater part of the large intestine are attached to the spinal column by a double layer of membrane called the mesentery, between the folds of which the blood and lymph vessels and nerves pass to and from the intestine. The mesentery also serves to prevent the intestine from kinking, as any unattached coil would be sure to do.

The interior of the upper part of the small intestine has its lining raised into transverse ridges, called *valvulæ conniventes*, which prevent the too rapid passing of the liquid food and form a large surface for digesting and absorbing it. The whole length of the small intestine has its inside covered with small projections called *villi* (see Fig. 120), which have inside them blood-vessels and lymphatics (lacteals), and are bathed in the digested food and suck it up as it passes along. There are also many small glands in the walls of the intestine. These produce a digesting juice, which acting with the pancreatic juice and the bile, continues the digestion of the contents of the intestine and turns them alkaline : they were acid on leaving the stomach. The digestion of meats is completed by the pancreatic and intestinal juices ; that of starches by the pancreatic juice ; and that of fat, principally by the bile.

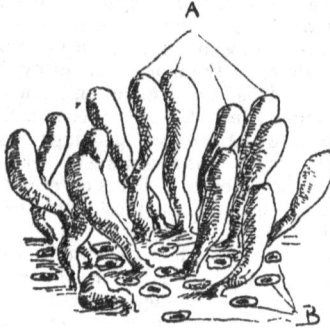

FIG. 120.

Diagram showing part of the interior of the small intestine with projections ("villi"), marked A, for absorbing digested matter, and recesses, marked B, for pouring out digestive fluid.

504. The intestines are furnished with circular bands forming a complete layer of involuntary muscular fibres, and also with a longitudinal layer. These contract slowly and in regular time ; waves of contraction proceeding from the upper towards the lower end of the tube, and squeezing the food onwards ; these movements are called *peristaltic* movements or *peristalsis*.

In the small intestine the fæces begin to acquire their foul smell ; and its contents cease to be antiseptic, as they were in the stomach.

505. Large Intestine.—The contents of the small intestine pass into the large intestine, which begins in the right iliac fossa. The large intestine, which is about five feet long, begins in a blind bag-like head, into the side of which the small intestine opens ; this head is called the cæcum. Attached to it is the vermiform appendix. It is this small, worm-like appendix which is affected in the disease called appendicitis.

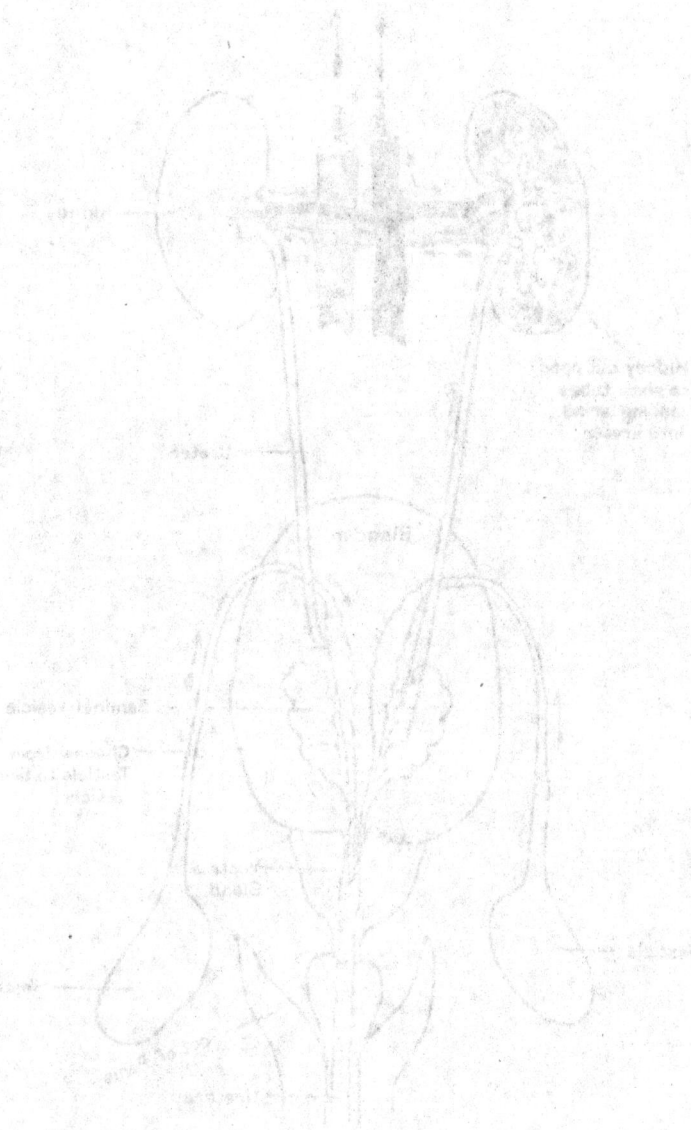
THE URINARY SYSTEM

THE URINARY SYSTEM

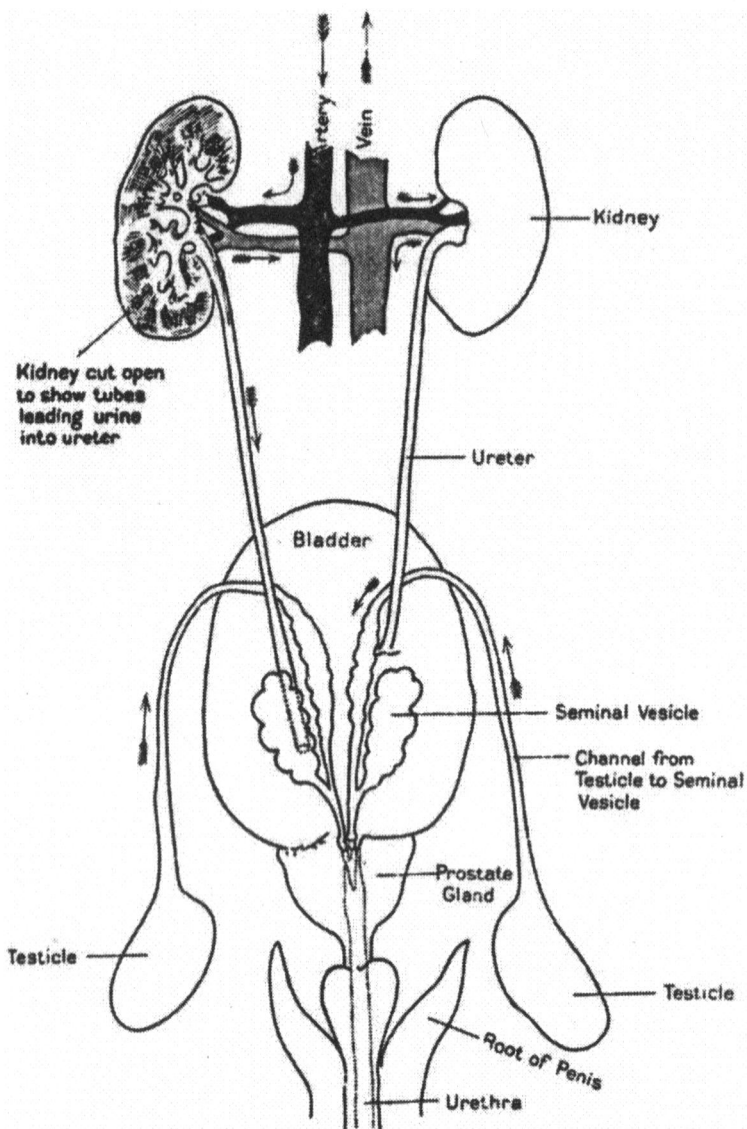

Artery

Vein

Kidney

Kidney cut open
to show tubes
leading urine
into ureter

Ureter

Bladder

Seminal Vesicle

Channel from
Testicle to Seminal
Vesicle

Prostate
Gland

Testicle

Testicle

Root of Penis

Urethra

Fig. 121.   *Diagrammatic sketch of genito-urinary organs*

The large intestine passes upwards in the right flank, then across the abdomen, then downwards through the left flank into the left iliac fossa, where it makes a double bend called the sigmoid flexure, and finally, the last part of it, called the rectum, goes downwards in front of the sacrum and coccyx and ends in the anus (see Fig. 119).

The process of putrefactive digestion is completed in the large intestine, and its contents become drier and formed in its lower end. The fæces are retained in the upper part of the rectum till it is convenient to void them.

The large intestine is provided principally with mucous glands whose secretion lubricates the passage of the fæces. In the lower part of the small intestines are masses of lymphoid glands called Peyer's patches, and single lymphoid glands. In the large intestine are single lymphoid glands. These lymphoid glands have no openings, and appear to have some connection with the lymphatic system.

506. The anus is kept closed by means of the sphincter muscles (of which there is an inner and outer one) until it is desired to defecate. These muscles act like purse-strings, being arranged circularly around the opening. The fæces are the undigested remains of food, mixed with the useless remains of the digesting fluids, and some matters excreted from the system ; and the whole mass is coloured by the bile and impregnated with foul gases.

The Urinary System.

507. This is one of vital importance to the body, inasmuch as it takes the largest share in the excretion (or getting rid) of waste products of the body, which would otherwise clog its organs and destroy life. This actually happens when the kidneys are destroyed by disease.

The urinary system consists of the kidneys, the ureters (two tubes which conduct the urine from the kidneys to the bladder), the bladder, and the urethra (a tube which conducts the urine from the bladder to be passed out of the body).

508. Kidneys.—The two kidneys are situated in the abdominal cavity (para. 461, Fig. 115), one on each side of the spinal column. They lie behind all the other contents of the abdomen, and their upper parts are as high as the last rib. They have each a very large artery passing in, and a vein passing out of them, on their inner and front edge ; the ureter comes out behind the vein and artery and goes down to enter the lower and back part of the bladder.

509. Bladder.—The bladder is situated in the pelvis (para. 461). It is a bag which is fixed at its base, and free to expand upward It will hold comfortably about one pint. It lies below all the intestines, and only rises into the abdomen when very full. It opens into the urethra at its lower part, and in the male at its neck has a gland called the prostate gland, through the middle of which the urethra goes. The receptacles for the semen lie behind the bladder at its base, and the tubes which conduct the semen from the testicles to the receptacles lie against its side.

The bladder has strong layers of involuntary muscle fibres which help the abdominal muscles to squeeze the urine out of it into the urethra, and which exercises pressure upon its contents at all times.

510. Male Urethra.—The urethra in the male (to which sex these remarks alone refer) is about $8\frac{1}{2}$ inches long and $\frac{1}{4}$-inch in diameter. It passes out from the base of the bladder through the prostate gland (see Fig. 122) in a downward direction, then curves forward to pass beneath the junction of the two pubic bones, joining with the two lateral roots of the penis along whose under surface it runs, ending in the orifice at its tip. Just after it has passed through the prostate gland, the openings of the seminal receptacles pass into the urethra. The rectum (lower end of large bowel) lies behind it as it passes the prostate. The situation of these parts is very necessary to know, as the introduction of the enema syringe's nozzle, and the passing of catheters properly, depends on such knowledge.

511. Action of the Kidneys.—The kidneys may be regarded as filters through which the whole blood of the body passes, and which remove from the blood a substance called *urea*, together with other impurities, dissolved in water, which together constitute the urine. The amount of urine passed off in a day is about 50 oz., or $2\frac{1}{2}$ pints. This quantity of urine contains about $2\frac{1}{2}$ oz. of solid matter. The urine is more watery and abundant in cold weather, as less water is then passed off by the skin than in hot weather.

As above stated, if the kidneys cease work from disease or other cause, the blood soon becomes poisoned by the accumulation of these matters in it, and "uræmia" with convulsions and insensibility results.

512. Structure of the Kidneys.—The kidneys consist of minute tubes which are folded and twisted, and end in small bags, each of which receives a tuft of capillary blood-vessels called vascular tufts. At their other ends the tubes open into the commencement of the ureters, in the "pelvis" or concave side of the kidney.

The water of the urine passes from the blood into the little bag at the ends of the tubes through the tuft of capillaries, and as it runs down the tube it is joined by the urea and other substances produced by the cells lining the tube walls, forming the urine. The cleansed blood passes on in its vessels, and the urine drains into the ureters and finally into the bladder.

The renal artery and vein are very large, and the blood passes through the kidneys rapidly.

513. Retention.—The urine is passed from the bladder as convenient, or when the bladder is full. When from any cause the water cannot be passed, "retention of urine" is said to occur.

To draw the water from the bladder an instrument called a catheter is used. It is a tube with a hole in the side near the end of it and is passed in at the orifice of the urethra until it reaches the bladder, the urine running through it.

To face page 300

"SECTION OF MALE PELVIS"

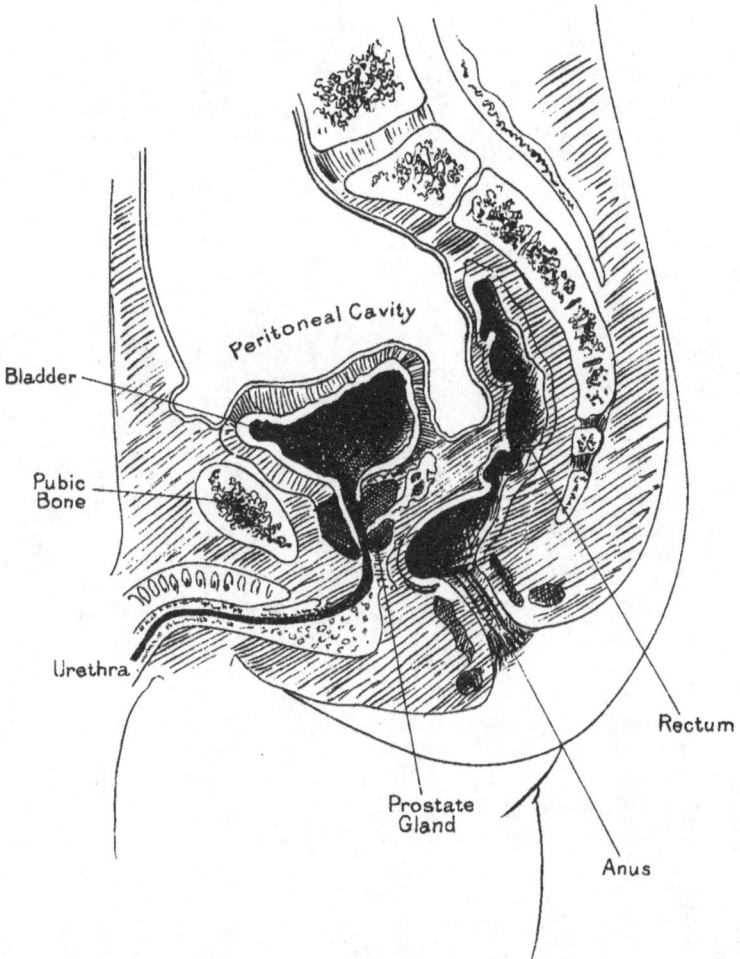

Peritoneal Cavity

Bladder

Pubic Bone

Urethra

Rectum

Prostate Gland

Anus

Fig. 122 Section from front to rear of a male pelvis
to show positions of bladder & rectum & the
course taken by the urethra, notice the direction
of the anus with view to passing nozzle of enema syringe.

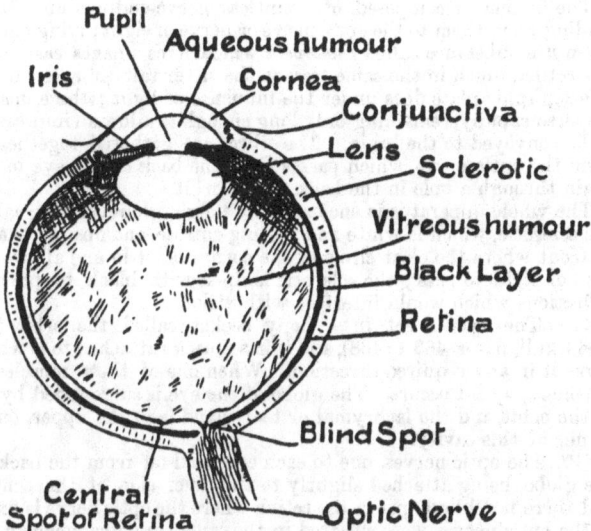

FIG. 123.—DIAGRAM OF SECTION THROUGH EYE (HORIZONTAL).

THE EYE.

514. The Eyes.—The eyes are delicate, optical organs, by means of which our brains are made aware of the shape, colour, size, and position of things within their range.

They consist principally of (1) the crystalline lens, commonly called the lens, a transparent refracting medium by which large things are reduced to a size small enough to be received as images upon the back of the eye ; (2) a sensitive screen called the retina, which is spread on the inside on the latter half of the globe of the eye, and on which any image thrown by the refracting medium is instantaneously photographed; and (3) the optic nerve, the fibres of which convey the impressions caused by the photographed images to the brain.

The cornea, which forms the clear part in front of the eye, aids as a refracting medium.

The lens is situated inside the globe of the eye near its front, and is about the size of a pea.

In front of the lens is a small chamber which is full of water (the aqueous humour), and behind it, filling out the shape of the eye, is a jelly-like substance called the vitreous humour.

515. The iris is a sort of diaphragm which covers the edges of the lens, and by its contraction and expansion regulates the amount of light admitted to the eye. It is coloured, and the aperture in its centre is called the pupil.

The retina is composed of countless nerve-endings and fibres leading from them to the optic nerve or nerve of sight; lying among them is a substance called *rhodopsin* which fixes images cast upon the retina, much in the same way as the silver salt in a sensitized photographic plate does under the influence of light ; these images disperse rapidly, remaining only long enough to allow an impression to be conveyed to the brain. The fibres are gathered together to form the optic nerve, which passes from the back of the eye to the brain through a hole in the back of the orbit.

The whole apparatus is enclosed in a tough, globular coat, called the sclerotic, which is white and shining outside, and opaque, except in front where the clear circle of the cornea is let in and allows the rays of light to pass ; the sclerotic is lined with black to prevent reflections which would interfere with vision.

516. The eye is set in a bony socket called the orbit (see The Skull, paras. 463 to 468), and it has muscles attached to it which move it in any required direction. When one of these muscles is too short, squint occurs. The globe of the eye is surrounded by fat in the orbit, and the lachrymal or tear-gland is in the upper, outer corner of this cavity.

517. The optic nerves, one to each eye, lead off from the back of the globe, being attached slightly to the inner side of the centre, and there is a blind spot in the retina where the optic nerve is fixed. If the optic nerves were situated in the centre any image which fell in the centre of the field of vision would be invisible, but as it is, the blind spots in the two eyes, not being in the centre, never have the same image cast upon them, and the centre of the retina is its most sensitive part.

518. The front and visible part of the globe of the eye is covered by a very sensitive membrane or skin called the conjunctiva, which is continued over the inner surface of the eyelids; it is transparent over the cornea, where it is closely fixed, and also over the sclerotic, but it is thicker and has more blood-vessels in it on the interior of the eyelids. The eyeball is kept always moist, so as to move without friction, by the tears which come from the lachrymal or tear-gland above mentioned, their surplus running down into the nasal passages by means of a tube called the lachrymal canal; the openings into this canal may be seen as two pinholes at the inner corners of the eyelids when they are pulled open, away from the eyeball. The tears only overflow when in grief, or when something irritates the conjunctiva and requires to be flushed out.

519. The eyelids are fringed with eyelashes, whose use is to prevent objects getting into the eyes.

520. **Errors of refraction.**—The refracting power of the eye is frequently imperfect, especially among people who do much reading or other work trying to the eyes, and instead of the picture being focussed as it should be exactly on the retina, it falls, in cases of short sight in front, and in long sight or old sight behind it. These "errors of refraction" are corrected by the use of concave and convex lenses or glasses. The exact degree or error is tested by means of test-

types and trial-lenses. Old sight is not really due to an error of refraction, but people with that condition need glasses to help them to read because the lens requires assistance to focus near objects.

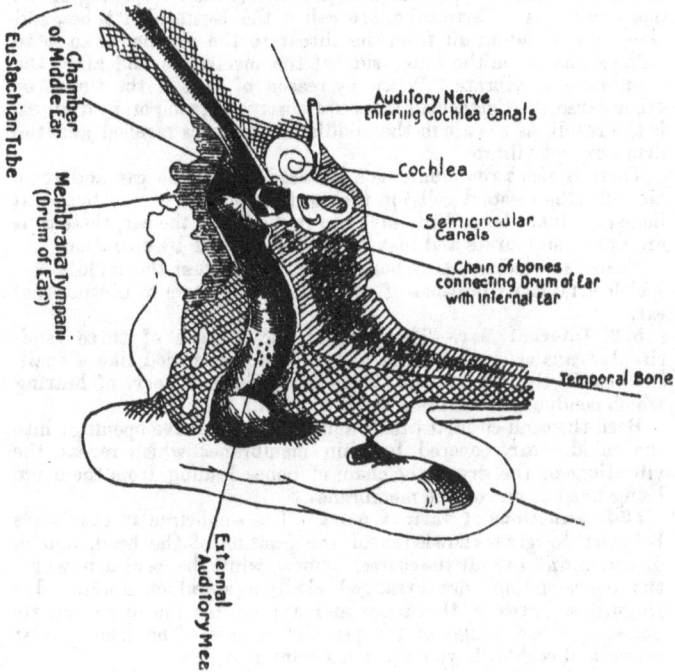

FIG. 124.—DIAGRAM OF SECTION THROUGH EAR.

THE EAR.

521. External Ear.—This organ consists of the external flap or *pinna*, which is made of cartilage, covered with skin, and shaped into ridges and depressions. It leads into the opening of the external meatus or ear-hole, a channel, the outer half of which is formed of cartilage prolonged from the pinna, while the inner half is a bony tunnel lined with thin skin. Hairs and wax-producing glands are found in the passage, which prevent small foreign bodies from reaching the delicate drum of the ear, placed obliquely at the inner end of the meatus. The passage is about one inch long and is slightly curved. The drum of the ear or membrana tympani is a thin membrane stretched across the inner end of the meatus, and kept in tension by a thin piece of bone, so as to cause it to vibrate.

522. Middle Ear.—The middle ear lies on the other side of the membrane, and in a small cavity hollowed out of the thickness of the temporal bone. It has a tube passing from it to the back of the throat where it opens on a level with the hinder opening of the nasal passages. These tubes are called the Eustachian tubes, and they serve to admit air from the throat to the middle ear so as to balance the air on the outer side of the membrane and allow the membrane to vibrate. When by reason of cold in the throat or other cause the Eustachian tubes are obstructed, temporary deafness is the result, as the air in the middle ear becomes rarefied and the drum cannot vibrate.

There is also a communication between the middle ear and some air-cells (the mastoid cells) in the mastoid process of the temporal bone (the lump behind the ear), and in disease of the ear, these cells are apt to suppurate and may have to be opened by operation.

There is a chain of tiny bones extending across the middle ear, which conducts vibrations of sound from the drum to the internal ear.

523. Internal Ear.—The internal ear consists of three semi-circular canals (on each side), a small chamber coiled like a snail-shell called the cochlea, and the auditory nerve or nerve of hearing which conducts the impressions to the brain.

Both the semi-circular canals and the cochlea have openings into the middle ear, covered by thin membranes which repeat the vibrations of the drum, the chain of bones leading from the drum being fixed to one of the membranes.

524. Functions of various parts.—The semi-circular canals are believed to give knowledge of the position of the head, and of direction, and to hear the coarser sounds; while the cochlea, in which the nerve-endings are arranged along a spiral membrane, distinguishes between the tones and appreciates the more delicate notes, and can judge of the pitch of sounds. The semi-circular canals and cochlea have fluid in their interior.

The external ear merely collects, and, by means of the column of air in the meatus, transmits the vibrations which constitute sound to the drum of the ear. The vibrations of the drum are conducted across the chamber of the middle ear to the membrane dividing the semi-circular canals from the middle ear, and are repeated by this membrane to the fluid on its other side and thus to the delicate nerve-endings spread out in the semi-circular canals and cochlea. The auditory nerve, as above stated, carries the impressions to the brain.

525. The external meatus sometimes gets stopped up either with wax or some foreign body ; these are usually dislodged by syringing, which must be done with great care, as the membrane has been ruptured by too hard syringing. The drum of the ear is often ruptured in artillerymen who stand near the muzzle of big guns when firing. This can be avoided by placing suitable plugs in the ear.

The Eustachian tube can be opened by blowing air into the pharynx with Politzer's bag which may be fitted to the Eustachian catheter.

NASAL PASSAGES &c.

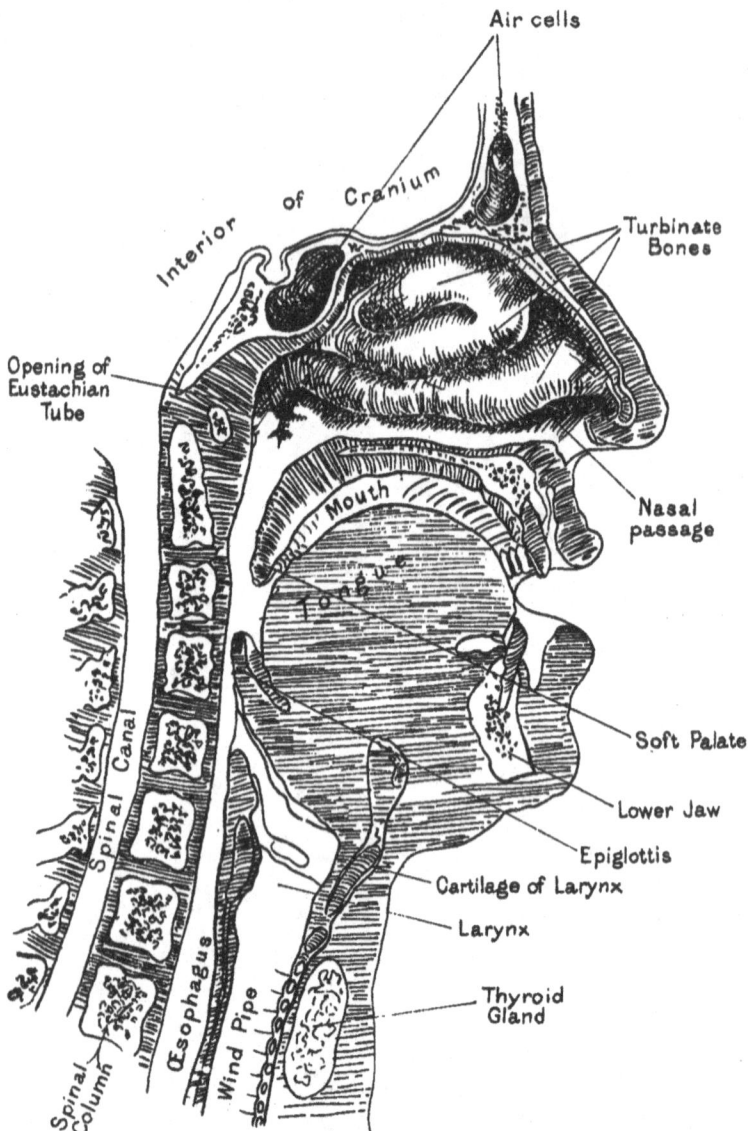

Fig. 125. *Section through head and neck to show positions of
nasal cavity, mouth, œsophagus & larynx
Slightly to left of mid-line.*

AIR AND FOOD PASSAGES.

526. The Nasal Passages.—The air before it reaches the lungs is warmed as it goes through the nasal passages, through which it is drawn during quiet breathing. During violent effort the mouth is also used.

These passages are formed by the bones of the face and palate (see under Skull). They are completed by cartilage in front and by the soft palate behind, and are lined with mucous membrane. The partition between the two sides is formed of bone and cartilage.

The outer sides have projecting from them three bones, called turbinate bones, which are curved downwards and which reach nearly to the partition or septum, thus partially dividing the passage into three channels on each side.

The floor of the passages is formed by the palate-plate of the upper jaw and by the palate-bone.

Several sets of air-cells communicate with the nasal cavities, and the tear-duct opens into the lower one.

527. The upper division of the passage and the upper pair of turbinate bones are the seat of the sense of smell, the branches of the olfactory nerves or nerves of smell being spread in the mucous membrane covering them.

The mucous membrane covering the rest of the passages is very fully supplied with blood, which warms the air on its passage to the lungs. Bleeding at the nose or epistaxis is caused by the rupture of one of these vessels.

528. The nostrils, which are the front openings into these passages, look downwards, and are provided with a number of hairs inside which intercept any foreign substance and stop it from being drawn into the air passages.

529. The posterior nares are the openings by which the air passes into the throat or pharynx after traversing the nasal passages; they are considerably larger than the nostrils.

In the operation of plugging the hinder nares and in passing the Eustachian catheter and the nasal feeding-tube, the instruments are put into the nostril and pushed along the floor of the nasal passage till they reach the pharynx, passing into it through the hinder nares.

In "cold in the head" it is the mucous membrane of the nasal passages which is inflamed, and the sense of smell is lost on account of the swelling up of the membrane which contains the nerve-endings of the olfactory nerve.

530. The Mouth.—The cavity of the mouth can be easily inspected, and needs little description. The teeth have been noticed (see under Skull).

The tongue is a muscular organ which is fixed at its base to the hyoid bone, a small curved bone which is to be felt just above the prominence of "Adam's Apple" (the larynx) under the skin in front of the neck. The tongue is covered with a rough skin on the top which has in it the nerves of taste, chiefly at the sides and back. Sweet, acid, salt, and bitter are the tastes perceived by the tongue and palate ; all other "tastes" are perceived by the organ of smell. The tongue can move in most directions, and is particularly active in the mastication of food, and in speech.

There are several glands which produce saliva and are called salivary glands, situated near and opening into the mouth; they are the parotid glands, which lie just below the ear, and near the angle or "corner" of the jaw; the sublingual glands, which lie under the tongue ; and the sub-maxillary glands, which are inside the angle of the lower jaw. There are also many glands which pour out mucus and keep the mouth moist.

531. The Fauces.—The epiglottis is a cartilaginous flap covered with mucous membrane, situated at the back of the tongue and immediately above the entrance to the larynx ; it is attached by ligaments to the back of the tongue, the side-wall of the pharynx, and the hyoid bone and thyroid cartilage. Near the back of the tongue on each side of the pharynx are seen the two pillars of the fauces enclosing the tonsil between them. The roof of the fauces is formed by the soft palate, attached to which is seen behind the pendulous part or uvula.

In swallowing, the larynx is drawn up by various muscles, the opening of the larynx being closed by the epiglottis ; the "bolus" or mass of masticated food is at the same time gripped by the muscles of the pharynx and gullet and so passed on to the stomach.

532. The Pharynx.—The pharynx is the cavity into which the mouth, and above it the posterior nares, open; it is like a "hopper" or funnel, and is suspended from the base of the skull, and continues down to the œsophagus behind and to the larynx in front. It has at its back the spinal column covered by muscle, and it is formed of muscles lined with mucous membrane ; the Eustachian tubes (see The Ear) open into it above the soft palate.

533. Distribution of air and food.—The pharynx receives both the air in breathing and the food in swallowing, and provision has to be made to direct them into their proper channels. In swallowing, it would be fatal if food found its way into the larynx, and most uncomfortable if it went up into the nose. To prevent the passage of food into the larynx, that organ is drawn up as before stated, the epiglottis covering its opening, and to prevent the food from passing up into the nasal cavity the soft palate acts as a valve, being flattened back against the back of the pharynx, the uvula filling up the central groove. The palate drops forward again against the back of the tongue when the food has passed.

During breathing, the muscles of the palate and epiglottis are inactive.

If any foreign body finds its way into the air passages, such as food or water, coughing is at once the result, and is Nature's method of expelling the substance, which would injure the air-passages.

"FOOD AND AIR PASSAGES."

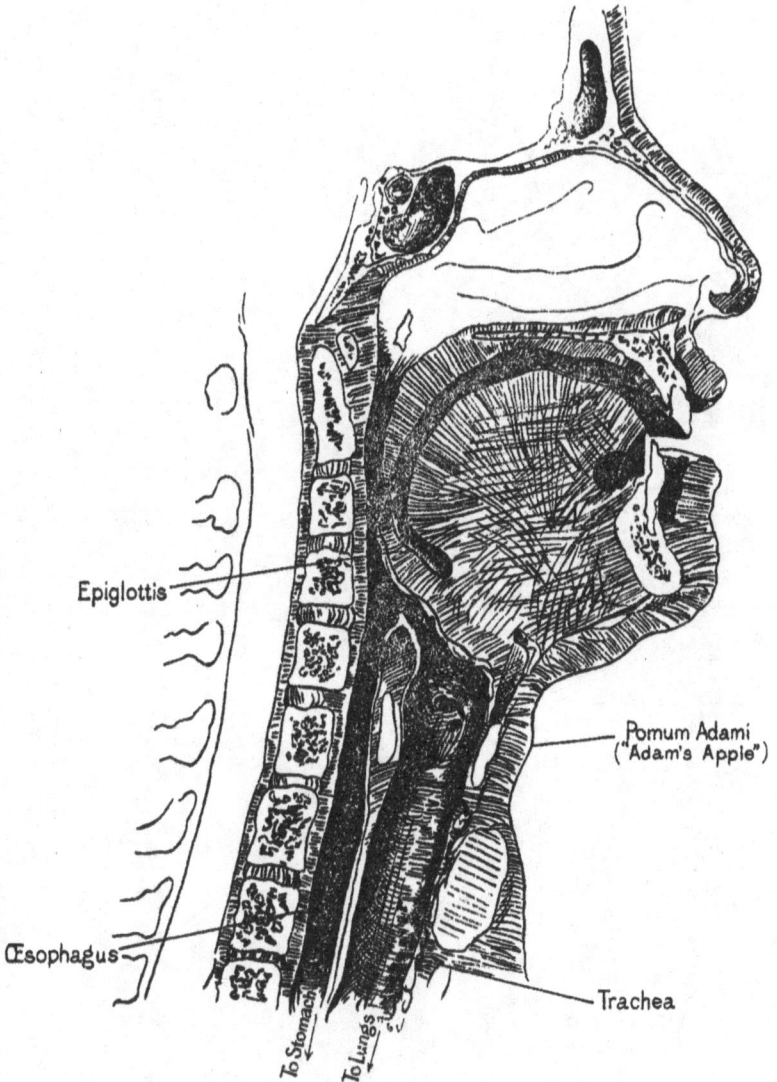

Epiglottis

Œsophagus

Pomum Adami
("Adam's Apple")

Trachea

To Stomach

To Lungs

Fig. 126. Section of head & neck to show food &
air passages.

CHAPTER XXX.

BANDAGES AND BANDAGING.

534. Instruction.—Great economy of time and labour will be effected in imparting instruction in bandaging, by practising one-half of the members of the class at a time in bandaging the other half. This can probably be best carried out by forming up the men in two ranks, and then causing the front rank to bandage the rear rank, and vice versa.

535. Bandages.—Bandages are used for many purposes, the chief of which are to fix splints or dressings, to apply pressure to a part, and to support the circulation. They may be divided into three classes, viz., triangular, roller, and special.

TRIANGULAR BANDAGES.

536. Description.—Triangular bandages, used chiefly on field service, are made by cutting pieces of calico or linen, 38 inches square, diagonally into halves ; each half then forms a triangular bandage. Of the three borders of the bandage, the longest is called the lower border, and the two others the side-borders. Of the three corners, the upper one, opposite the lower border, is called the point, and the remaining corners the ends.

Stowage.—To fold the bandage for stowage, it should be folded perpendicularly down the centre, placing the two ends together, the right end on the left ; then the ends and the point should be brought to the centre of the lower border, thus forming a square ; fold in half from right to left, and in half again from above downwards, twice.

I.

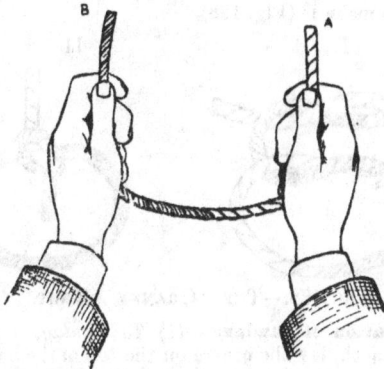

II.

III.

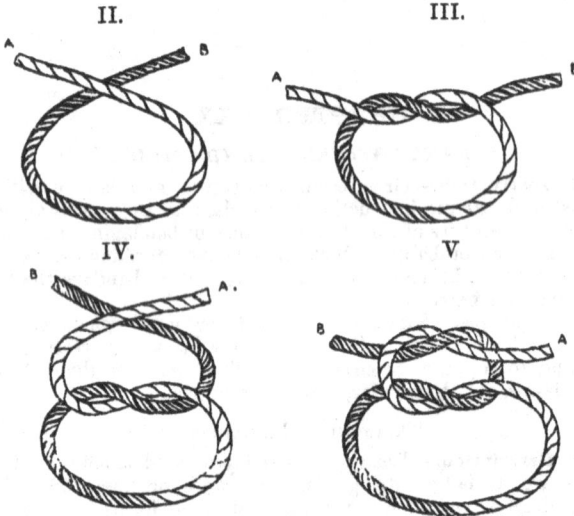

IV.

V.

FIG. 127.—How to Tie a "Reef-Knot."

Three modes of application.—The bandage is applied as (*a*) a whole cloth, (*b*) broad-fold, (*c*) narrow-fold. The whole-cloth is the bandage spread out to its full extent. The broad-fold is made from the whole-cloth by carrying the point to the centre of the lower border, and then folding the bandage again in the same direction. The narrow-fold is made by folding the broad-fold once lengthwise.

587. Reef-knots.—In every case where a knot has to be tied, a reef-knot will be used, the formation of which is best explained by the accompanying diagrams showing how to make it (Fig. 127), and how not to make it (Fig. 128).

I.

II.

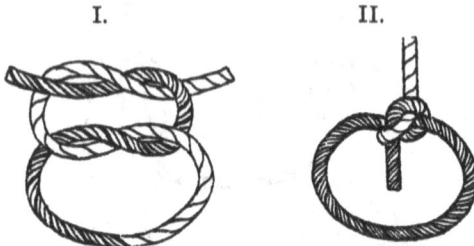

FIG. 128.—The "Granny" Knot.

588. Application of bandage.—(1) *To bandage top of head.*—Take a whole-cloth, lay the centre on the top of the head, the lower border lying along the forehead just above the eyebrows; fold in the edge, pass the end round behind, leaving the ears free ; cross below the occipital protuberance over the point of the bandage, bring the ends to the front again, and knot off on the centre of the forehead. Place the hand on the top of the head to steady the dressing, draw the point down to tighten and fit the bandage to the head, then turn it up and pin off on the top.

(2) *Side of head.*—Place the centre of a narrow-fold over the dressing, pass the ends horizontally round the head, cross, and knot off over the dressing.

(3) *Both eyes.*—Place the centre of a broad-fold between the eyes, carry the ends backwards, cross, and knot off in front.

(4) *One eye.*—Place the centre of a narrow-fold over the injured eye, pass one end obliquely upwards over the forehead, the other downwards across the ear ; cross below the bump at back of head and knot off above the eye-brow on injured side.

(5) *Chin and side of face.*—Place the centre of a narrow-fold under the chin, pass the ends upwards, and knot off over the top of head, tucking in the ends.

(6) *Neck.*—Place the centre of a narrow-fold over the dressing, cross the ends, bring back and knot off over the wound.

(7) *Chest.*—Apply the centre of a broad-fold over the dressing, pass the ends round, and knot off on the other side, leaving a long end ; take a narrow-fold, tie to long end, bring it over the shoulder, and pin off to broad-fold over the dressing.

(8) *Abdomen.*—Place the centre of a broad-fold over the wound and knot off on the side.

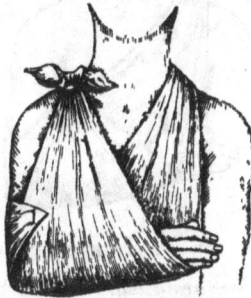

Fig. 129.—Greater Arm-sling.

(9) *To apply the greater arm-sling.*—Take a whole-cloth, throw one end over the shoulder on the sound side, carry round the neck so as to lie over the opposite shoulder ; place the point behind the elbow of the injured arm, allowing the other end to fall down in front of the patient ; bend the injured arm carefully, and place it across the chest on the middle of the bandage, thumb pointing towards the chin ; bring up the lower end in front of the forearm and knot off to the end lying over the shoulder on the injured side ; draw the point forward round the elbow and pin off.

(10) *In broken collar-bone.*—There is one exception to the above method of applying the greater arm-sling, viz., in fracture of the clavicle, where it is not advisable to allow anything to press on the injured bone. To avoid this, the lower end, which is brought up in front of the forearm, should be passed between the arm and the side of the injured shoulder, and knotted off to the upper end behind the neck (Fig. 130).

The triangular bandage may be also used to secure the arm temporarily in cases of fractured clavicle. Having placed a small pad in the arm pit, apply the centre of a narrow-fold bandage to the outer surface of the arm of the injured side, and carry the front-end horizontally across the chest ; bring the back-end forwards between the arm and chest (on the injured side), over the upper margin and front of the horizontal end, then pass it upwards and backwards through the loop thus formed to the back of the chest, and exercise steady traction, so as to draw the arm backwards ; then secure the two ends on the opposite side of the chest. The arm-sling depicted in Fig. 129 can then be applied.

Instead of triangular bandages an ordinary roller bandage may be used, taking care to place a pad between the upper arm and the chest, to draw the upper arm well back, and to support the elbow, as shown in Fig. 131.

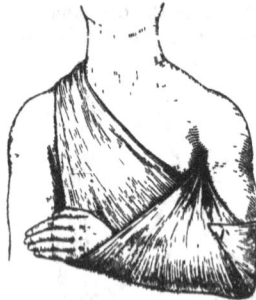

FIG. 130.—ARM-SLING FOR FRACTURED COLLAR-BONE (CLAVICLE).

(11) *To apply the lesser arm-sling.*—Take a broad-fold, place one end over the shoulder on the sound side, carry it round the back of the neck so as to lie over the opposite shoulder, allowing the other end to fall down ; bend the arm carefully and place the wrist across the middle of the bandage with the hand a little higher than the elbow, bring up the lower end, and knot off to the upper end over the shoulder on the injured side.

(12) *To bandage the shoulder.*—Lay the centre of a whole-cloth on the top of the shoulder, point-upwards, the lower border lying across the middle of the arm. Fold in the lower border, carry the ends round the arm, cross them, and knot off on the outer side.

Apply the lesser arm-sling, draw the point of the first bandage under the arm-sling, fold it back on itself, and pin off over the shoulder.

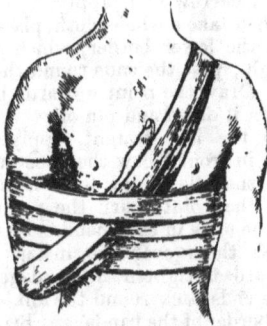

Fig. 131.—Roller Bandage for Fractured Collar-bone.

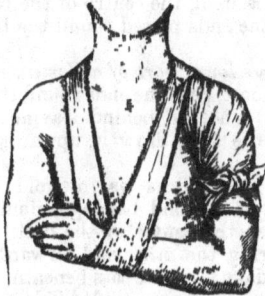

Fig. 132.—Shoulder Bandage and Lesser Arm-sling.

(13) *Elbow.*—Place the centre of a whole-cloth over the back of the bent elbow, point-upwards, turn in the lower border, pass the ends round the forearm, cross them in front, pass up round the arm, cross behind, and knot off in front. Tighten the bandage by drawing on the point, which is then brought down and pinned off. Apply greater arm-sling.

(14) *Hand.*—Take a whole-cloth, place the hand palm-downward on the centre of the bandage, fingers towards the point, bring the point over the back of the hand to the wrist, pass the ends round the wrist, crossing them over the point which is then folded towards the fingers, and covered by another turn of the bandage round the wrist. Knot off the ends in front of the wrist.

(B 10977)

x

Or a figure-of-8 bandage (narrow-fold) may be used. Place centre of bandage over dressing, bring ends round to opposite side of hand, cross and take two or three turns round the wrist, and knot off. Apply the greater arm-sling.

(15) *Hip.*—Take a narrow-fold, apply it round the waist, and knot off in front ; then take a whole-cloth, place the centre over the hip, point-upwards, the lower border, which should be folded in, lying across the thigh ; pass the ends round the thigh, and knot off on the outer side. Draw the point upwards beneath the bandage round the waist, turn it down and pin off.

(16) *Knee.*—Keep the leg straight, apply a broad-fold, cross behind, and knot off in front below the knee-cap.

(17) *Foot.*—Place the sole of the foot on the centre of a whole-cloth, toes towards the point ; turn the point upwards over the instep, take one of the ends in each hand close up to the foot, bring them forward, cross them over the instep covering the point. Draw the point upwards to tighten the bandage and fold it towards the toes. Carry the ends back round the ankle, cross them behind catching the lower border of the bandage. Bring the ends forward, cross them again over the instep, covering the point, carry them beneath the foot, and knot off on the inner side.

(18) *Other part of limbs.*—When applied to any other part of the limbs, a broad-fold is used, the centre of the bandage being placed over the dressing, the ends passed round the limb, and knotted off over the wound.

(19) *Perinœum and lower part of abdomen.*—Take a whole-cloth, lower border uppermost, pass the ends round the waist immediately above the hips, and knot off behind leaving one long end ; pass the point between the legs, draw it upwards, and knot off to the long end behind.

Another method :—Apply a narrow-fold bandage round the waist ; pass the end of a second bandage, similarly folded, beneath the waist-bandage at the centre of the back, fold over and secure with safety-pin ; bring the other end forward between the thighs up to the waist bandage in front, pass beneath, turn over and secure with safety-pin. This forms a modified T-bandage.

(20) *To fix splints.*—Take a narrow-fold bandage, double it upon itself, and place the loop thus formed upon the splint on the outer side of the limb ; pass the free ends round the limb from without inwards, and one of them through the loop ; tighten the bandage by steadily drawing on the two ends, and then knot them in the usual way.

ROLLER BANDAGES.

539. Varieties.—Roller bandages are made of calico, linen, flannel, loose-woven material, gauze impregnated with some antiseptic, or of elastic webbing. The rollers ordinarily in use for bandaging the head or limbs are made of loose-woven material. Flannel bandages are used for special purposes, for warmth, or after inunctions. Loose-woven bandages are used with plaster of

Paris. Gauze bandages are used in antiseptic dressings. Elastic web bandages are used to support the circulation, or exercise pressure on a limb.

540. Sizes.—Roller bandages consist of long strips, varying in length and width according to the part to which they are to be applied, thus :—For the head and upper limbs, 2½ inches wide, and from 3 to 6 yards long ; for the fingers, ¾-inch wide, and 1 yard long ; for the trunk and lower limbs, 3 or more inches wide, and 6 to 8 or more yards long.

They are tightly rolled on themselves in a compact, cylindrical form ready for use.

541. Instruction in rolling.—The class will first be instructed in the proper methods of rolling a bandage, single and double-headed, and at the conclusion of the exercises the bandages will invariably be inspected, to see that each man hands his in properly rolled.

542. Application of Bandage.—To apply the bandage, the operator stands or sits opposite the patient. The limb is placed in the position it is to occupy when bandaged, and care must be taken that the bandage is not put on so tightly as to cause discomfort, or swelling of the limb below ; a bandage too tightly applied may produce gangrene of the limb, by cutting off its blood supply. If, on squeezing the tips of the fingers or toes of the bandaged limb, it is observed that the colour returns much more slowly than when this is done on the unbandaged limb, it may be assumed that the bandage is too tight.

The roller is taken in the right hand when bandaging the left limbs, and in the left hand when bandaging the right. The outer surface of the bandage is applied to the inner side of the wrist or ankle, and two turns taken straight round the limb from its inner to its outer side, to fix it.

(1) *Simple spirals.*—From this point the bandage may be taken up the limb in simple spirals, that is, evenly put-on turns of the bandage, each overlapping for one-third the width of the bandage below, taking care to have the lower edges of the turns of bandage parallel with each other.

(2) *Reverse spirals.*—When the swell of the limb is reached, the edges can no longer be maintained parallel, the bandage will not lie evenly, and gaps occur between the turns if the simple spiral is used. It therefore becomes necessary to use the reverse.

To make the reverse, the thumb of the disengaged hand is placed on the lower border of the bandage on the outer side of the limb, the bandage is slackened and turned over, reversed downwards, and passed round the limb to the opposite side, its lower edge parallel with that of the turn below. On reaching the outer side the reverse is again made, and so on up to the joint. The angles formed by the successive reverses must be kept in a straight line.

(3) *Figure-of-*8.—On reaching the joint, neither the spiral or reverse will lie evenly, so that the figure-of-8 has to be resorted to. This, as its name implies, is applied by passing the

(B 10977)   X 2

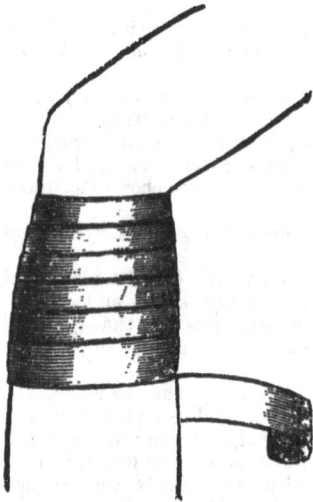

FIG. 133.—SIMPLE SPIRAL.   FIG. 134.—REVERSE SPIRAL.

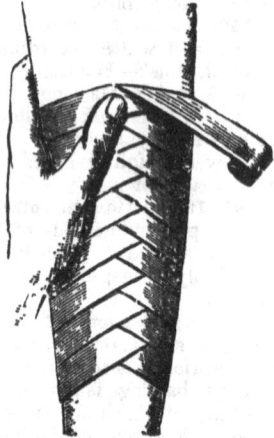

roller obliquely round, alternately upwards and downwards, the turns resembling the figure 8, each figure overlapping the one below by one-third the width of the bandage. The crossings of the figures should be kept in the same line as the reverses below.

(4) *Removal of bandage.*—To remove a bandage it should be unrolled from the top, and the slack gathered into a ball and passed from hand to hand round the limb.

(5) *To bandage a finger.*—Take two turns round the wrist, carry the bandage across the back of the hand to the root of the injured finger, up the finger by an open spiral to the top, whence it is brought by an evenly-laid close spiral to the root ; then across the back of the hand to the opposite side of the wrist from that which it started from, round the wrist once or twice, and pinned off.

(6) *To bandage the hand or foot.*—Two turns are taken round the wrist or ankle, the bandage carried across the hand or foot to the opposite side, passed across the palm or sole, and brought back to the opposite side of the wrist or ankle, over the back of the hand or foot, thus forming a figure-of-8, which may be repeated as often as required.

(7) *To bandage the chest.*—A roller 6 inches wide and from 6 to 8 yards long is used. It is applied from below upwards, in a single spiral, each spiral overlapping the one below for one-half its breadth. On completing the last spiral, the bandage is pinned off behind, leaving about a yard and a half free ; this end is brought over one shoulder as a brace, carried obliquely down over the bandage in front to the lowest turn, to which, as well as to the upper turns, it is fastened, thus preventing the bandage from slipping down.

(8) *To bandage the abdomen.*—A bandage to the abdomen is similarly applied to that for the chest, except that it may be put on from above downwards, and that it is kept in position by the free end being carried from behind forward between the thighs, and fastened in front.

(9) *To bandage the head.*—To keep a dressing on an ordinary wound of the head a few circular turns of a bandage are sufficient.

The knotted bandage.—To exert pressure on a graduated compress applied over a bleeding wound the knotted bandage is used. This is made with a single-headed bandage. The bandage should be unrolled for about a foot, and the end held in the left hand, which is kept close to the temple, the roller is then carried round the forehead and occiput, so that it comes back to the unrolled end at the wound. At this point the roller is twisted round sharply and then carried down below the chin and over the vertex. On coming to the temple again the same twist is made, and the roller is once more passed round horizontally; when sufficient pressure is obtained the bandage is fixed by knotting the two ends together.

(10) *To bandage the groin, shoulder, or thumb.*—*The spica bandage:*—A roller bandage may be applied to the groin, shoulder, or thumb in the following manner, which is known as the spica bandage.

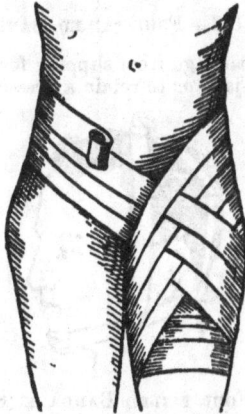

FIG. 135.—SPICA BANDAGE.

It is made by applying the bandage in a series of figure-of-8 turns, overlapping from below up. Take two turns of a single-headed roller round the thigh from within outwards as a point of attachment; carry the bandage upwards over the groin above the hip, and round the back to the opposite hip, then across in front of the abdomen, passing round the other side of the thigh and upwards between the thighs to complete the figure-of-8.

The turns are to be repeated as often as necessary.

Special Bandages.

543. Varieties.—(1) *The T-bandage.*— The T-bandage is specially prepared by taking a piece of bandage 3 inches wide and 1½ yards long and sewing to it another similar strip 1 yard long, so as to form a T, the free end of the short portion of the T being split sufficiently to enable one piece to be brought up on each side of the scrotum. It is applied by passing the long strip round the hips so that the attached part is at the sacrum; pin off in front. Bring up the short piece between the thighs, and fasten to the first piece in front. It is used to keep a dressing on the perinæum.

(2) *The four-tailed bandage.*—To prepare the four-tailed bandage, take a yard and a half of 3-inch roller bandage, make a slit in its centre about 3 inches long, and then slit up the ends so as to leave 6 inches in the centre. In applying it, place the central slit on the point of the chin, tie the two upper tails behind the neck, and the two lower tails on the top of the head; the ends of the upper and lower tails should then be tied together behind the

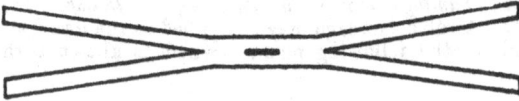

FIG. 136.—FOUR-TAILED BANDAGE.

head to prevent the bandage from slipping forward. It is used for fracture of the lower jaw, or to retain a dressing on the chin.

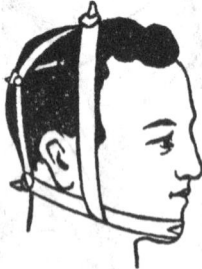

FIG. 137.—FOUR-TAILED BANDAGE (SIDE VIEW).

CHAPTER XXXI.

WOUNDS.

544. Definition.—A wound may be defined as the forcible solution of continuity of any of the tissues of the body; but the term is more commonly limited to injuries of the soft parts, involving the skin or mucous membrane.

Injuries in which the skin is not involved, and in which the deeper structures, such as bones and ligaments, etc., do not participate are usually spoken of as contusions. Therefore wounds may be described as (1) subcutaneous, *i.e.*, contusions, (2) open.

545. Classification.—Open wounds are usually classified under the following headings:—

(1) *Incised.*—These wounds are made by sharp-cutting instruments, such as a knife, razor, or a sharp sword. They have clean cut edges, and their length is usually greater than their depth. They frequently bleed freely, because the vessels are cleanly divided Bruising of the margins of the incision is absent, and, when properly treated, they generally heal rapidly, leaving simply a line-like scar.

(2) *Lacerated.*—Such injuries are caused by blunt instruments, by machinery, by the wheels of vehicles, or by fragments of shells.

As the name implies, these wounds have usually ragged edges, and there may be actual loss of substance. They do not as a rule bleed much, because the vessels are torn rather than cleanly divided. Bruising of the margins of the wound may occur, and they do not usually heal so rapidly as incised wounds, and the resulting scars are more marked.

(3) *Punctured wounds and stabs.*—These may be produced by any form of penetrating instrument, from a hat-pin or needle, to a sword or bayonet.

The wound is deep and narrow. The skin-wound may in itself be insignificant, but the chief danger of this class of wound is due to the liability of the deeper structures being injured; thus, blood-vessels and nerves may be divided, or the abdominal or thoracic contents injured. They do not usually bleed much externally, but may give rise to serious internal hæmorrhage. When the inflicting instrument is clean, they frequently heal without trouble.

(4) *Contused wounds.*—These are usually caused by injuries from blunt instruments, such as a stone, or kick from a boot. The edges are always more or less bruised. Contused and lacerated wounds are practically the same.

(5) *Gunshot-wounds*, whether caused by small-bore bullets or shells, are simply modifications of one or other of the above.

Small-bore bullet-wounds.—If the bullet has not struck anything before hitting the patient it usually causes a clean wound of the punctured variety, penetrating right through the body. Accordingly, two or more skin wounds will be noticed, one where the bullet enters (called the wound of entrance), and a second where the bullet leaves (called the wound of exit). Four or more skin-wounds may thus be caused by one bullet, as, for instance, when the arm and chest, or both thighs, are perforated. The entrance-wound is usually circular in form, slightly smaller than the bullet that made it, and the edges of the skin may be slightly inverted or tucked in. The exit-wound is frequently larger than the wound of entrance, and may be circular or irregular in shape, depending upon the structures injured in the body; the edges of the skin may be slightly everted or turned outwards. Between the wounds of entrance and exit there is injury to the tissues in the track along which the bullet has passed. This bullet-track (taking into consideration the position of the body when struck) is usually a straight line from the wound of entrance to the wound of exit. Thus, a wound which has apparently involved the chest or abdomen may, on putting the patient into the position he was in when struck, be found not to have done so, and vice versa.

A bullet may strike a stone before hitting the patient and become altered in shape, and the resulting wound may then be lacerated in character as well as punctured; and, moreover, the bullet may lodge in the body instead of passing through it as usual. Again, owing to the angle at which it strikes the body, a bullet may cause a deep groove with actual loss of tissue, instead of a wound of the punctured variety.

Shell-wounds generally produce considerable laceration of the parts, and may lead to the total destruction of a limb, etc. They have no peculiarities beyond their severity, but, being open ragged wounds, they are more liable to septic infection.

(6) *Poisoned wounds.*—By these are meant any of the above class of wounds which have become infected with septic matter, that is to say, germs. They are of a serious nature, as the germs growing in the wounds produce poisonous substances, which are absorbed into the body and produce constitutional symptoms, such as fever, etc.; moreover, if unchecked, blood-poisoning may be set up and death result. The great importance of keeping all wounds aseptic (or germ free) must therefore be obvious.

Snake bite, etc.—Under poisoned wounds may be included special wounds, such as the bites from poisonous snakes and the stings of insects; wounds from poisoned arrows or spears must also be mentioned.

In bites from poisonous snakes the poison is injected into the wounds at the moment they are made. They are very dangerous, because the poison rapidly reaches the blood, often causing the death of the patient in a very short time.

Treatment of snake-bite.—It is most important to endeavour to allay the anxiety of the patient. The *first* thing to do is to prevent the poison from reaching the heart through the veins. This is done by immediately tying a piece of string, or a strong strip of shirt or handkerchief, very tightly round the limb some distance above the wound, between it and the heart, so that the part below is strangled. *Next*, if any brandy or other stimulant be at hand, give a good dose, as the snake-poison has the effect of stopping the circulation. Then, if possible, cut freely into the wound and encourage bleeding, and until this has been thoroughly done do not take off the band.

If permanganate of potash crystals are available, make a cross-shaped incision over the bite and rub some of the crystals in thoroughly.

If the breathing is bad or has stopped, use artificial respiration.

Should the wound be in a part of the body where a band cannot be placed, then at once make a crucial incision to encourage it to bleed, and give stimulants.

Treatment of stings of venomous insects.—The stings of bees, wasps, hornets, etc., should, if found, be removed ; ammonia, or bicarbonate of soda, if available, should be applied.

CHAPTER XXXII.

THE DRESSING AND HEALING OF WOUNDS.
(INCLUDING THE FIRST FIELD DRESSING.)

546. General remarks.—Absolute cleanliness in the dressing of wounds is imperative. By absolute cleanliness is meant *surgical cleanliness*, and this means much more than ordinary cleanliness.

We have seen in the preceding chapter that poisoned wounds are caused by their becoming infected with germs, and a poisoned wound may lead to the death of a patient.

The hands are great carriers of germs, and so may easily infect a clean wound.

A dresser should take the utmost care of his hands, especially as regards the nails and the folds of skin surrounding them. This care of the hands should be a daily duty.

547. Rules to be followed in applying dressings.—(1) Never begin to change a dressing until everything that is to be likely to be required for the new dressing is ready close to hand.

(2) Arrange the bed-clothes so that no part of them can touch the wounded area ; the bedding, etc., should be protected from damp, etc., by means of jaconet or mackintosh.

(3) Remove the bandages, but do not touch the actual dressing at present.

(4) Scrub your hands most thoroughly with soap and a stiff nail-brush which has been soaked in antiseptic solution, or preferably, previously boiled.

(5) Rinse off the soap, and, without drying your hands, soak them for some minutes in antiseptic solution.

(6) Having thus cleaned your hands as thoroughly as possible, do not on any account allow them to touch anything such as your clothing, your face, or the patient's bedding or person. Do not dry them unless a sterilized towel is available to dry them on.

(7) Never touch either dressings or wound with the fingers : use a pair of sterilized forceps instead.

(8) Remove the old dressing with the forceps, having first loosened it, if it has stuck, with warm antiseptic solution. Be careful to wipe from the wound outwards, so as not to carry germs from the surrounding skin into the wound.

(9) Place the fresh, sterilized dressing gently in position with the forceps and then re-bandage the wounded area.

(10) Before dressing any wound or assisting at an operation which might produce infection, it is advisable to protect any cuts or scratches on the hands, covering them with a couple of layers of gauze and painting that over with collodion, so as to make a waterproof coating.

(11) If the necessary means of purifying the wound are not at hand, do not attempt to wash it or wipe its surroundings ; simply apply a dry, antiseptic dressing.

(12) All old dressings should be at once removed and destroyed, preferably by burning.

548. First field dressing.—A field dressing forms a component part of every British soldier's kit on active service, so as to be available, at all times and in all places, as a first dressing for wounds.

When officers and men go on active service the first field dressing will be placed in the pocket on the right side of the skirt of the frock (see Clothing Regulations),and thus the quantity of material required to be carried as medical stores is reduced. It should never be carried in the trouser-pocket or stitched in the helmet.

The field dressing, pattern 1911, consists of an outer packet of sewn khaki cotton cloth, containing two small separate dressings, each complete in itself. Each single dressing consists of :—(1) A loose-woven bleached cotton bandage, $2\frac{1}{2}$ yards long by $2\frac{1}{2}$ inches wide ; (2) a piece of bleached cotton gauze, 36 inches by 23 inches, weight not less than 260 grains, folded into a pad 4 inches by $3\frac{1}{4}$ inches and stitched to the bandage 18 inches from one end ; (3) one safety-pin.

The bandage and gauze pad are enclosed in waterproof jaconet, the edges cemented with rubber solution so as to render the packet air-tight, having a portion of one of the corners turned back and not cemented. The pin is wrapped in waxed paper and attached outside the jaconet.

The gauze contains 1 per cent. by weight of sal alembroth and is tinted with aniline blue.

The gauze pad is folded once, so that the bandage lies outside the gauze. The short end of the bandage is folded in plaits ; the long end is also folded in plaits for 18 inches from the pad and then loosely rolled for the remainder of its length. The rolled portion of the bandage is secured by a stitch to prevent unrolling.

The contents are compressed so that the outer packet does not exceed $4\frac{1}{4}$ inches in length, $3\frac{1}{8}$ inches in width, and $\frac{7}{8}$ of an inch in thickness.

Printed directions for use are upon the outside cover, and a printed label of directions for use is placed upon each of the two inside covers.

Printed directions for outer cover :—

WAR OFFICE, MEDICAL DIVISION.

First Field Dressing.

To open. { Outer cover.—Pull tapes apart.
Inner waterproof cover.—Tear apart the uncemented corners as indicated by the arrow.

*Contents :—*Two dressings in waterpoof covers, each consisting of a gauze pad stitched to a bandage, and a safety-pin.

Directions for use :—Take the folded ends of the bandage in each hand, and, keeping the bandage taut, apply the gauze pad to the wound and fix the bandage. One dressing to be used for each wound. *Do not handle the gauze or wound.*

(Maker's name, date, month and year.)
(*sic*) S. MAW, SON & SONS, LONDON,
February,
1911.

Printed label of directions for inner cover :—

WAR OFFICE, MEDICAL DIVISION.

First Field Dressing.

Tear apart the uncemented corners as indicated by the arrow. Take the folded ends of the bandage in each hand, and, keeping the bandage taut, apply the gauze pad to the wound and fix the bandage. *Do not handle the gauze or wound.*

(Maker's name, date, month and year.)
(*sic*) S. MAW, SON & SONS, LONDON,
February,
1911.

549. How to apply first field dressing.—In applying the first field dressing the points to be attended to are—Expose the wound by cutting open the clothing, never by dragging it over the wound. Never wipe the wound or attempt to clean it while on the field. Open the packet, taking care not to drop the contents on the ground, and not to handle the gauze that will touch the wound. Apply a dressing as directed on the covers, putting the gauze straight on the wound.

For a second wound, use the second dressing as instructed in the directions on the outer cover.

550. Healing of wounds.—The way in which a wound heals is as follows :—

(1) The blood escapes.

(2) The ends of the divided blood-vessels draw back, contract, and clots of blood form in them, thus stopping the bleeding.

(3) The fluid part of the blood continues to ooze out, finally gets jelly-like, and sets, glueing the edges together ; a little of the fluid part of the blood which escapes forming a scab or crust on the surface. At no time is there any discharge beyond a small quantity of blood-stained serum in the first twenty-four hours.

(4) New blood-vessels gradually make their way from side to side of the wound, and the circulation is thus restored : new tissue is produced and unites firmly the cut surfaces. At the end of ten days or a fortnight the wound has completely healed, a thin red scar being all that remains of it. This is what happens in a cut when the surfaces of the wound touch one another, and is called " healing by first intention."

When the wound is large and the raw surfaces cannot touch one another, small, red, rounded projections, called granulations, grow from the bottom and sides of the wound until it is filled up, and a new skin is gradually formed over them. In the end a scar forms, which, when the wound is quite healed, is slightly drawn in ; this is called " healing by granulation." Wounds which heal by granulation are much more difficult to keep free from infection.

The main object in the dressing of a wound is to protect it from the entry of small bodies, called germs. These not only prevent healing, but lead to the formation of matter, and, possibly, to blood-poisoning. A wound into which these germs have entered is called a septic wound, and the treatment which is directed against these germs is called the antiseptic treatment. A wound free from germs is called an aseptic wound.

CHAPTER XXXIII.

ANTISEPTIC TREATMENT OF WOUNDS.

551. Germs.—Germs, sometimes called microbes, and scientific-ally called bacteria, belong to the vegetable world. They are to be found everywhere, especially in dust or dirt. They are on the skin, in all dressings which are not specially prepared, in clothing, on instruments, and in water which has not been recently boiled. They are extremely small, and cannot be seen by the naked eye. One of them alighting on a wound, where, owing to the warmth and moisture, it becomes active, can in twenty-four hours produce seventeen millions of like germs. The growth of these germs irritates the wound, causes it to form matter (or to suppurate) and produces poisonous substances, which, being drawn into the blood, cause fever and even blood-poisoning. The wound is then said to become septic or poisoned. The killing of these germs which have already reached a wound, and the cleansing of the hands, skin, instruments, and dressings, constitute the antiseptic treatment of wounds.

552. Antiseptics.—Antiseptics are chemical substances, some of which have the power of killing germs, whilst others are only able to prevent their growth. There are both liquid and solid anti-septics, most of which are dangerous poisons. For dressing wounds and cleansing the hands, etc., they are commonly employed in the form of "lotions" made by dissolving some of the substance selected in water. The strength of the lotion is always known, for instance, 1 in 20, 1 in 40, 1 in 1,000, which means that 1 part of the anti-septic has been mixed with 19, 39, or 999 parts of water-respectively.

The following are the antiseptics in common use :—

(1) *Carbolic acid.*—This is, ordinarily, a liquid, and is generally used in the form of a solution or lotion of a strength of 1 in 20, 1 in 40, or 1 in 60. The 1-in-20 lotion is used for disinfecting instruments ; 1 in 40 and 1 in 60 may be used for dressing wounds or disinfecting the hands. Solutions stronger than 1 in 20 should not be used for this purpose, as they irritate wounds and make the skin of the hands rough and numb.

(2) *Perchloride of mercury.*—This is a heavy, solid, white substance. It is used as solutions varying between 1 in 1,000 and 1 in 10,000, and is a very powerful antiseptic. Steel instruments should not be placed in this lotion, as it turns them black and makes cutting instruments blunt.

(3) *Biniodide of mercury*, employed in the form of a 1-in-500 solution in methylated spirit. It is used for purifying the hands, or the skin of a patient, before operation.

(4) *Boric or boracic acid* is generally seen as flat, colourless, glistening crystals, or as a white powder. It is used either as the powder or as a lotion made by dissolving the acid in water (as a saturated solution). It is a non-irritating and weak antiseptic.

(5) *Iodoform*, a yellow powder of characteristic and unpleasant odour. It is used for dusting on septic wounds.

(6) *Permanganate of potash* occurs as dark-purple crystals. It is used in solutions of varying strength (generally expressed as grains to the pint). Strong solutions stain the hands brown.

553. Order in which dressings should be done.—Suppose a dresser has in his wards various kinds of wounds, some that are clean, such as operation wounds, and other that are suppurating, and, accordingly, contain germs as explained above. In which order should they be dressed? Clearly, the clean, aseptic wounds should be first attended to, and after these are all dressed the suppurating wounds may be done ; any other course will lead to infection of the clean wounds from the dirty ones.

An aseptic wound must be kept aseptic by exercising the strictest cleanliness, and a septic wound may, by antiseptic measures, be brought into a healthier condition. These two points should be the aim of every dresser.

554. The necessity of thoroughly cleansing the hands between each dressing must now be obvious ; if this be not done, one wound will surely be infected from another. After finishing all the dressings, the hands should be cleansed again ; this is for the dresser's own protection, as if omitted he may well infect his own hands through small scratches or un-noted skin abrasions.

555. How antiseptic dressings are used.—The method of using these antiseptic dressings to wounds is as follows :—

(1) *In hospital*, in the case of an operation, where everything is at hand for thoroughly carrying out the antiseptic treatment after all blood has been wiped away by means of antiseptic swabs, the edges of the wound are drawn together by the surgeon by means of stitches, a drainage-tube, if necessary, having been inserted. Pieces of dry, antiseptic gauze are next placed over the wound, and over the top of these antiseptic wool is laid—much if the wound is large, less if small. Over the wool is placed a bandage to keep the dressing in its place.

(2) *In the field*, or where all precautions as to sterilizing hands, skin, etc., cannot be carried out, it is best not to handle the wound at all, but simply to apply the first field or other dry, antiseptic dressing, taking care to handle it as little as possible, and not to touch with the fingers the part of the dressing which is to come next to the wound.

After having applied the dressing, and splint if necessary, steps may be taken to remove the patient to a place of safety ; but there is one exception to this, namely, bullet-wounds penetrating the abdomen. Experience has shown that the chance of recovery in these cases depends very largely on the patient not being moved at all, but being treated for a time, if possible, where he has fallen. The reason is that the small-bore bullet makes such a small hole in the intestines that little or none of its contents may escape through it, but if the patient be moved, the contents of the gut are much more likely to escape, and set up fatal inflammation. Starvation is the best treatment, not even water being given. Dress the wounds, disturb the patient as little as possible, erect an improvised shelter for him, remove or empty his water-bottle, impress upon him the importance of lying absolutely still, and leave him lying there until a medical officer can see him.

556. Dressings.—Materials used for dressings must be sterilized previously to use. In the case of dry antiseptic dressings such as gauze or wool, these have been specially prepared by being saturated in antiseptic solution, then dried, and afterwards wrapped up in waterproof paper, which has also been sterilized. They are done up in small packages, which can be considered safe for use in the field provided they have been freshly opened. The materials for stitches and drainage tubes have also been sterilized, and are usually kept ready for use in an antiseptic fluid in closed, glass bottles or tubes.

557. Trays and Instruments.—All boxes, trays, basins, etc., used for holding dressings or instruments are made of some hard, smooth material, such as glass, china, or vulcanite, and are sterilized by heat before and after use. Instruments such as scissors, forceps, etc., are sometimes so made as to be able to be taken to pieces, and they, as well as knives, are made as smooth as possible, without crevices, so that they can be easily cleaned and do not harbour germs.

558. Antiseptic baths and fomentations.—When a wound has become infected with germs and is inflamed and discharging, it is usual to treat it with antiseptic baths or antiseptic fomentations. Boric acid is the usual antiseptic in such cases. An antiseptic bath consists of boric acid dissolved in warm water (strength, 5 grains to 1 ounce of water). The limb, or other part, is held in a special vessel containing this warm lotion for such a length of time as may be directed.

An antiseptic fomentation is made in exactly the same way as any other fomentation, except that several folds of boric lint are used instead of the ordinary fomentation-flannel or spongiopiline.

CHAPTER XXXIV.

BLEEDING OR HÆMORRHAGE.

559. Varieties.—Bleeding or hæmorrhage occurs when any portion of the system of blood vessels gives way, or is opened into by injury or disease.

There are three varieties of hæmorrhage : (*a*) arterial, (*b*) venous, and (*c*) capillary.

These three varieties may furthermore occur (1) externally, when the blood can be seen escaping, such as from a cut ; (2) internally, when the blood escapes in the tissues or organs of the body and cannot be seen. This variety may be recognized by the symptoms of the patient, as will be subsequently described. Bleeding in moderate quantity into the tissue of the body is often spoken of as an " extravasation."

INTERNAL HÆMORRHAGE.

560. This, as the name implies, is bleeding from a vessel or vessels inside one of the cavities of the body, *e.g.* chest, abdomen or skull. The condition is one which can only be recognized by the symptoms presented by the sufferer, no blood being visible as in the case of external hæmorrhage.

Internal hæmorrhage occurs as the result of injury or disease.

561. Symptoms.—The symptoms of internal hæmorrhage are as follows :—Great prostration and weakness. The surface of the body is blanched and white. The lips lose their colour, becoming ashy-grey. A cold clammy sweat breaks out on the patient's forehead, and his features assume an aspect of intense anxiety. His breathing becomes shallow, hurried, and sometimes laboured. At times he yawns and sighs. His pulse is weak and may be imperceptible. Later the patient gasps for air and struggles to obtain it, gradually becomes weaker and unconsciousness sets in.

562. Treatment.—Send for a surgeon. Try and ascertain the cause of the bleeding. If from disease of, or injury to, any part of the body where ice can be applied, at once apply it. Loosen anything tight about the neck or body. Give small pieces of ice to suck. Do not give stimulants. Raise the foot of the bed three or four inches from the ground. Apply hot-water bottles to the patient's feet. Keep him *absolutely quiet.* Avoid all conversation with him. Try and gently restrain him should he become restless. Do everything to allay anxiety should he become nervous about his condition, as this is a most important duty in connexion with the treatment of these cases.

563. Treatment of an extravasation.—This is generally seen in a form of a bruise, or black eye, etc. The treatment consists simply of rest and the application of soothing lotions.

EXTERNAL HÆMORRHAGE.

564. Arterial hæmorrhage.—In arterial hæmorrhage the blood escapes from the arteries. It may be known by (1) the blood escaping in jets or spurts, because it is pumped out by the heart ; (2) its bright red colour (3) that it may be stopped by pressing on the artery between the wound and the heart.

565. Venous hæmorrhage.—In this case the blood escapes from the veins. It may be known by (1) the blood being of a dark, purplish-red colour, (2) its flowing in a continual stream and not escaping in spurts, (3) that pressure applied on the side of the wound furthest from the heart stops it, while pressure applied between the wound and the heart does not do so. A dependent position, muscular exertion or straining, or any obstruction to the veins above a wound, greatly increases venous bleeding. Hence it is much greater after accidents than at operations.

566. Although the above account of arterial and venous hæmorrhage gives the usual signs by which they may be distinguished, certain exceptions may occur. In some instances arterial blood may appear as venous ; for example, when it comes from the bottom of a deep and narrow wound, it may flow continually instead of in spurts ; or when a patient is partly suffocated it may become of a dark colour. On the other hand, venous blood exposed to air in its passage from a deep wound, may, owing to its taking up oxygen, become bright and red in colour.

567. Capillary hæmorrhage.—The blood escapes from the capillaries, and oozes from all parts of the wound, trickling down to the deeper parts, where it forms a little pool.

568. Occurrence of hæmorrhage.—Hæmorrhage may occur as (1) primary, (2) reactionary, and (3) secondary.

(1) *Primary hæmorrhage.*—Is that which occurs at the time when the artery is wounded.

(2) *Reactionary hæmorrhage.*—Is that which occurs after the primary hæmorrhage has ceased, and within twenty-four hours of the injury or operation. It appears when the patient is recovering from the shock of the injury.

(3) *Secondary hæmorrhage.*—Is that which occurs any time after the first twenty-four hours following an injury or operation, but seldom before about ten days or a fortnight afterwards. It is now rare because its chief cause (septic infection of the wound) is now also rare.

569. Arrest of external hæmorrhage.—The means of temporarily arresting external hæmorrhage until more permanent means can be resorted to by the surgeon are (1) pressure, (2) application of heat or cold, and (3) position of the patient.

(1) *Pressure.*—If the bleeding point be within reach, hæmorrhage need cause no alarm, as pressure will control it, however big the vessel may be.

THE ARTERIES OF THE BODY

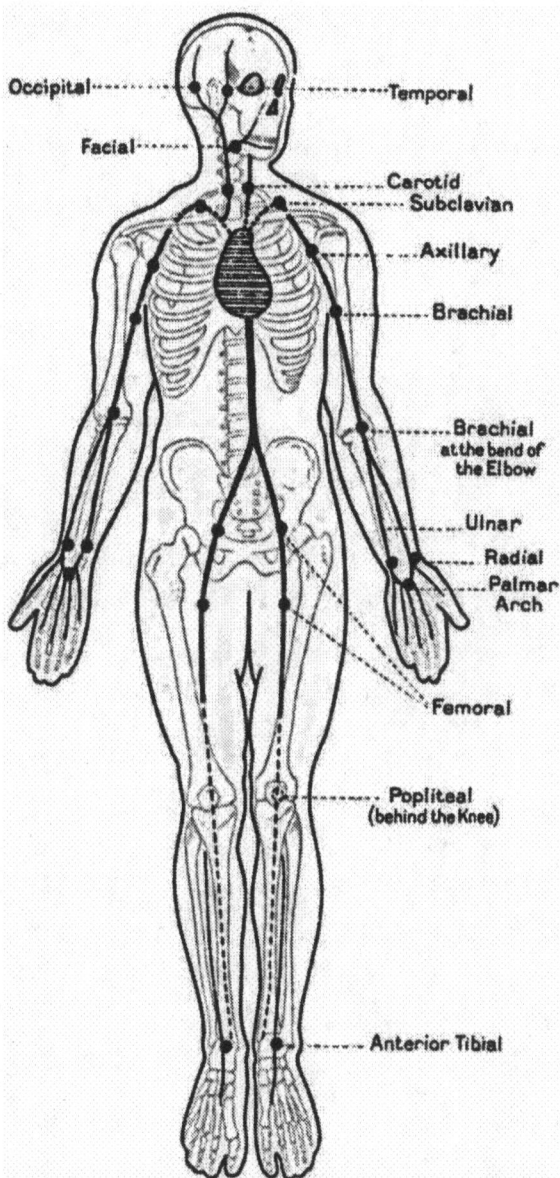

Occipital

Temporal

Facial

Carotid

Subclavian

Axillary

Brachial

Brachial
at the bend of
the Elbow

Ulnar

Radial

Palmar
Arch

Femoral

Popliteal
(behind the Knee)

Anterior Tibial

Fig. 138.   *The black dots indicate the point where
to apply compression*

It may be applied :—(*a*) Directly on the bleeding point, if necessary by means of the finger or thumb (digital compression) ; but preferably by plugging the wound with a piece of antiseptic gauze. (*b*) Close to the wound, between it and the heart (if the bleeding is from an artery) ; or below the wound, that is on the side distant from the heart (if from a vein). It may be applied by the finger, or, in case of the limbs, by means of a tourniquet. It should be made in such a direction as to press the vessel against some resisting structure, such as a bone. (*c*) In bleeding below the knee or elbow, pressure may be applied by placing a pad in the bend of the joint and flexing the limb.

(2) *Heat or cold.*—Of these, heat is the more effective, but neither are so certain as pressure properly applied. Heat may be applied by means of hot water at a temperature of from 140 to 160 degrees Fahrenheit, that is to say, rather hotter than the hand can comfortably bear. Warm water is worse than useless, as it tends to increase rather than diminish the bleeding. Cold water is not so effectual as hot ; it is also liable to increase shock.

(3) *Position of the patient.*—This is often of great importance. Rest, and absolute rest, is essential. Lay the patient down, and try to keep him as quiet as possible and to allay his alarm. While keeping the patient lying perfectly still, if the bleeding is from a limb, raise it and keep it elevated.

As a rule, pressure combined with elevation (in the case of a limb) will always check the bleeding until means can be obtained for permanently arresting it.

The application of styptics (such as perchloride of iron, etc.) to stop bleeding should never be done without orders from a surgeon. Other methods of permanently arresting hæmorrhage, such as tying the vessels, can only be done by him.

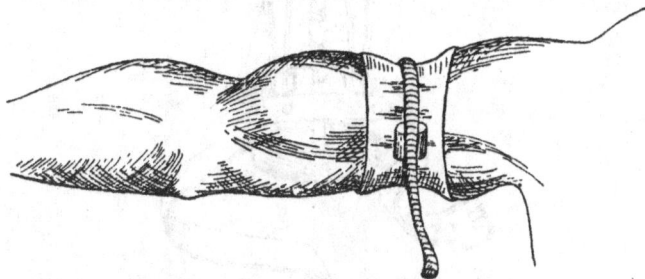

FIG. 139.—COMPRESSION OF THE BRACHIAL ARTERY BY AN ELASTIC TOURNIQUET.

570. Compression by tourniquet.—Compression by means of a tourniquet is only applicable in the case of the arteries of the limbs where the pad takes the place of the thumb and finger as described in digital compression.

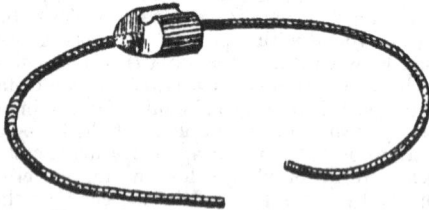

Fig. 140.—Elastic Tourniquet.

571. Kinds of tourniquets.—There are three kinds of tourniquets in common use—the elastic, the screw, and the field.

(1) *Elastic tourniquet.*—The elastic tourniquet consists of thick, elastic tubing which is wound tightly round the limb, and is then fixed by hooks or other appliances.

(2) *Screw-tourniquet.*—The necessary parts of the screw-tourniquet are a pad, a band, and a means of tightening the band so as to press the pad against the artery and so compress it against the bone.

The pad is placed over the main artery, the strap is passed round the limb and buckled. Care must be taken that the pad does not shift from its position over the artery. The screw is then turned until the bleeding stops.

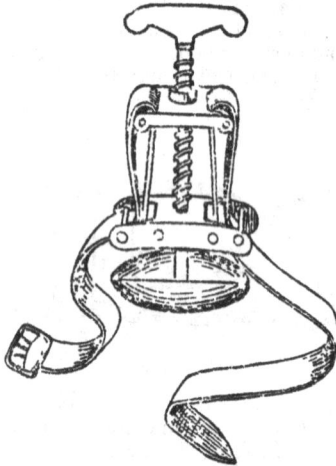

Fig. 141.—Screw-tourniquet.

(3) *Field tourniquet.*—This consists of a pad fitted to a strap and buckle; it is applied in a similar manner to the screw-tourniquet.

(4) *Improvised tourniquets.*—Place some hard substance or a

graduated compress over the trunk of the bleeding vessel. Over this lay the centre of a folded handkerchief or bandage, and tie the ends together on the side of the limb opposite the pad. Then place a stick, or any piece of wood which may be at hand, such as a tent-peg, in the loop thus formed, and twist it until sufficient pressure is made to stop the bleeding. The piece of stick, or whatever is used for tightening the handkerchief or bandage, is kept in position by means of a second handkerchief or bandage, applied below and fastened round the limb. (See Figs. 142 and 143.)

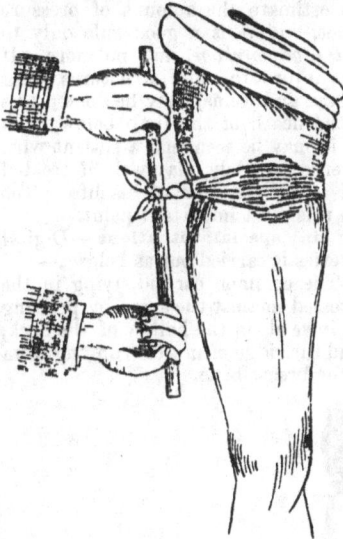

FIG. 142.—IMPROVISED TOURNIQUET FOR COMPRESSION OF WOUND OF THE FEMORAL ARTERY.

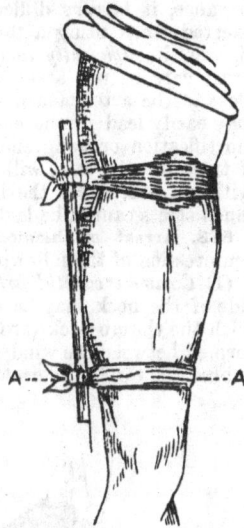

FIG. 143.—THE TOURNI-QUET FIXED BY A BANDAGE AT " A."

The most readily and easily made pad for a tourniquet is obtained by tying a knot in the centre of a pocket-handkerchief or triangular bandage, placing the knot over the bleeding vessel ; then pass the ends round the limb and tie them together, and tighten by means of a stick as described above.

In selecting the substance for making a pad, it should be specially kept in mind that it should have a smooth surface and round edges. A properly applied compress, which can be quickly made from strips torn from the clothing of the individual under treatment, is preferable to any other form of improvised pad. Experience has shown that not only does it fulfil the purpose for which it is applied more effectually, but it is less painful than a stone or other hard substance used as a pad. Irregularly shaped stones or other hard material used as substitutes for a pad, cannot be borne for long owing to the great pain they cause. If a stone or hard substance has to be used it should always be carefully wrapped in a handkerchief or bandage before being applied.

The pugarees of helmets, putties, and the straps and belts of a man's equipment may often be used with success in dealing with the arrest of hæmorrhage.

572. Caution in use of tourniquets.—Digital compression, or compression through a pad of antiseptic material, is greatly to be preferred to compression by tourniquets. Being a mechanical contrivance, it is very difficult to estimate the amount of pressure exerted when using a tourniquet, and it is a good rule only to tighten it *sufficiently to check the hæmorrhage*, and no more. If great care be not taken, serious injury to other structures lying close to the artery (such as nerves and veins) may be done ; this may easily lead in the end to the death of the limb below, from mortification or gangrene. So it may be seen that a patient who, if treated with care, will recover completely, may well, if treated without care, suffer the loss of a limb or even of his life. Too much stress cannot be laid upon this most important point.

573. Arrest of hæmorrhage in special situations.—Digital compression of the following arteries is carried out as below :—

(1) *Common carotid artery.*—The common carotid, lying in the side of the neck, may be compressed against the spine by pressing with the thumb backwards and inwards in the hollow of the neck, formed between the windpipe and the ridge of muscle running from behind the ear to the centre of the breast-bone.

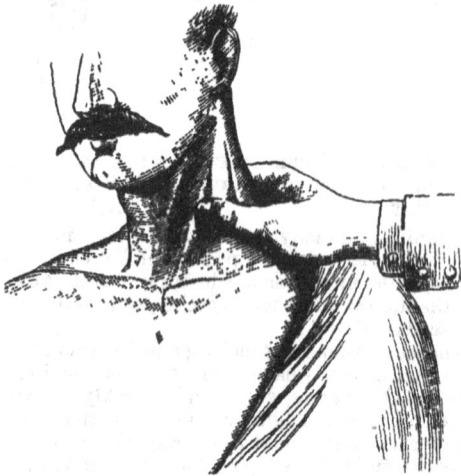

Fig. 144.—Digital Compression of the Carotid Artery Against the Spine.

(2) *Subclavian artery.*—The subclavian artery may be compressed at the base of the neck opposite to the centre of the collarbone. By drawing forward the shoulder, the artery will be more easily reached by the thumb pressing downwards against the first rib behind the clavicle. Compression can also be effected with the handle of a key wrapped in soft cloth, in the same way as with the fingers.

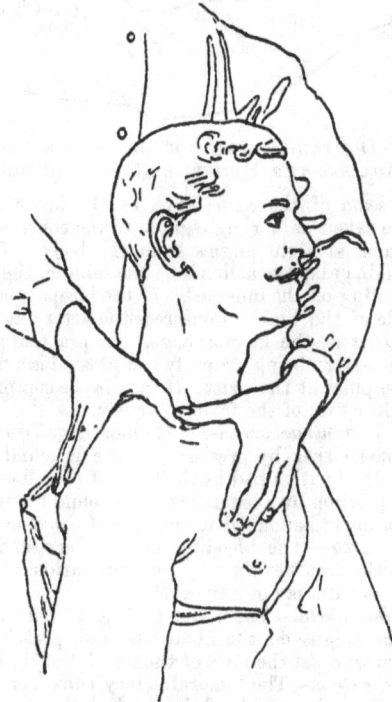

FIG. 145.—DIGITAL COMPRESSION OF THE SUBCLAVIAN ARTERY AGAINST THE FIRST RIB.

(3) *Axillary artery.*—To compress the axillary artery, raise the arm, place the fingers in the arm-pit and press upwards against the head of the humerus.

The vessels of the upper and lower limbs are those to which, in case of hæmorrhage either from them or their branches, tourniquets and digital compression can best be applied.

(4) *Brachial artery.*—The brachial artery may be compressed with the fingers against the inner side of the middle of the humerus.

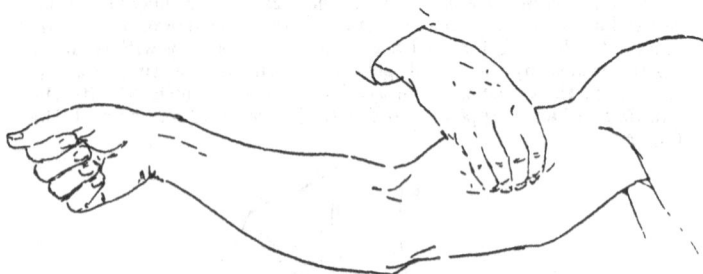

FIG. 146.—DIGITAL COMPRESSION OF THE BRACHIAL ARTERY
AGAINST THE HUMERUS. (BEST METHOD.)

The inner seam of the coat-sleeve, or the inner margin of the
biceps may be taken as a rough guide to the course of the artery.
Extend the arm at right angles from the body. Then, standing
behind the limb, grasp the arm about the middle, the fleshy part of
the fingers resting on the inner edge of the biceps muscle, thumb on
the outer side of the limb. Compress the artery against the bone
sufficiently to arrest the hæmorrhage. In practising this method
the fact of the artery being properly compressed is evidenced by the
absence of the pulse at the wrist. It can also be compressed by both
thumbs as in the case of the femoral artery.

(5) *Radial and ulnar arteries.*—Hæmorrhage from these vessels
may be checked either by pressure on the brachial artery or by
the flexion-method with a pad in the bend of the elbow, the forearm
being kept in position by a bandage passed round the wrist and arm ;
the limb then being bandaged to the side of the chest.

(6) *Palmar arch*—The bleeding may be arrested as described
above under the last heading. The application of a graduated
compress to the palm is not advisable.

(7) *Abdominal aorta.*—The abdominal aorta may be compressed
by flexing the thighs on the abdomen, and pressing backwards
against the vertebræ at the level of the navel, but slightly to its left.

(8) *Femoral artery.*—The femoral artery runs from the centre of
the groin down the inner side of the thigh to the centre of the back
of the knee-joint. The artery may be compressed against the hip-
bone by pressing at the fold of the groin, or against the upper end of
the thigh-bone by pressing backwards and outwards on the line of
the artery, some four fingers' breadth below the fold of the groin.

(9) *Arteries of leg and foot.*—Direct pressure on the bleeding
point, or in the course of the artery above the wound, should first
be tried. If unsuccessful, compress the femoral artery as above
described.

(10) *Temporal artery.*—Bleeding occurring from this vessel is
best controlled by an antiseptic pad applied directly to the bleeding
spot.

(11) *Scalp.*—Hæmorrhage from wounds of the scalp and forehead can be controlled by an antiseptic pad and bandage.

(12) *Tongue.*—Hæmorrhage from the tongue, if the wound is sufficiently far forward to permit of it, can be controlled by pressure with a pad of gauze. If this is not successful, pass the finger to the back of the tongue and press it forwards against the lower jaw-bone.

(13) *Lips.*—Hæmorrhage from the lips can be controlled by a pad in a similar manner, or by grasping the lip on each side of the wound.

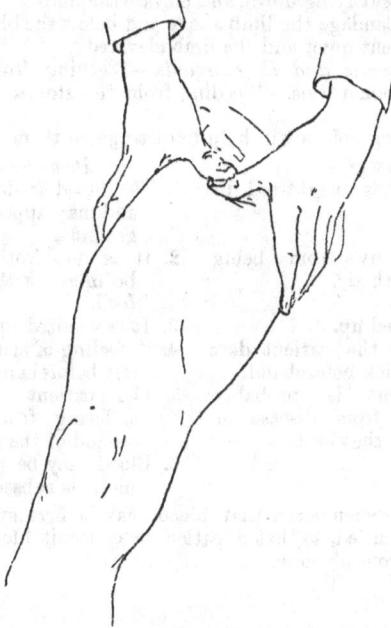

Fig. 147.—Digital Compression of the Femoral Artery Against the Femur.

(14) *Cheek.*—Hæmorrhage from the cheek may be controlled by compressing the wound between a pad of gauze placed on the wound and the forefinger, which is placed inside the mouth.

(15) *Throat and Palate.*—Hæmorrhage from the throat or palate can be most readily dealt with by giving ice to suck. Hæmorrhage from the cavity from which a tooth has been recently extracted may be arrested by pressing into it a small plug of antiseptic gauze or wool.

(16) *Nose.*—This is called epistaxis; it may be treated by making the patient lie down and holding a piece of ice, if available, to the bridge of the nose; or the patient may be directed to sniff ice-cold

water up the nostrils. The application of cold to the nape of the neck is often effectual. Keeping both arms fully extended above the head is also of value.

These methods being unsuccessful, a surgeon should be sent for, as the nasal passages may require to be plugged before the hæmorrhage can be controlled.

(17) *Varicose veins.*—This generally occurs as the result of an ulcer, from the floor of which the blood will be seen to be issuing. Place the patient lying down, and elevate the limb. Apply an antiseptic pad. Bandage the limb above and below the bleeding point. Keep the patient quiet and the limb elevated.

(18) *Hæmoptysis and Hæmatemesis.*—Bleeding from the lungs is known as hæmoptysis. Bleeding from the stomach is known as hæmatemesis.

The following points will help to distinguish them :—

Hæmoptysis.	*Hæmatemesis.*
1. The blood is bright-red in colour.	1. The blood is dark in colour, and may appear like coffee-grounds.
2. It is frothy from being mixed with air.	2. It is not frothy, but may be mixed with particles of food.
3. It is coughed up.	3. It is vomited up.
4. As a rule the patient does not feel sick beforehand.	4. A feeling of sickness is often felt beforehand.
5. The patient is probably suffering from disease or wound of the chest.	5. The patient is probably suffering from disease or wound of the stomach.
	6. Blood may be passed in the motions subsequently.

It must be remembered that blood may be first swallowed and afterwards vomited, so that a patient may vomit blood which has really come from his nose.

CHAPTER XXXV.

FRACTURES AND THEIR TREATMENT.

574. Definition and causes.—When a bone is broken it is said to be fractured.

The causes of a fracture may be (1) injury, (2) disease.

The violence may be applied (*a*) directly, or (*b*) indirectly to the bone, or it may be broken by (*c*) muscular action.

Disease of the bone itself may so weaken it, that it breaks much more easily than it naturally would.

575. Fracture by direct violence.—The bone breaks at the spot struck or crushed; the violence may be caused by a kick, a bullet, the passage of a wheel over the part, etc.

576. Fracture by indirect violence.—The bone does not give way at the point struck, but, owing to the shock being transmitted, it is broken at some distance from the actual seat of violence. As examples may be mentioned the frequency of fractures of the collar-bone from falls on the hand, and fracture of the base of the skull from a fall from a height on to the feet. In the first instance, the violence is applied to the hand, and the shock travels up the arm to the clavicle and breaks it; and in the second instance the shock is transmitted from the feet, through the legs and spine to the skull.

577. Fracture by muscular action.—This is caused by violent contraction of the muscles. It is not so common a cause of fracture as the above. Fractures of the patella or knee-cap are not uncommonly caused in this way.

578. Varieties.—Fractures are described as (1) simple, (2) compound.

Skin not broken.

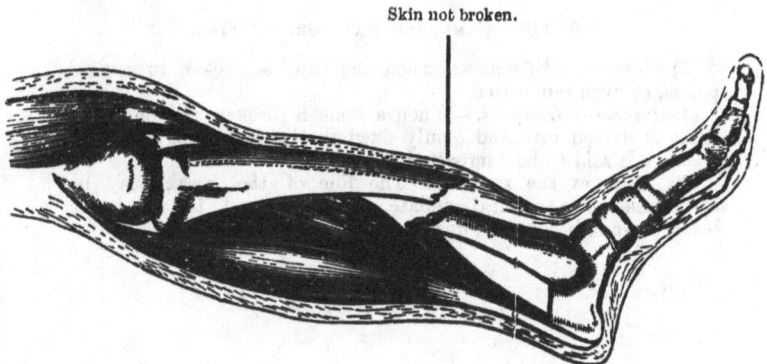

Fig. 148.—SIMPLE FRACTURE OF TIBIA.

(1) *Simple fracture.*—When the skin over the bone is not broken, the fracture is said to be simple.

(2) *Compound fracture.*—When a wound through the skin and soft parts leads down to the break in the bone, the fracture is said to be compound. Sometimes, but not always, the bone protrudes through the skin, as in Fig. 149. Compound fractures are much more serious injuries than simple fractures.

579. Complicated fracture.—A fracture (either simple or compound) is said to be complicated when, in addition to the break in the bone, the arteries, veins, or nerves of the limb are injured ; or when the lung or the brain are damaged by a broken rib or skull ; or a fracture may be complicated by a dislocation of the bone in addition.

580. Other forms.—Fractures are further described as :—

(1) *Complete fractures,* when the bone is broken right across.

(2) *Incomplete* or *greenstick-fractures,* when the bone is partially broken or bent. This variety is most commonly seen in children, because their bones are softer than those of adults.

Wound in the skin and soft part, leading down to the bone which is protruding.

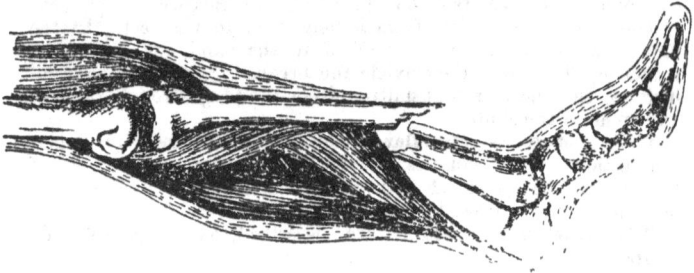

FIG. 149.—COMPOUND FRACTURE OF TIBIA.

(3) *Comminuted fractures,* when the bone is broken in several pieces, or even pulverized.

(4) *Impacted fractures.*—When a bone is broken and one fragment is driven into and firmly fixed in the other fragment, the fracture is said to be " impacted."

581. Line of the fracture.—The line of the break may be transverse, oblique, spiral, stellate, or wedge-shaped ; the two latter being commonly seen in gunshot injuries.

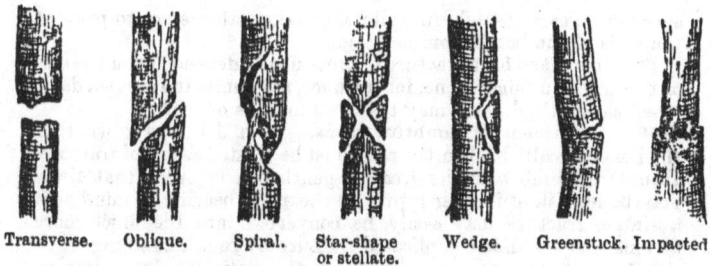

Transverse.   Oblique.   Spiral.   Star-shape   Wedge.   Greenstick. Impacted
                                      or stellate.

FIG. 150.—DIAGRAMS OF FRACTURES.

582. Signs of fracture.—It may be known that a bone is broken by the following signs :—

(1) Pain ; which is generally referred by the patient to the point at which the bone is broken.

(2) Loss of power, *i.e.*, the limb cannot be put to its proper use; for instance when a leg is broken a man cannot stand upon it ; when an arm is broken the hand cannot be raised to the back of the head.

(3) Alteration in shape ; the limb may be bent, twisted, or shortened, and, when compared with the sound limb, it appears of an unnatural shape.

(4) Unnatural mobility ; that is, when the limb is handled (which should not be unnecessarily done), it gives way where, if sound, it would not be movable.

(5) When handled (see (4)), there is generally a grating sensation, caused by the broken ends of the bone grating against one another. This is known as " crepitus."

(6) Swelling of the limb is generally present.

(7) The patient may have experienced the sensation of a sudden snap or giving way of the bone.

583. Mode of repair.—The repair (or union as it is called) of a fractured bone is a similar process to that already described under the Healing of Wounds, but it is modified owing to the process taking place in a different kind of tissue. A bone has its blood-vessels just as any other portion of the body; it must not be looked upon as a hard, bloodless structure, but as a portion of the living body which is itself alive. The blood poured out at the time of the injury sets into a jelly-like mass, which in time becomes formed into new bone. This soft mass which is going to become bone is called " callus," and it surrounds the broken ends of the bone, and in hardening holds them firmly together. After the lapse of months a large portion of the callus at first formed becomes absorbed, and in the end, there may be very little trace to be seen where the fracture has been.

In order to allow the process of repair to proceed naturally, it is necessary that the broken ends of the bones remain completely at rest. Nature attempts to ensure this by causing pain when the limb is moved, and to assist Nature, and secure immobility the surgeon fixes the limb in splints, or takes other steps to prevent the ends of the bones from moving.

The time taken for a fracture to unite firmly depends upon the size of the bone ; a finger-bone, for instance, may unite in fourteen days, whereas the thigh-bone may take two months or more.

584. Treatment of doubtful cases.—If in doubt as to whether the bone is really broken, the case must be treated as one of fracture. Handle the limb with the greatest gentleness in order that there may be no risk of further injury to the part, bearing in mind that a simple fracture may easily be converted into the much more serious compound or complicated fracture by rough handling.

585. Early treatment: *Removing the clothing.*—In removing the clothing the greatest gentleness must be used. In the case of a fractured thigh or leg, the outside seam of the trousers should be split right up. Braces must be unfastened all round. There must be no dragging on taking off the clothing. The leg of the cut trousers should then be very carefully drawn to the inside of the injured limb, and the leg of the trousers on the sound limb can then be pulled off. The sock should be cut off, after the boot has been slit up the back-seam, fully unlaced and removed. In fracture of the arm the coat-seam and shirt must be ripped up.

Application of splints.—Apply splints round the limbs, so as to render the fragments immovable. In doing this there need be no effort made accurately to replace the fractured parts, but merely in a general way, to reduce the deformity by first fastening the lower bandage round the carefully-applied splints, pulling gently and slowly in the line of the limb, and then securely fastening the upper bandage. To support the limb effectually the splint should extend beyond the joints above and below the fracture.

586. Splints.—Splints consist of supports made of some unyielding material (wood, iron, perforated zinc, pasteboard, etc.), varying in length, width, and shape with the part to which they are to be applied. Before being applied they should be padded with some soft material, to protect the limb from the hard surface and edges of the splint.

587. Pads for splints.—These are usually made of soft linen or calico stuffed with cotton-wool mixed with tow, or with tow alone. Care must be taken that the pads are quite even, and contain no lumps of tow or wool, which should be well teased out. Pads should be large enough to protect the limb from the edges of the splint. Some splints are covered with jaconet to keep them clean and the pads dry.

Splints are bound to the limb by bandages or tapes, so that when fixed the limb is protected and held firmly in its proper position.

588. Moving a patient.—In moving a patient all disturbance of the limb should be prevented as much as possible. In the upper extremity the arm may be supported in a sling and tied to the side. In the lower extremity the limbs should be tied together at the knees and ankles.

In no case should a man with a broken limb, or supposed broken limb, be moved until splints have been applied.

589. After-treatment.—The subsequent treatment of fractures, that is, the setting of the bones and final application of the splints, is carried out by the surgeon ; but it is necessary that men should be familiar with the apparatus in general use in military hospitals, in order that they may render intelligent assistance.

Examples of apparatus are :—Rattan-cane splints for the limbs ; japanned iron-wire arm-splints; sheets of perforated zinc, with shears, hammer, anvil, and rivets to shape and join them ; strips of aluminium made up as splints ; plaster of Paris ; sheets of pasteboards ; and gutta-percha, poroplastic felt, and leather, which have to be cut to shape and softened in water. There are special splints for certain parts of the body :—For the thigh-bone, Liston's long thigh-splint (generally jointed for packing); for the lower part of the thigh-bone, McIntyre's splint ; for the leg, the same splint or a metal back splint.

590. Fracture-bed.—For cases of fracture it is necessary that the bed should be even and firm, so that in a case of fractured thigh or leg, for instance, the limb can be kept quite straight and immovable. Boards are also used for this purpose. These can be placed under the limb, leaving the rest of the bed free. A six-foot barrack-table can be used.

591. Sand-bags.—Bags filled with sand are very useful to steady a limb. They are placed on each side to steady it and prevent movement.

592. Danger of tight bandages.—After a splint has been applied, there may be much pain and swelling of the parts, due to the bandages being too tight. The orderly should at once inform the sister or non-commissioned officer.

593. Plaster of Paris splints.—For a plaster of Paris splint there are required : One or two pounds of fresh plaster of Paris, which, after the tin has been opened, should be put on the hob, near the fire, for twenty minutes ; one or two flannel bandages ; three or four loose-wove or muslin bandages ; two clean basins, one for the dry plaster, and the other for cold water ; and a newspaper spread under the limb to protect the bedding. Method of applying : The muslin bandages are soaked in water ; the flannel bandage is wrapped round the limb, which is then covered with one layer of the wet, muslin bandage ; a handful of dry plaster is taken, dipped into the cold water, and smeared on ; another bandage is applied, and covered with more plaster, and so on. The limb is kept carefully in position till the plaster sets. Salt in the water quickens setting, gum-mucilage delays it. To remove the plaster of Paris from the hands, wash in water to which a little soft sugar has been added.

594. Improvised splints.—On the battlefield, or in cases of emergency, specially-made splints may not be at hand, and it therefore becomes necessary to contrive an apparatus which shall take their place. Such splints are called improvised splints, and can, with a little ingenuity, be made out of parts of the man's equipment and accoutrements, e.g., rifle, bayonet, scabbard, etc. ; padding for the same can be conveniently made out of his clothing. In addition to these, ample material for making splints is found around all farm houses, villages, etc., in the shape of the wood from doors, shutters, tables, gates, hurdles, floorings, or provision boxes ; also brushwood, telegraph-wire, corrugated iron, etc. ; while padding for them is usually at hand in the form of corn-sacks, shavings, newspapers, hay, straw, leaves, ferns, and grass. Materials for fastening the splints in position are available in the shape of rifle-slings, straps, belts, braces, boot-laces, etc. ; putties and helmet pugarees form useful bandages, or strips for that purpose can be torn from shirts. The rifle-splint is described in para. 595 (9).

595. Special fractures.—Under this heading only the more common fractures will be discussed.

(1) *Fracture of the spine.*—This injury may result from falling from a height on the back across a bar, or on to uneven ground ; or from a fall upon the head. In this fracture the vertebræ are broken and displaced ; the spinal cord and nerves are damaged according to the amount of displacement present. The result being complete or partial paralysis of the parts below the seat of fracture.

Treatment.—(*a*) Do not attempt to move the patient until a medical officer arrives ; but,

(*b*) If no surgeon is available within a reasonable time, proceed to render first aid yourself.

(*c*) Pass some form of support beneath the patient; for example, a blanket, sheet, roll of canvas, etc., taking care in doing so that the sufferer is disturbed as little as possible, and that he himself makes no attempt to roll over.

(*d*) After this has been done, poles must be fixed on to the support on each side.

(*e*) The patient is then slowly and with the utmost care placed upon a stretcher, board, gate, etc., and carried, if possible, by four people to the nearest place of shelter, where he is kept absolutely quiet until the arrival of a surgeon.

(2) *Fracture of the skull.*—The patient may be quite unconscious or only dazed; there may be bleeding from the mouth, ears, or nose.

Treatment.—Keep the patient absolutely quiet until he can be seen by a surgeon. Do not give stimulants. Take special care of the ears, etc., so that no dirt or septic matter may get in. This is very important, as bleeding externally means that the fracture is compound, and if septic matter gets in, it may lead to inflammation of the brain. If available, plug the ears and nostrils with a piece of gauze or wool moistened in antiseptic solution.

(3) *Fracture of the pelvis.*—This is nearly always due to severe, direct violence, such as the passage of a whe l across the body.

As a rule there is little displacement of the bones ; and the treatment consists in keeping the parts at rest by means of a broad bandage.

(4) *Fracture of the lower jaw.*—In addition to the usual signs of fracture the following are often present :—

(*a*) Inability to speak or move the jaw with any degree of freedom.

(*b*) Irregularity of the teeth, noticeable on looking into the mouth, or passing the finger along them.

(*c*) Bleeding from the gums.
(*d*) Salivation.

Treatment.—Apply the four-tailed bandage as described under the heading of "Special bandages," and remove the case to hospital forthwith.

(5) *Fracture of the ribs.*—When a rib is broken the patient complains of severe pain on taking a long breath, and crepitus may be detected on placing the hand over the injured part. In addition to these signs, when the lung is injured, as is often the case, blood may be coughed up.

Treatment.—Apply two broad-fold bandages firmly round the chest, in such a manner that the centre of one bandage is immediately above, and that of the other directly below, the seat of fracture ; the upper half of the lower bandage overlapping the lower half of the upper. The bandages should then be tied off on the opposite side of the body to the injury, knots slightly to the front. When the ribs are crushed in and the lung is severely injured do not apply bandages to the chest, as great damage may be inflicted by the fragments being still further pushed into the lung. In this case lay the patient down, slightly inclined towards the injured side, loosen all clothing, give small pieces of ice to suck, and place an ice-bag over the injured area. Apply the greater arm-sling in either case, and remove at once to hospital.

(6) *Fracture of the collar-bone.*—This is caused either by a fall on the shoulder or outstretched hand, or by direct violence applied to the collar-bone itself. The arm on the injured side is helpless : the patient generally supports it at the elbow with his other hand, and the head is inclined towards the injured side. On examining the injured side, a deformity in the line of the collar-bone will be at once apparent, and to this point the patient will refer most of the pain from which he suffers.

Treatment.—After having removed the coat and all necessary clothing, place a pad about the size and thickness of the palm of the hand in the axilla of the injured side, and apply the bandages for fractured clavicle as described under "Bandaging."

(7) *Fracture of the upper arm.*—The upper arm may be broken (*a*) near the shoulder, (*b*) about the centre of the bone, or (*c*) near the elbow-joint. The usual signs of fracture are present.

Treatment.—(*a*) If the fracture is near the shoulder, first put a pad along the inside from the arm-pit to the elbow ; then bandage the affected arm to the side by means of a broad-fold bandage, the centre over the centre of the arm and the ends passed round the body and tied on the opposite side. Apply the lesser arm-sling.

(*b*) If the fracture occurs in the shaft or middle portion of the bone, four short splints must be applied to the arm, in front, behind, and on either side. Care must be taken that the front splint is not too long to prevent easy bending of the elbow, and that the bandages retaining the splints in position are applied above and below (*i.e.*, not over) the seat of the fracture. Apply the lesser arm-sling.

(*c*) If the arm bone is broken in its lower part near the elbow, the forearm should be bent up, the splint about to be described applied, and the arm supported by the greater arm-sling. Take two pieces

z

of moderately thin wood about three inches wide ; one long enough to reach from the arm-pit to the elbow, and the other from the elbow to the finger tips ; tie these together so as to form a right angle or sort of capital L, and apply the splint thus formed on the inner side of the arm and forearm by means of bandages above and below the fracture. Keep the thumb pointing upwards. A ready-made angular splint, if available, may of course be used in place of the above.

(8) *Fracture of the forearm.*—One or both bones of the forearm may be broken ; the signs of fracture not usually being so evident in the former as in the latter case. There is generally in all cases loss of power and acute pain on moving the limb, and deformity at the seat of fracture. A transverse fracture at the lower end of the radius is known as a " Colles's fracture " ; it is very frequently of the impacted variety.

Treatment.—Is the same whether one or both bones are broken. Bend the forearm at right angles to the arm, keeping the thumb uppermost and the palm of the hand towards the body. Then apply two broad splints on the inner and outer sides of the forearm respectively, the former being long enough to reach from the elbow to the fingers, and the latter from the elbow to the back of the hand. Bandage, if possible, above and below the fracture, steadying the hand by another bandage. Finally apply the greater arm-sling.

(9) *Fracture of the thigh-bone.*—The thigh-bone may be broken by direct violence, the bone giving way in this case where the force was applied ; or by indirect violence. There is usually well-marked shortening of the limb, and the foot of the injured side is often turned outwards.

Treatment.—(*a*) Bring the foot of the injured side into line with the sound side, by gently and steadily pulling upon it. If an assistant is at hand, after the foot has been drawn into its proper place, give it to him to keep in position until splints, etc., have been applied ; or, pending the application of splints, the feet may be tied together at the ankles.

(*b*) Apply a splint on the outer side of the injured limb, long enough to reach from the axilla to beyond the foot. A broom-handle, or any piece of wood long enough, may be used, or a rifle, although short for this purpose, may be used in the special manner to be described under " rifle-splint."

(*c*) Apply a second splint on the inside of the fractured thigh reaching from the fork to the knee.

(*d*) Secure the splints in position by bandages as follows : The first is passed round the chest just below the axillæ, and the second round the pelvis ; both these should be broad-fold bandages. The third and fourth, which are narrow-fold bandages, should be applied round the thigh above and below the fracture, so as to enclose the thigh and both splints. Another bandage should be passed round the leg enclosing the long splint. Fasten the ankle to the lower end of the long splint. Finally the injured limb should be bandaged to its fellow.

Rifle-splint.—The following are the rules for the application of a rifle-splint (Fig. 151) :—Remove the bolt and see that the rifle or magazine contains no cartridges.

Take a narrow-fold bandage, place it over the heel plate of the butt in such a way that two-thirds of its length are in what will be the outer side, and one-third on the outer side of the butt; take

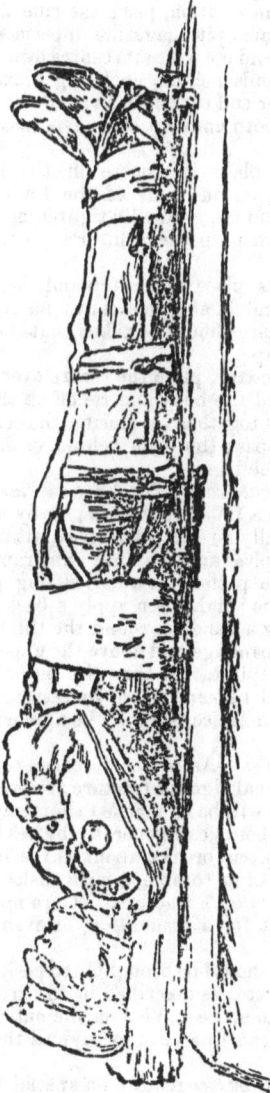

FIG. 151.—RIFLE-SPLINT APPLIED.
(Short rifle (Lee-Enfield) applied.)

a half-hitch round the butt with the long end, making a half-knot on the outer side above the D for the sling. Tie the ends so as to form a loop about two inches long. This is for the perineal bandage to pass through, and is called the butt-loop.

Leave the magazine in position, place the rifle along the injured limb, butt towards the arm-pit, magazine uppermost.

Take a narrow-fold bandage, place its centre over the ankle of the injured limb, pass the ends behind, enclosing muzzle of rifle, cross behind. With the outer end take a turn round the muzzle in front of the foresight, bring both ends up, cross over instep and tie off on the inside of the foot.

Take a narrow-fold, place its centre in the fork, bring one end out behind, the other in front of the limb; pass one end through the butt-loop and tie, gradually tightening the knot as the limb is gently drawn to its proper length. Pass both ends round the butt and tie off.

Take two long splints, place one on top and the other along the inner side of the thigh and fix at each end by a narrow-fold bandage tied off over the rifle : care should be taken that the top splint does not press on the knee-cap.

Take a broad-fold bandage, place the centre over the butt of the rifle, pass the ends round the body and tie off on the opposite side.

Tie the patient's legs together by placing the centre of a broad-fold over both ankles, pass the ends behind, cross, bring up, and tie off on top between the legs.

(10) *Fracture of the knee-cap.*—The knee-cap may be broken by direct violence, such as a fall on the knee ; or by muscular action. The fragments will usually be easily detected and are generally well apart. The limb is helpless and the knee joint rapidly swells.

Treatment.—Place the patient in a half-sitting position so as to relax the muscles of the thigh, then apply a back-splint from the hip to the heel, fixed by a bandage round the thigh and above the ankle. A narrow-fold bandage laid above the upper fragment may be crossed behind the splint, and then tied off in front below the lower. The heel should be kept raised by resting it on the sound foot or a folded coat, and an ice-bag may be applied over the knee-joint.

(11) *Fracture of the leg.*—As in the forearm, one or both bones may be broken. The usual signs of fracture are present, but if only one bone is broken there will be no marked shortening of a limb. A break of the tibia (shin-bone) can generally be readily felt beneath the skin. The fibula often breaks about three inches above the ankle ; fracture at this point, combined with dislocation of the foot outwards, is known as "Pott's fracture." Care must be taken not to mistake this accident for a dislocation, or even a sprain, of the ankle.

Treatment.—The limb should be brought into position and steadied by drawing on the foot, etc., as described in the treatment for fractured thigh. Splints should be applied on the outer and inner sides of the limb, reaching from the knee to beyond the foot, and both legs bandaged together.

(12) *Fractures of fingers or toes* require no special mention. They are treated on ordinary lines.

596. Compound fractures.—Any of the above fractures may be compound. They are much more serious injuries than simple fractures because of the wound in the soft parts leading down to the bone. The greatest precautions must always be taken against septic infection of the wound; as if this occurs, inflammation of the bone may arise, leading perhaps to general blood-poisoning and death.

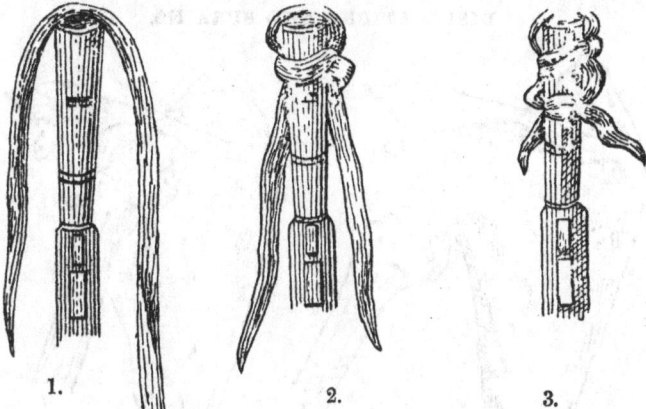

1. Narrow-fold laid on.

2. Half-hitch and half-knot above "D" for sling.

3. Butt-loop formed.

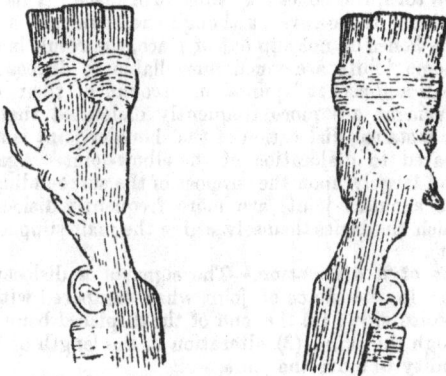

FIG. 152.—FORMATION OF BUTT-LOOP.

CHAPTER XXXVI.

DISLOCATIONS AND SPRAINS.

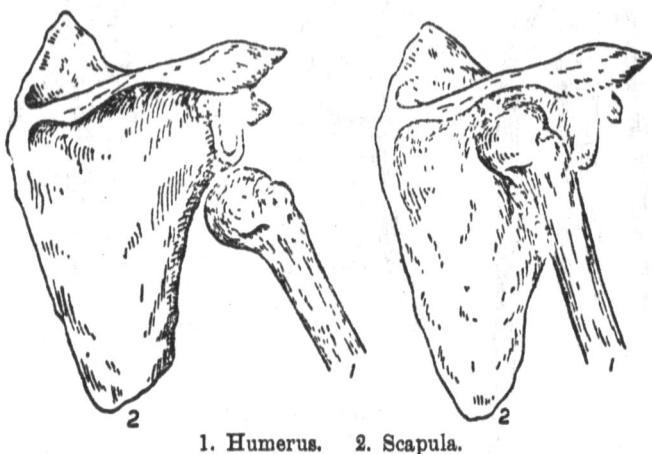

1. Humerus. 2. Scapula.

FIGS. 153 AND 154.—DISLOCATION OF THE SHOULDER-JOINT.

Dislocation of the head of the humerus downwards into the arm-pit.

Dislocation of the head of the humerus backwards on to the scapula.

597. Definition.—When an injury to a joint occurs and the ligaments are torn, the bones may slip out of place. This is known as a dislocation. If, however, although the ligaments are torn or stretched, the bones do not slip out of place, the result is known as a sprain. Some joints are much more liable to dislocation than others : " ball-and-socket " joints on account of their extensive range of movement are more frequently dislocated than " hinge-joints " ; for instance, dislocation of the shoulder-joint is a common injury compared to dislocation of the elbow-joint. Again, joints which depend largely upon the support of the surrounding muscles (such as the shoulder-joint) are more frequently dislocated than joints in which the bones themselves give the main support (such as the hip-joint).

598. Signs of a dislocation.—The signs of a dislocation are : (1) alteration in the shape of joint when compared with the one on the opposite side ; (2) the end of the displaced bone can often be felt through the skin ; (3) alteration in the length of the limb ; and (4) inability to move the joint.

A dislocation can be distinguished from a fracture by : (1) it always happening at a joint ; (2) the limb, instead of being unnaturally movable, as is the case in a fracture, is unnaturally stiff ; (3) if the end of the bone can be felt it is found to be smooth and rounded in dislocation, sharp and angular in fracture ; and (4) by there being no grating.

It must be remembered, however, that a dislocation may be combined with a fracture ; as, for instance, fracture of the humerus with dislocation of the shoulder-joint.

A dislocation may also be compound ; the meaning of this and need for special care has already been mentioned.

599. Signs of a sprain.—The signs of a sprain are : (1) severe pain, increased on movement ; (2) inability to bear weight on the limb ; (3) swelling round the joint ; and (4) absence of special signs of fracture or dislocation.

600. Treatment.—The reduction of dislocation must be left to a surgeon. Any attempts at reduction by one unacquainted with the necessary manipulations may lead to severe injury to the patient.

Sprains require, as a rule, rest and the application of evaporating lotions.

CHAPTER XXXVII.

BURNS AND SCALDS.

601. Immediate treatment of burns.—The damage to the body occasioned by burns varies with the degree of heat applied to the part burnt : the more intense the degree of heat the more severe the burn. As regards immediate treatment, it should be remembered that severe burns, more particularly those situated on the head, neck, and trunk, and those which occupy a great extent of surface, are likely to be attended from the outset by serious constitutionl disturbances described under the head of " Shock," and from which alone the patient may sink unless properly supported.

Burning clothing should be extinguished by laying the person on the ground and rolling him up in a rug, blanket, coat, curtain, or anything of this nature that is handy.

As the danger to life in severe burns comes from shock, the sufferer's general condition should receive attention first of all ; this is important.

The charred surface is temporarily protected from septic infection owing to the germs in the skin having been destroyed by the heat. The treatment of shock should be carried out as described hereafter.

602. Dressing of burns.—The points to be aimed at in all cases are protection of the injured surfaces from the air, and relief of pain. A burn or scald must be covered up as quickly as possible, and should on no account be exposed to the air longer than is absolutely necessary. This will be best accomplished by removing burnt clothing which is not adherent to the charred surface ; never attempt to pull it off, but cut it. Any clothing, etc., adherent to the burnt surface should not be touched, but allowed to remain where it is. The injured part may then be immersed in, or be bathed with, warm water to which some bicarbonate of soda has been added This will float off any charred clothing, etc., sticking to the part. The scorched or burnt surfaces may be dressed with lint covered with aseptic vaseline and boric acid powder. After the part has been dressed it should be enveloped in cotton-wool and put in the position most comfortable to the patient. The dressing had best be applied in a number of strips rather than in one large piece. This renders their subsequent removal easier to the sufferer ; also, where a large surface has been burnt, by dressing in this manner and so exposing only a small portion at a time to the air, the tendency to shock is lessened. Boric ointment spread on strips of lint can be used in the same manner. Deeper burns destroying the skin are liable to become septic and require such antiseptic treatment as may be ordered by the surgeon. Burns should, after the first dressing, be dressed as seldom as possible.

During the subsequent treatment, the chief danger is sepsis and its results. Also, when the parts beneath the skin have been burnt the formation of disfiguring and deforming scars is frequent. To prevent and diminish these results the sufferer requires very careful nursing. Inflammatory affections, such as pneumonia, may follow after burns.

For burns of the face the dressings should be applied on a mask of lint or linen, in which holes are cut for the eyes, nose, and mouth.

603. Scalds and their treatment.—Scalds (which are caused by the application of hot fluids to the body) should be treated on the same lines as burns. When blisters form they may be pricked to permit the escape of their contents, but every endeavour should be made to avoid breaking the skin more than is necessary. If, after the first pricking (which should be done at the margin), the blister becomes again distended and is painful, a fresh outlet should be made and the fluid allowed to escape.

604. Convalescence.—The convalescence from extensive burns or scalds may be prolonged and tedious, and after the first ten days a generous diet with tonics will be necessary.

605. Suffocation from swallowing very hot water, or by inhaling steam.—This is rather a common accident among children, and is always serious. It may become rapidly fatal from swelling of the upper part of the larnyx causing obstruction to respiration. Treatment in such cases must be prompt, and the sufferer constantly watched.

Treatment.—Apply fomentations to the front of the neck, from the chin to the top of the breast-bone (sternum). Keep the patient sitting up and give ice to suck. It is best to have the sufferer at once seen by a surgeon, as surgical treatment may be required at any moment.

CHAPTER XXXVIII.

SHOCK, LOSS OF CONSCIOUSNESS, AND FITS.

606. Shock is a condition produced by any severe injury or emotional disturbance. It is usual as the result of pain, or of injuries such as extensive burns or serious mutilation of the body. The sufferer becomes pale and cold, he lies in a semi-conscious and helpless state, the face pinched, the lips ashy, the temperature subnormal, the pulse feeble or almost absent. He often breaks out into a cold sweat, and may have fits of shivering, or be restless.

Treatment.—Restoration must be attempted by placing the patient in bed with the head low. Restore warmth to the body by warm bed-clothing, hot-water jars to the extremities, or the application of a mustard-poultice over the heart. Administer hot drinks and stimulants in small quantities, but take care that the patient is conscious enough to swallow or he may be choked by the fluid passing into the larnyx.

607. Insensibility or loss of consciousness is due to various causes which damage or interfere with the action of the brain. It may be produced by pressure on the brain, as when bleeding takes place within the skull ; by actual damage to the brain-substance, as results from a blow on the head, from a fracture of the skull, or from a bullet-wound ; or, as is often the case, by interference with the circulation of the blood within the brain. It frequently happens as the result of the blood not being properly aerated in the lungs, either because the lungs do not act properly, or because the air supplied is impure, as when suffocation occurs in a room containing coal-gas, or other poisonous gases.

Treatment.—Send at once for medical assistance. Lay the patient on his back, and as a general rule, if the face is flushed keep the head high : if pale, keep the head low. Loosen all tight clothing round the neck, chest, or stomach. If there is any inclination to vomit, place the head on one side, so that the contents of the stomach may not get into the larynx and cause suffocation. Avoid all crowding round the person, and admit free access of fresh air. Give no food or stimulants, unless by direction of a medical officer. Do not leave the patient alone, but stay with him till help comes.

608. Concussion is a variety of shock caused by injury to the brain, generally from a blow or fall on the head. The symptoms resemble those of shock, but are generally accompanied by a more confused and bewildered state of the patient, or by complete unconsciousness.

The treatment is as for shock, but stimulants are not to be given without orders.

609. Fainting may be caused by over-exertion in hot weather or heated rooms, or by getting into the upright position when weak from disease, or it may result from hæmorrhage, or starvation, or from seeing some revolting sight, or it may follow fear or great grief. A fainting-fit is distinguished by the patient falling down in a helpless condition, generally insensible, without convulsions. The face and lips are pale and the surface of the body cold, often covered with a clammy perspiration.

Treatment.—Lay the patient on his back with his head low, and loosen the clothes about the neck and chest. Sprinkle cold water on the face and neck. Apply smelling-salts to the nose, and, when the patient is able to swallow, administer stimulants in very small quantities. Fresh air is a necessity. If hæmorrhage be the cause it must be arrested immediately, and stimulants should not be given without orders. If it results from starvation, fluid nourishment, such as strong beef-tea, should be given, but only in moderate quantities at first. Leave the patient lying down for some time after he recovers.

610. Epileptic fits are due to constitutional, or local, causes. The patient falls down insensible, and has convulsions affecting part or the whole of the body, foams at the mouth, and often bites the tongue, making it bleed.

A fit may be divided into three stages :—

1st stage.—This is often commenced by a peculiar cry. The patient then falls down quite unconscious. He becomes rigid all over, every muscle being contracted ; he holds his breath ; his face becomes pale and then livid. This stage lasts from 30 to 40 seconds.

2nd stage.—Unconsciousness continues ; but instead of rigidity, convulsions come on ; the eyes roll ; the tongue may be bitten ; and urine and fæces may be passed involuntarily. This stage lasts from one to four minutes and passes slowly into :

3rd stage.—Consciousness is gradually regained. The muscular spasms cease ; the patient gradually comes to himself, but is very exhausted and confused mentally. He then frequently sleeps for some hours.

Treatment.—Lay the patient on his back with his head slightly raised ; loosen the clothes about the neck and chest, and prevent him biting his tongue by placing something (such as a spatula, or handle of a tooth-brush) between his teeth as a gag. Employ only sufficient restraint to prevent him injuring himself, and avoid pressing on the chest ; it will be sufficient if one man restrains the patient's legs—kneeling by his right side and placing the right arm across the knees to do so ; a second attendant lightly restrains the patient's right arm, and a third the left arm and also watches the head. Treatment will not cut short an epileptic fit.

611. Apoplectic fits occur mostly in elderly persons. The patient falls suddenly insensible. The face is red, the breathing loud and snorting, and the pupils frequently of unequal size.

Treatment.—Raise and support the head and upper part of the chest. Loosen the clothes about the neck. Apply cold water to the head. Do not give stimulants.

612. Compression of the brain is the result of severe injuries to he head, such as fracture to the skull ; the symptoms resemble those of apoplexy, and the same precautions should be taken.

613. Sunstroke, or *heatstroke* which is the result of excessive heat, occurs in hot climates or summer weather. The patient falls suddenly, generally insensible, sometimes in convulsions, the skin feeling burning-hot to the hand.

Treatment.—Carry the patient at once into the shade or the coolest available place. Provide plenty of fresh air. Raise the head and remove the clothes from the neck and upper part of the body. Douche the head, neck, chest, and spine, or the whole body with cold water. Avoid crowding round the patient. Do not give stimulants. Give enemata of ice-cold water.

614. Drunken fits are caused by the drinking of a large quantity of alcohol. They occur suddenly, but may not come on for some time after the liquor has been taken. The patient falls into a deep stupor ; there is a vacant expression of the countenance, which is sometimes red. The lips are livid and pupils dilated, and the breath smells strongly of liquor.

Treatment.—Place the patient on his side with head slightly raised and do not allow him to lie on his back, or on his face. Remove all constrictions from the neck and induce vomiting. Have the stomach-tube ready in case the medical officer on his arrival should decide to use it.

CHAPTER XXXIX.

SUFFOCATION, CHOKING, &c.

615. General symptoms.—These are as follows :—Violent attempts to breathe ; staring eyeballs ; distended, prominent veins in the neck ; purple countenance ; convulsive movements of the body, etc. If the condition causing the suffocation or choking be not speedily removed, insensibility follows and death results. Such a condition is called *asphyxia*.

616. Choking.—This may be caused by pieces of meat, coins, false-teeth, or any other body lodging over the entrance to the wind-pipe, and so causing obstruction to respiration. Treatment must be prompt. Forcibly open the mouth and pass the forefinger to the back of the throat and endeavour to hook up the obstructing body. In the case of children, hold them legs-uppermost and thump the back between the shoulder-blades. This should also be attempted in adults if the first-mentioned remedy is ineffectual. In all cases send for a medical man at once.

617. Suffocation by smoke or gas.—Remove the person into the fresh air, and at once proceed to restore breathing by artificial respiration. In mild cases respiration may be stimulated by freely douching the chest with cold water.

Poisonous gases are dangerous to life by replacing the oxygen in the blood.

618. Rescue from fire.—Before entering a building on fire, with a view to rescuing from the smoke and heat any individuals within, tie a wet handkerchief over the nose and mouth. Take off any superfluous clothing, and if possible have a bucket of water thrown over one. It is imperative to work quickly ; avoid being overcome by the smoke by bending low beneath it—the air is clearest near the floor. When carrying persons out from burning buildings, the rescuer must try especially to protect from the flames the head and neck of those he carries.

619. Electric shock.—Contact with an electric cable may produce very severe shock, insensibility, and death. The sufferer is unable to extricate himself owing to the current depriving him of all power of moving.

It is imperative at once to get the sufferer away from the cable, and the person going to his assistance does so at great risk of being himself caught by the current. If the current can be switched off this should, of course, be done, but if this cannot be done endeavours to extricate the person must be made. The rescuer must insulate himself from the current, otherwise on touching the sufferer with naked hands the electricity will also hold him. There is no time to search for india-rubber gloves or mats to stand on, as the sufferer must be got away immediately. A dry, wooden broom-handle may be utilized to shove the person away from contact ; or an empty, india-rubber tobacco pouch may be improvised as a glove. A coat held by the sleeves, or a belt or puttee may be thrown over the head or round the body of the victim to drag him away from the contact. All the common metals are good conductors of electricity, iron, copper, brass, etc., and should be avoided ; water, also, is a good conductor, and in dealing with electricity damp clothing should be avoided.

After rescuing the patient, the general treatment for insensibility must be carried out, and artificial respiration begun if breathing has ceased ; any burns being left for treatment until the grave condition of shock has been overcome.

CHAPTER XL.

EFFECTS OF COLD.

620. Frost-bite is the result of exposure to excessive cold. It affects the nose, ears, fingers, or feet ; the part tingles and becomes blue ; and, in the more severe cases, white and free from pain. The treatment is to rub the affected part with snow or cold water, avoiding taking the patient into a warm room until the part has been thoroughly, but very gradually, thawed. All application of heat should be avoided, as it might produce gangrene.

621. Chilblains are local congestions of the skin, usually of the fingers and toes, caused by exposure to cold and wet. Damp and ill-fitting boots are a common cause. If the parts have become damp they should be thoroughly dried with a soft towel, then rubbed gently with some fine bran. Keep the parts warm and protected from the cold with woollen gloves or socks worn day and night.

The chilblain may be painted with tincture or liniment of iodine. If the surface is broken, apply zinc or boric ointment, and protect with cotton-wool. Exercise, good food, and warm clothing are the best preventives, and are necessary for the cure of this affection. Young people and those with a poor circulation are the chief sufferers.

CHAPTER XLI.

FOREIGN BODIES IN THE EYE AND EAR.

622. Foreign bodies in the eye.—Foreign bodies lodged in the eye, either on the eye-ball or under the lids, cause severe discomfort, and if not quickly removed give rise to inflammation and great pain. Eye-lashes sometimes get turned in and act as foreign bodies.

Treatment.—Prevent the patient rubbing the eye, and carefully examine it in a good light by pulling down the lower lid and gently pushing up the upper. If the foreign body is now visible, it may be removed by gently brushing it away with the folded corner of a handkerchief.

The patient may himself, by adopting the following simple methods, rid his eye of a foreign body :—(1) By blowing the nose violently several times in rapid succession, at the same time looking downwards and inwards. (2) By immersing the face in water, and at the same time opening the eye and moving it about to wash out the foreign body. (3) By taking hold of the edge of the upper eyelid, and drawing it downwards and forwards over the lower lid. On letting go the upper lid, the foreign body may be brushed off it on to the lower lid, from which it may easily be removed. (4) By smelling any pungent substance, such as ammonia, which, by causing a free secretion of tears, may wash the body out.

Should, however, these methods fail, the following treatment should be adopted :—Let the patient sit down facing the light; stand behind him and steady his head against your chest. Tell the patient to look down. Place a probe, or wooden match, or other similar object lengthwise on the upper eyelid about half an inch above the edge. Now lay hold of the edge of the lid with the forefinger and thumb (left hand for the right eye and the right hand for left eye), draw it gently downwards and outwards, then turning it quickly upwards, fold it over the probe, which at the same time must be withdrawn with a downward and outward sweep. The eyelid having been everted, the foreign body may be seen and should be wiped off with a camel-hair brush, or the corner of a handkerchief. The lid should then be pulled forward to let it resume its normal position, the patient at the same time being told to look up.

A piece of grit, cinder, or iron, sometimes becomes embedded in or sticks on the surface of the eye-ball, causing great pain and intolerance of light. Such a foreign body may be recognized as a dark spot on the clear part of the eye-ball (cornea). Its removal should be left to a medical officer. Pending his arrival, or until assistance can be obtained, the eye should be filled with olive oil, and a pad of cotton-wool or folded handkerchief bandaged gently over it.

623. Lime in the eye.—This is a very serious accident, and may cause rapid destruction of the eye. Remedies must be prompt.

Treatment.—Fill the eye at once with olive or castor oil. Remove the pieces of lime as quickly as possible and with the greatest gentleness ; but make no attempt to pick off any particles which have become adherent to the conjunctiva or eye-ball; this should be left to the medical officer.

Or the eye may be bathed with a warm solution of vinegar and water (about two table-spoonsful to a pint). By directing a stream of this on to a piece of the adherent lime, it may be washed off. In no circumstances should force, ever so slight, be used in endeavouring to remove the pieces of lime.

624. Foreign bodies in the ear-passages.—In these cases, at once bring the patient to hospital, or send for medical assistance.

Never attempt, when the foreign body cannot be seen, to probe for it, or even syringe the ear, with a view to its removal. If an insect gets into the ear passages and becomes fixed, pour in some olive oil so as to float it out; but it is best in all cases to wait until a medical officer can examine the case. Should there be great pain, fomentations should be applied to the ear and side of the head.

CHAPTER XLII.

DROWNING.

625. Restoration of the apparently drowned. — Send immediately for medical assistance, blankets, stimulants, and dry clothing, but proceed to treat the patient instantly on the spot, in the open air whether ashore or afloat. The points to be aimed at are :— (1) The removal of all obstructions to the passage of air into the lungs ; (2) the restoration of the breathing ; (3) after breathing is restored, the promotion of warmth and circulation. The efforts to restore life must be persevered in for one or two hours, or until a doctor has pronounced life to be extinct. Efforts to promote warmth and circulation, beyond removing the wet clothes and drying the skin, must not be made until the first appearance of natural breathing; for if the circulation of blood be induced before breathing has recommenced, the restoration of life will be endangered.

626. Schäfer's method of resuscitation of the apparently drowned.—If breathing has ceased, immediately on removal from the water, place the patient face-downwards on the ground, with the arms drawn forward and the face turned to the side.

Then, without stopping to remove or loosen clothing, commence respiration, as every instant of delay is serious.

To effect artificial respiration put yourself astride, or on one side of the patient's body, in a kneeling or squatting position, facing his head. Placing your hands flat on the small of his back, with the thumbs parallel and nearly touching, and the fingers spread out over the lowest ribs, lean forward with the arms straight and steadily allow the weight of your body to fall on the wrists, and so produce a firm, downward pressure, which must not be violent, on the loins and lower part of the back. (Fig. 155.) This part of the operation should occupy the time necessary to count, slowly—*one, two, three.*

By this means the air (and water, if there be any) is driven out of the patient's lungs. Water and slime from the air-passages may also run out.

Immediately thereafter, swing backward, rapidly releasing the pressure, when air will enter the lungs. Do not lift the hands from the patient's body. (Fig. 156.) This part of the operation should occupy the time necessary to count, slowly—*one, two.*

Repeat this forward and backward movement (pressure and relaxation of pressure) twelve or fifteen times a minute, without any marked pause between the movements. In other words, sway your body forwards and backwards upon your hands once in every four or five seconds.

Whilst the operator is carrying out artificial respiration, others may, if there be opportunity, busy themselves with applying hot flannels to the limbs and body, and hot bottles to the feet, or with promoting circulation by friction; but no attempt should be made on the part of the operator to remove wet clothing, or give restoratives by the mouth, till natural breathing has re-commenced.

When this has taken place, allow the patient to lie on the right side, and apply friction over the surface of the body by using handkerchiefs, flannels, etc., rubbing legs, arms, and body, all towards the heart, and continue after the patient has been wrapped in blankets or dry clothing. As soon as possible after complete recovery of respiration, remove the patient to the nearest shelter. On restoration, a teaspoonful of warm water may be given, and, if power of swallowing has returned, small quantities of wine, warm brandy and water, beef-tea, or coffee. Encourage the patient to sleep, but watch carefully for some time and allow free circulation of air round the patient.

627. Further instructions.—Prevent unnecessary crowding round the patient, especially if in an apartment. Avoid rough usage and do not allow the patient to remain on his back unless the tongue is secured. In no circumstances hold the patient up by the feet. On no account place the patient in a warm bath unless under medical orders.

Artificial respiration must also be resorted to in cases of suffocation either from the fumes of charcoal, or *choke-damp* in mining accidents; or from hanging; also in cases of lightning-stroke; severe electric shock; chloroform poisoning, etc.

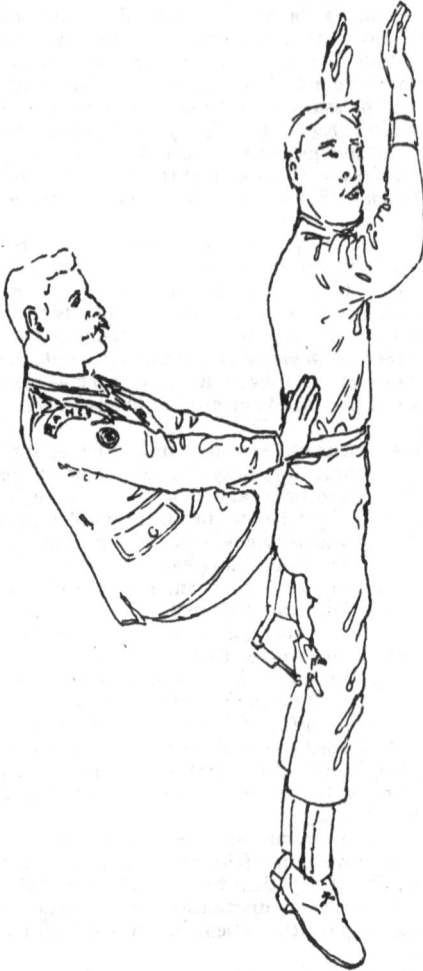

Fig. 155.—Expiration in Schäfer's Method.

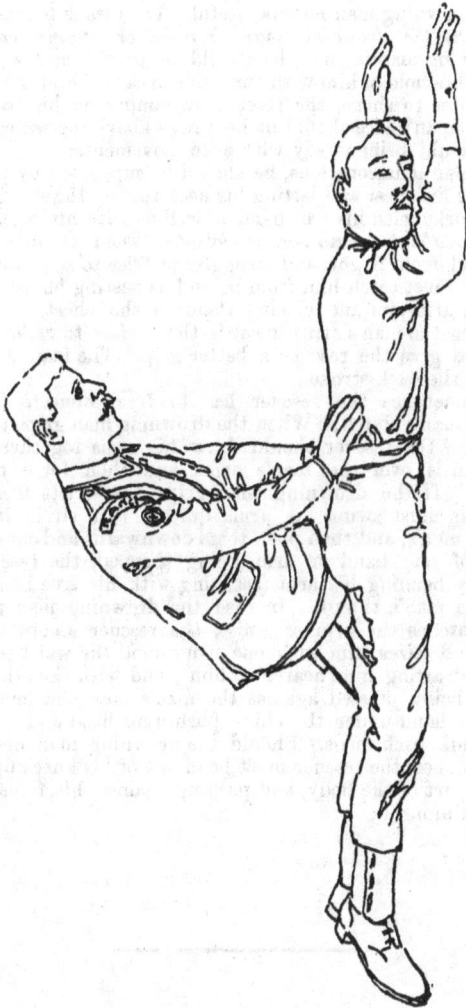

Fig. 156.—Inspiration in Schäfer's Method

628. Rescuing a drowning person.—Although it is not necessarily the work of the medical corps, a description of how to rescue a drowning man may be useful. The means to adopt are :—

(a) *When the drowning man is quiet or unconscious.*—When the drowning man is quiet, he should be turned on his back ; the rescuer takes hold of him with one hand on each side of the head, and conveys him to shore, the rescuer swimming on his back. The drowning man's face should be held high above the water, and the rescuer should swim slowly with even movements.

If the man is unconscious, he should be supported by placing an arm under his chest and letting his neck rest on the shoulder. The rescuer works with his free hand as well as with his legs.

(b) *When the drowning man is violent.*—When the man has lost self-control from fright, and struggles or tries to seize the rescuer, the latter must catch him from behind, thrusting his hands under the man's arm-pits and placing them on the chest, at the same time lifting the man's arms towards the surface to make him float higher and give the rescuer a better grip. The man is conveyed ashore by the back-stroke.

629. Sometimes the rescuer has to free himself from the drowning man's clutch. When the drowning man grips the wrists from above, the rescuer should draw his arms together inwards and upwards over the man's arms, and then force them out sideways. If the drowning man grips the wrists from below, the rescuer must swing his arms quickly in a circle inside the drowning man's, and then push them downwards and out sideways. In case of one hand or arm being gripped, the rescuer frees himself by bending his arm (assisting with his free hand) in the line of the man's thumb. In case the drowning man grips the neck or catches the arm or waist, the rescuer stoops over him quickly, and seizes him with one arm round the waist just above the hips, drawing him nearer to him ; and with the other arm— the hand being pressed against the man's nose and mouth, the butt of the hand under the chin—pushes his head and upper part of the trunk backwards. Should the drowning man not release his grip at once, the rescuer must bend one of his knees up against the lower part of the body, and pushing against this, force the man away from him.

CHAPTER XLIII.

POISONING.

630. Definition.—A poison is any substance which on being absorbed into the organs of the body, or by chemical action on the tissues, injures health or destroys life.

631. Suspected cases.—A case of poisoning may be suspected by (1) the sudden appearance of the symptoms in a person otherwise healthy, (2) the symptoms coming on soon after food or drink has been taken. (If after a meal of which many have eaten, the symptoms will be complained of by several or all who have partaken of it.) The symptoms vary in character, and the treatment will depend upon the poison taken.

632. How poisons act.—Poisons injure health or destroy life in various ways, according to their nature; e.g., (1) By actually burning the parts they touch, i.e., the mouth, throat, and stomach, and causing shock; or by making the parts swell up so as to suffocate the patient. These poisons are called *corrosives;* they may be acids or alkalies—oil of vitriol is an example of an acid, and caustic potash of an alkaline corrosive.

(2) Others by so irritating the parts they touch, such as the throat, stomach, and bowels, as to cause inflammation, often severe in degree; this inflammation gives rise to pain, vomiting, and later on to diarrhœa which may kill the patient by exhausting him. These are called *irritant poisons*, examples of which are arsenic, phosphorus, decomposed foods, etc.

(3) By being absorbed into the blood and producing their poisonous action on the brain, nerves, heart, blood, or other important organ, and so interfering with their function that death ensues. Examples of these are opium, chloroform, strychnine, prussic acid, snake-poison, arsenic. These are called *systemic (i.e.,* constitutional) *poisons.* Some poisons of this group are also called *narcotic poisons*, as they cause insensibility, e.g., alcohol and opium. It is not unusual to find that certain irritant poisons produce dangerous results on vital organs, when they become absorbed into the blood, in addition to their local irritant effects, e.g., arsenic and carbolic acid.

633. Treatment.—In all cases of suspected poisoning, medical assistance should be sent for immediately, and the directions here given should be followed at once by the orderly, as no time must be lost.

Two main principles must be borne in mind in the treatment of cases of poisoning :—

First.—Try to remove the poison already taken, if possible or advisable.

Second.—Try to lessen the poisonous effects by giving the proper remedy, sometimes called the antidote.

Any poison remaining, all vomited matter, or anything likely to prove of importance in the inquiry which is sure to take place subsequently, should be carefully preserved for inspection.

When a poison, of which the nature is unknown, has been swallowed, the following combination may be administered :—

$$\left.\begin{array}{l}\text{Carbonate of magnesia} \\ \text{Powdered charcoal} \\ \text{Hydrated peroxide of iron}\end{array}\right\} \text{equal parts.}$$

To be given freely in a sufficient quantity of water.

This preparation is harmless, and is an antidote to many of the most common and active poisons.

Hydrated peroxide of iron may be obtained by precipitating tinct. ferri perchlor. by liquor ammoniæ. Milk, or flour and water, may also be given.

(1) *Corrosive Poisons.*

Symptoms.	*Treatment.*
Great pain, immediately after taking the poison, in the mouth and throat, which look as if scalded ; mouth and lips stained and blistered. Shock and perhaps difficulty in breathing. Breath may smell very sour, or of hartshorn.	*Do not give emetics.* If the smell is sour, probably the poison is an acid, in which case magnesia-mixture, lime-water, or chalk and water, linseed or olive oil poured into the mouth help to stop further action by neutralizing the acidity. If the breath smells of hartshorn or does not smell acid, probably the poison is an alkali, in which case some weak vinegar and water or limejuice should be administered. Apply hot-water bottles to the feet and other means for restorating from shock. Use remedies as soon as possible. Have the tracheotomy instruments in readiness.

Scrapings from white-washed wall or ceilings may well be used in emergency as an antidote for acids. Use weak liquor ammoniæ (liquid ammonia), or aqua calcis (lime-water), to neutralize acids preferably to the carbonates, as the latter produce so much gas on combination that it may burst the stomach open.

Vinegar is the safest acid to administer.

The following are the most common corrosive poisons :—

Oil of vitriol (sulphuric acid), spirits of salts (hydrochloric acid), nitric acid, caustic soda, caustic potash, strong ammonia, oxalic acid (salts of sorrel), and carbolic acid.

(2) *Irritant Poisons.*

Symptoms.	*Treatment.*
Pain not at first very great; generally a sensation of burning, or a strong taste in the mouth and throat, coming quickly if the poison is liquid, and less quickly if it is solid when taken. The parts touched by the poison are not burned, and the pain is not so great as in the case of a corrosive poison, but it gradually increases and vomiting sets in, with pain in the stomach, diarrhœa with straining, and sometimes blood in the stools. Much can be learned by looking at the vomited matter. Shock and exhaustion set in generally.	*Give emetics.* Give warm water and encourage vomiting until the water returns clear; then milk or white of egg, oil or melted butter to allay the irritation. Get the stomach-tube ready. In phosphorus and cantharides poisoning, butter or oil should *not* be given.

The following are the most common irritants :—

Copper, stale or badly-tinned fish or meat, arsenic, antimony (tartar emetic), perchloride of mercury, zinc, iodine, cantharides, and powdered glass.

(3) *Systemic Poisons.*

Symptoms.	*Treatment.*
No sign of burning, redness, or pain, but there may be giddiness, dimness of sight, drowsiness (gradually increasing), difficulty in breathing, irregular or weak pulse, delirium, cramps, convulsions. The pupils of the eyes either widely open or tightly closed, according to the particular system of the body affected—nervous, vascular, respiratory, etc.	*Give emetics.* The stomach must be emptied by means of emetics or the stomach-tube. Symptoms must be treated: that is, in case of drowsiness, the patient must be kept awake by being walked about, cold water being freely used, and hot coffee given. If the drowsiness becomes greater, or the breathing threatens to fail, artificial respiration should be resorted to sometimes for hours; if the pulse is weak, give ammonia (sal volatile); if there are cramps, gentle rubbing of the limbs; if delirium or convulsions are present, the patient should be carefully watched and kept as quiet as possible, and administered the special antidotes in the case of each poison. If the case is prolonged, nourishment should be given by the mouth or the rectum.

Emetics.—The following may be administered to produce vomiting :—

1. Mustard ⎫
2. Salt ⎭ One tablespoonful to a tumbler of water.

3. Sulphate of zinc, grs. 30 in ℥i of water.
4. Ipecacuanha, grs. 20 to 30 of the powder ; *or*
   ℥ss to ℥i of the wine.
5. Ammonium carbonate, grs. 20 to 30 in ℥i water.

Remember that an emetic promptly given may save the patient's life, but one must not be given in a case of corrosive poisoning.

CHAPTER XLIV.

IMPROVISATION.

634. In dealing with this subject it is not possible or desirable to lay down any hard and fast rules. Force of circumstances as well as general surroundings and geographical position at the time, all enter largely into these matters. For instance, the occasions on which we may require to improvise dressings, surgical appliances, methods for the carriage or disposal of sick and wounded, may be in peace or war, in winter or summer, in sunshine or rain, by road, rail, or sea, at home or abroad.

Much of the success attending the efforts to carry out any scheme for improvisation will depend largely on the ingenuity of those dealing with it. They must be guided not only by the immediate conditions and surroundings, but by the material at their disposal.

In this manual improvisation has been dealt with under various headings, it being an extremely necessary part of military medical training. For example, improvised tourniquets are dealt with in para. 571, Chap. XXXIV, improvised splints in paras. 594 and 595, Chap. XXXV, improvised carriage of wounded in Chap. XVIII, improvised shelter for housing wounded in para. 210, Chap. XV, and para. 256, Chap. XVI, and shelters generally are referred to in Chap. XXIV. Improvised methods of field sanitation are dealt with in Part II.

Further directions for improvisation not dealt with elsewhere are given in this chapter.

635. Dressings.—Linen, cotton, flannel, blankets, clothing, teased-out wool and tow, can be all used for improvised dressings. Any material used should be selected from as clean a source as possible. If time and circumstances allow, they should be thoroughly washed and boiled, then baked or sun-dried, and when cool used at once. When not required for immediate use they should be preserved in covered receptacles, which have themselves been previously sterilized as far as practicable, for instance, in tin biscuit-boxes, earthenware jars, etc., hermetically sealed with resin or strips of rubber-plaster, wax, or similar substance placed round the lid.

Bark-cloth, made from the bark of a species of fig-tree, such as is worn by the natives in the interior of Africa, has been used with success in improvisation of surgical dressings. It was baked in earthen pots and soaked in water in which eucalyptus leaves had been boiled ; then dried and kept ready for use in stoppered and air-tight earthenware jars, which had been previously sterilized by heat.

636. Sterilization.—Heat is the readiest and most desirable method of sterilization of all improvised dressings and instruments. It may be moist or dry. If moist heat be selected, any utensils which can be used for boiling purposes, such as large meat-tins, biscuit-boxes, earthenware native cooking-pots, or kettles and pans, can all be used for boiling the instruments or dressings in. Dry heat can be obtained in the oven of a cooking-range, in which dressings must be thoroughly baked.

Moist heat is greatly preferable to dry, as it kills germs much more easily ; it should always be selected if possible. Instruments can be quickly sterilized by being held in a flame.

637. Antiseptic lotions.—The best substitute for these is water which has been thoroughly and recently boiled. It should be used fresh if possible, and not stored. But if storing is unavoidable, the vessels should themselves be sterilized by having water boiled in them, and they should be kept closely stoppered.

Weak solutions made of " Jeyes' fluid " or " Izal " have with success been used as substitutes for the better-known antiseptics.

CHAPTER XLV.

SURGICAL INSTRUMENTS AND APPLIANCES.

638. Description of instruments.—The following are brief descriptions of the instruments and appliances in most common use :—

Aspirator.—An instrument for drawing off fluids by means of an exhausting air-pump.

Bistoury.—A long, narrow knife, which is either straight or curved, sharp or blunt-pointed.

Bistoury, Hernia.—A long, narrow knife, blunt except for about the space of an inch from the point, which is also blunt, used in the operation for rupture.

Bougie.—An instrument used for dilating strictures.

Catheter.—A tube for passing through the urethra into the bladder to draw off the urine. Catheters are either made of silver or silver-plate, or of gum-elastic, or india-rubber ; they contain a wire called a *stylet*. French olivary catheters and soft rubber catheters are flexible and have no stylets. In the metal and gum-elastic catheters the eye is near the point. In French catheters it is $1\frac{1}{2}$ inches from the point. English catheters are numbered from 1, the smallest, to 18, the largest ; and French catheters, from 1 to 30.

Caustic-holder.—A little case for holding caustic, usually made of vulcanite or silver.

Director.—An instrument with a groove in which to guide the point of a knife.

Drainage-tubes.—India-rubber or glass tubes used after operation for draining a wound.

Elevator.—An instrument for raising depressed pieces of bone.

Enema-apparatus.—An instrument for administering enemata.

Forceps, Dental.—An instrument used for extracting teeth.

Forceps, Dissecting.—Plain forceps used for dissecting purposes.

Forceps, Dressing.—Forceps with scissor-handles, used for removing old dressing, etc., from wounds and sores.

Forceps, Ferguson's Clawed or Lion-forceps.—A strong forceps with claws, used for gripping bone where much force is required.

Forceps, Gouge.—A strong forceps, cutting at the points, so as to gouge bone.

Forceps, Liston's Bone.—A strong forceps for cutting bone in operations.

Forceps, Phimosis.—Forceps for holding the foreskin in the operation of circumcision.

Forceps, Polypus.—Forceps for grasping small tumours usually in the nasal cavity.

Forceps, Sinus.—Forceps for introduction into a sinus, which is a tubular cavity.

Forceps, Spencer Wells' or Pressure-forceps.—Forceps for the compression of bleeding vessels during operations.

Forceps, Tongue.—Forceps for holding the tongue, generally used in giving chloroform.

Guillotine, Tonsil.—A sliding knife for slicing the tonsil.

Hernia-director.—Made of steel, and broader than the ordinary director, used for the operation for strangulated hernia or rupture.

Insufflator.—A tube used for blowing powder into some cavity, such as the throat.

Irrigator or Douche.—A metal or glass vessel to which a tube is attached fitted with a nozzle and stop-cock, used for flushing or washing wounds with boiled water or antiseptic lotion.

Laryngoscope.—An instrument for examining the throat and larynx.

Lenses, Test—Glasses of various powers used for testing the eyes.

Ligatures.—Threads of sterilized silk, catgut, or tendon used for tying up blood-vessels.

Needle, Aneurysm.—A curved, blunt instrument with an eye near the end, used for passing a ligature under an artery.

Needle, Cataract.—A needle, without an eye, in a handle, used in the operation for cataract.

Needle-holder.—A strong, special forceps for holding a needle to put in stitches during operations.

Needle, Surgical.—Curved and straight needles of various sizes.

Ophthalmoscope.—An instrument for examining the eyes.

Post-mortem case.—A case containing the instruments used in the examination of bodies after death.

Probang, or Œsophageal bougie.—A flexible instrument for passing down the gullet.

Probe.—A silver instrument for probing wounds.

Retractor.—A blunt hook or flat piece of metal, bent at an angle for holding apart the edges of a wound during operation.

Saw, Amputating.—A saw used for sawing the bone in amputation of a limb.

Saw, Butcher's.—A framed saw, the invention of Mr. Butcher, used for the same purposes as the amputating-saw, but more especially for excision of joints.

Saw, Hey's.—A small saw for cutting a piece out of a bone used in operations on the skull.

Scalpel.—A short knife with a curved edge, made in different sizes and used for cutting and dissecting.

Scoop.—A spoon-shaped instrument used for scraping various growths, etc.

Shears, Rib.—A large scissors-like instrument used for cutting the ribs.

Sound.—An instrument for feeling what is beyond the reach of the fingers.

Spatula.—A blunt knife for spreading ointments; also an instrument used for depressing the tongue when an examination is being made of the throat.

Sterilizer.—An apparatus for killing germs on instruments or in dressings, by means of heat.

Stethoscope.—An instrument with which to listen to the sounds in the chest.

Stomach-tube.—An apparatus used for washing out or emptying the stomach.

Sutures.—Threads of wire, silk, catgut, silkworm-gut, horse-hair, or tendon used by the surgeon for stitching wounds.

Syringe.—An instrument made of glass or metal, used for injecting fluids.

Syringe, Higginson's.—An apparatus consisting of an india-rubber pump to be squeezed by the hand, and two pipes, one fitted with a nozzle to pass into the anus, and one with a pewter end to slip into the basin for giving enemata.

Syringe, Hypodermic.—A graduated glass or metal syringe fitted with a hollow needle, employed in the injection of morphia and other medicines beneath the skin.

Thermometer, Clinical.—A closed, glass tube containing a bulb and a fine column of mercury for registering the temperature of the human body.

Tourniquet.—An instrument for making pressure on an artery to stop the flow of blood through it. (See Figs. 140 and 141.)

Tracheotomy-tubes.—Two curved, silver tubes, one fitting inside the other, used for putting into the windpipe when it has been opened by an operation called tracheotomy.

Trephine.—A tubular saw, used in operations on the skull.

Trocar and Canula.—A sharp-pointed instrument and sheath for tapping collections of fluid. Large, for tapping the belly or chest; small, for tapping hydrocele.

Truss.—An appliance used to keep the bowel in its place in cases of rupture.

Wools, Holmgren's.—Coloured wools of various shades used for testing for colour-blindness.

Lists of contents of the various articles of Field Medical Equipment will be found in the Appendices of the Regulations for the Army Medical Service, and in the Field Service Manual, A.M.S.

CHAPTER XLVI.

ATTENDANCE ON INFECTIOUS CASES.

639. Spread of infection.—Infection is caused by the entry into the body from without of a living thing, a germ or microbe. These germs produce such infectious diseases as enteric fever, cholera, smallpox, plague, dysentery, malaria, etc. In nursing such cases, care must be taken to guard against the spread of infection by destroying the germs which leave the patient's body in the breath, discharges, and excretions, and are able to start the disease afresh in another individual.*

640. Personal precautions.—It is the duty of the orderly to guard himself by all reasonable precautions against infection.

He should never go on duty fasting.

The finger-nails should be kept short, a nail-brush should always be used before taking a meal, and the hands washed and rinsed in some disinfectant immediately after touching the patient. As much fresh air as possible should be obtained, and no food should be eaten in the wards.

641. Disinfectant.—A *disinfectant* is something that "frees from infection." The most reliable disinfectant is heat in the form of boiling water, steam, or hot air of a temperature of 250° F. Articles that are disinfected by heat are said to be "sterilized," *i.e.*, they are rendered absolutely free from every kind of germ.

For articles that cannot be subjected to the action of heat, chemical disinfectants have to be used. These are very much less satisfactory than heat. Of chemical disinfectants the best are carbolic acid 1 in 20 (5 per cent.), or perchloride of mercury 1 in 1,000. If used in weaker solutions than these they cannot be relied upon to kill germs. Milk of lime and chloride of lime are also used for disinfecting stools. (See Regulations for the Army Medical Service, for disinfectant solutions.)

642. Ventilation of wards.—Constant and free ventilation is the only method of purifying the air of a ward. Noxious emanations are given off by the patient's body, which are hurtful not only to himself but to his attendants ; the risk of the latter catching disease is much diminished by free ventilation.

The window should be kept constantly open at the top, care being taken to guard the patient from draughts. When not too cold, the windows should be opened top and bottom two or three times a day, and the room thoroughly flushed with fresh air, the patient being carefully covered up. A fire is an aid to ventilation (see para. 732).

643. Disinfection of linen.—A supply of bedding and clothing distinctively marked with an " I " should be set apart for the use of patients suffering from infectious diseases. (See Regulations for the Army Medical Service.) Both bed and body linen should after use be at once placed in a disinfecting solution as laid down in

---

* " The Control of Infection," Chap. VII, Part II, Sanitation, or the Prevention of Disease, should be read in conjunction with this chapter by orderlies and others after their first year of training.

Regulations for the Army Medical Service, unless specially directed to be dealt with in any particular way.

Especial care is necessary in the treatment of soiled linen from enteric-fever patients. All excretal matter should be rinsed out before placing the articles to steep in the cresol solution. Hands must be carefully scrubbed after touching soiled linen.

644. Disinfection of stools and urine.—In enteric fever the infectious germs are contained in the stools and urine of the patient.

Unless otherwise ordered, a small quantity of cresol solution or other disinfectant should be put in the bed-pan and care should be taken that no moisture from the disinfectant remains on the outside of the bed-pan. After use it should be covered up with a china cover and removed at once from the ward, enough cresol being added completely to cover the stool, at least 8 fluid ounces being used, the whole being well mixed by stirring with a piece of stick.

Where water-closets or slop-sinks do not exist, the best method of disposing of enteric stools is to boil or burn them. Where a water-closet or slop-sink is available for their disposal, before emptying the stools into these they should be mixed with an equal quantity of cresol solution and allowed to stand for one hour to allow the disinfectant to act.

While the stool is standing, the bed-pan with the china cover should be covered with a cloth soaked in cresol solution. This should also be done when a stool is being kept for inspection.

The urine should also be well mixed with an equal quantity (at least 4 ounces) of the cresol solution and allowed to stand for an hour before being emptied, if no special method is arranged for its disposal.

All utensils (*e.g.*, feeding-cups, bed-pans, urinals, etc.), intended to be used by enteric patients must be marked with an " E." (See Regulations for the Army Medical Service.)

645. Disinfection of sputum.—Cresol solution should be placed in the spit-cup before use.

Rags or special handkerchiefs which can be burnt should be used to wipe away all discharges from the mouth and nose.

646. Disinfection of patient's body.—The patient should be carefully sponged from head to foot daily, care being taken that he is not unduly exposed.

In scarlet fever the flakes of skin which become detached from the body during the process of desquamation may convey the infection. Some medical officers therefore have their scarlet-fever patients, during the peeling stage, anointed daily from head to foot with some disinfectant dissolved in olive oil. This prevents the escape of dust and particles of skin from the patient. In addition, warm baths are frequently given during convalescence.

647. Dusting of patient's room.—The dusting of a ward should be done with a duster damped with some disinfecting solution, to prevent the dust, in which infectious germs may be present, being scattered about ; after use the duster should be at once placed in the tub containing the disinfecting solution.

All crockery used by infectious cases should be specially marked and kept for this use only.

CHAPTER XLVII.

MEDICINES AND THEIR ADMINISTRATION.

648. Methods of giving drugs.—Drugs may be introduced into the system in several ways. They may be swallowed, inhaled, injected under the skin, rubbed into the skin, injected into the rectum, or administered by means of medicated baths (see Chap. L.).

649. By the mouth.—The great majority of medicines are given by the mouth. Drugs given in this way may be administered in the forms of liquids, pills, powders, or in capsules.

Liquids.*—Before a dose of mixture is given the label must always be read, the bottle shaken, and the exact dose poured into a graduated measure-glass. The quantity must never be guessed, and spoons are not reliable measures.

When a certain number of drops are to be given a minim-measure should if possible always be used, since drops vary very much in size with the character of the fluid and the shape of the bottle. When one or two minims of a medicine are ordered, measure ten minims and then add enough water (unless any special vehicle is ordered) to bring it up to ten drachms. Each drachm of the mixture will contain one minim of the medicine.

While pouring out the medicine the bottle should be held with the label uppermost, that this may not be soiled if any drops should run down the side, and so obliterate the directions.

Pills.—These contain drugs in a solid form. The patient should take a small mouthful of water, then put the pill in the mouth and drink a little more water.

Powders.—When small, these should be shaken on to the back of the tongue and then washed down with a drink of some fluid ; when too large to do this, they must be mixed with water.

Capsules.—These are small pear-shaped receptacles made of gelatine, which are sealed up after having a dose of the drug placed in them.

Tablets.—In addition, certain drugs are often compressed into tablets, and these may be given in the same way as pills.

650. By the lungs.—Drugs given in this way are inhaled. Medicines which are inhaled, *i.e.*, drawn in with the air at each inspiration into the lungs, are usually intended to act upon the lungs, and are therefore almost entirely reserved for cases in which these organs are affected. Inhalations are also used for sore-throats and when the larynx is inflamed. Lastly, certain drugs, such as chloroform, ether, etc., are inhaled for the purpose of producing general anæsthesia.

Oxygen is often employed in cases of pneumonia, and in other diseases of the lungs. The gas is contained in a metal cylinder which is brought to the bedside. The flow is regulated by means of a stop-cock, and the gas is conducted from the cylinder through rubber tubing. If the patient is strong enough, he inhales the gas through a glass funnel (which is attached to the rubber tubing) held before the mouth and nostrils. The effect is carefully watched, the

---

* Medicines intended for external use are so labelled, and if containing a poison are dispensed in fluted bottles and labelled " Poison."

flow of gas being restricted, or the funnel removed further away, if any distress becomes apparent.

651. Hypodermic injections.—By this method the drugs to be administered are injected under the skin. " Under the skin " is the meaning of both " hypodermic " and " subcutaneous." Absorption into the circulation is very much more rapid by this way than any other, the drug taking effect within from one to five minutes. Being such a potent method, it is as a rule used only in cases of emergency, *e.g.*, for the relief of pain, to induce vomiting, or to stimulate the heart.

Intra-muscular injection is when the injected drug is pushed much deeper, *i.e.*, into the muscles, as in the intra-muscular administration of mercury.

652. Inunction means the rubbing of an ointment into the skin. The portion of the skin to be treated should first be washed with soap and water, and then dried. This stimulates the circulation in the skin and enables it more quickly to absorb the medicament. This method of introducing drugs into the system is practically reserved for the administration of mercury. The chief point to be remembered is that the ointment must be rubbed into the skin and not left on it, the part being thoroughly massaged with the palm and finger-tips. It should take from twenty minutes to half an hour to rub in the usual dose of mercurial ointment. The orderly should carefully wash his hands immediately afterwards. The same spot should not be selected each day, as the skin may become inflamed.

653. Rectal medication.—Drugs may be introduced into the rectum in either a liquid or a solid form. They are given in this way when the patient is unconscious or vomiting, or for the relief of diarrhœa or rectal pain, or for stimulating a patient who is collapsed after operation. Liquid preparations should be slowly run in through a glass funnel and rubber tube.

Suppositories are solid preparations of a conical shape and of varying sizes, according to their contents. The suppository is oiled and slowly passed well into the rectum.

654. Accuracy in giving medicines.—Full directions are, as a rule, given as to the time of administration of each dose of medicine. It should always be punctual to the minute. Three-times-a-day medicines are usually given at 10 a.m., 2 p.m., and 6 p.m. ; twice-a-day, at 10 a.m. and 6 p.m.

A medicine that is ordered to be taken " before meals " should be given a quarter of an hour before food, and one to be taken "after meals," immediately after the meal is finished.

A double dose of medicine should never be given at one hour because the previous dose has been forgotten.

After each dose of medicine the measure-glass must be washed.

All medicines should be carefully labelled. All poisons should be kept in a separate, locked cupboard. The liniments and lotions should stand on a shelf by themselves.

Fluid Measure :—

60 minims	(m. lx)	= 1 fluid drachm.	(℥ i)
8 drachms		= 1 ounce.	(℥ i)
20 ounces		= 1 pint.	(O i)
8 pints		= 1 gallon.	(C i)

CHAPTER XLVIII.

ENEMATA.

655. An enema is a liquid preparation which is injected into the rectum. It is chiefly given to produce an action of the bowels, to relieve pain, to stimulate, or to feed the patient. Its composition and size vary with the purpose for which it is used. Nutrient enemata and those prescribed to allay pain are usually small in quantity, those intended to clear out the bowels are large.

656. Method of administration.—The patient is usually placed on the left side or on the back. It is the more convenient to have the patient lying on his left side, since the large intestine runs backward from the anal aperture in the direction of the left hip; but it sometimes happens that it is impossible to put him in that position—as, for instance, after an abdominal operation, or injury to the pelvis. In such a case the enema must be given with the patient lying on his back. This is more difficult, and it is wise to practise giving it in this position so that when necessary it may be done easily and not cause the patient discomfort.

When the enema is given with the patient lying on his side, the hips must be brought to the edge of the bed and flexed, also the knees. A warmed mackintosh covered with a towel is then placed under the patient, and the bed-clothes, with the exception of one blanket, turned back. The vessel containing the fluid to be injected should be placed in a convenient position, and the catheter or nozzle of the syringe oiled. The index finger of the left hand should be passed between the buttocks, and laid lightly on the anus, and the tube passed below the finger into the rectum, directing it upwards and backwards. No force must be used, the tube must be carefully passed over the small tongue of integument which is found at the anterior angle of the anus.* If the Higginson's syringe is used the fluid must be pumped in with the right hand. Five minutes should be occupied in injecting one pint. There should be no attempt at hurrying, otherwise the enema may be instantly returned.

If the patient may not be turned on his side, he should, lying on his back, be brought as near to the edge of the bed as possible, the right knee flexed, and the anus found as before with the index finger of the left hand. The tube is then gently passed with the right hand, being directed backwards and slightly downwards. When the injection has been given the tube should be gently and slowly removed from the rectum, and firm pressure at once applied upon the anus with a folded towel to assist the patient in retaining the enema. The buttocks being pressed together also assists in this way.

657. Purgative enemata.—Purgative enemata are given either with the object of assisting an easy action of the bowels, e.g., before and after operations, or for the relief of constipation.

---

* Almost immediately the muscle will relax and the tube slip in.

Soap-and-water enema.—This is made by dissolving one ounce of soft soap in a pint of warm water. Ordinary yellow soap can be used. One pint is the usual quantity. This is generally administered with a Higginson's syringe, often with a No. 12 catheter attached to the nozzle. The temperature of the fluid should be about 100° F. The air should be expelled from the tube before it is inserted. The enema should be retained for from eight to ten minutes. When giving any sort of purgative enema, a warmed bed-pan should be ready at hand for use, to prevent accidents.

Glycerine enema.—This is usually given by means of a special vulcanite syringe holding half an ounce, the usual quantity given being from one to two drachms.

Turpentine enema.—When given as a purgative, one ounce of oil of turpentine is mixed with fifteen ounces of thin starch.

When given for the relief of abdominal distension, half an ounce is usually given in two ounces of thin starch.

Olive oil enema.—An olive oil enema consists of four ounces of oil with eight ounces of thin starch, or four ounces of olive oil, run into the bowel by means of a glass funnel and a long piece of rubber tubing, followed in half an hour's time by an ordinary soap-and-water enema ; or four ounces of oil can be beaten up with sixteen ounces of soap and water and injected.

Castor oil enema.—This consists of one ounce of castor oil mixed with ten ounces of thin starch, or one ounce of castor oil mixed with three ounces of olive oil, warmed and injected, and followed in half an hour by a soap-and-water enema.

658. Nutrient enema.—This is given when a patient is taking insufficient food by the mouth, or when it is desired that the stomach should be kept completely at rest. The powers of digestion possessed by the rectum being limited, any food given in this way must be thoroughly digested by means of " peptonizing powders " before use. The size of the enema, together with the frequency of injection, will be as ordered ; four ounces four-hourly being the usual quantity for an adult. Peptonized milk is usually the chief constituent of these enemata. The enema should be strained before administration and be at a temperature of 100° F.

Patients who are being systematically fed by the bowel should have a plain-water enema once in every twenty-four hours, and in addition, before each enema is given, the rectum should be gently washed out with warm water or warm boric lotion. To do this a soft catheter, well oiled, to which a piece of rubber tubing with a glass funnel at the other end is attached, is passed into the bowel By pouring warm water or boracic lotion slowly into the raised funnel, and then lowering it before it is quite empty, to allow it to run out again, the bowel is well washed. The enema is given by means of the same apparatus. The time taken in administering four ounces should be at least five minutes.

A large nutrient enema containing as much as one pint is sometimes ordered. This is more difficult of administration. The tube, which must be fairly large, must be passed for some distance, not more than seven inches, into the rectum in a backward and upward direction. The enema is given in the same way as the smaller one, but half an hour at least must be expended in giving one pint.

A large quantity can also be given by means of an irrigator suspended above the bed, and connected by means of rubber tubing with a catheter in the rectum. The tubing is compressed by a clip so that fluid from the irrigator can only be passed through it very slowly and thus enter the rectum drop by drop, where it is absorbed before any quantity can accumulate.

659. Starch-and-opium enema.—This is given for the relief of pain, or to check excessive diarrhœa. Two ounces of thin starch are mixed with the prescribed amount of laudanam and heated to a temperature of 100° F. It is then slowly injected into the bowel by means of a glass syringe and a rubber tube.

660. Rectal tube.—A long rectal tube is sometimes passed for the relief of abdominal distension. A stout, rubber tube, well oiled, is passed into the rectum for about seven inches, and left in position. The other end of the tube should be placed in a small basin of carbolic lotion. If any gas escapes from the bowel it will be heard bubbling through the fluid.

CHAPTER XLIX.

EXTERNAL APPLICATIONS, COUNTER-IRRITANTS, POULTICES, &c.

661. A gargle is used as a wash for the mouth and throat. A tablespoonful is to be taken into the mouth, the head then thrown slightly back and the fluid set in motion by breathing through it, at the same time taking care not to swallow any. This should be repeated two or three times on each occasion.

662. Eye-lotions are used for washing away discharges from the eye. They are applied by means of a vessel called an "eye-bath," by a special irrigator, or by allowing a steady stream from a pledget of cotton-wool, held about two inches above the eye, to run over as much of the inner surfaces of the lids as possible. This is most effectually done by everting the eyelids (see para. 622). This done, retaining the upper lid in position by means of the thumb, the lower lid is now easily everted by placing the forefinger on the skin below the eye and drawing it downwards, the patient at the same time looking upwards.

663. Eye-drops are applied in different ways according to the purpose for which they are used. When they are intended to act upon the conjunctiva, the lids must be everted in the usual way and the drops allowed to fall vertically upon the inner surfaces. When drops are used with the object of dilating or contracting the pupil, the lower lid is drawn downwards and one or two drops allowed to fall on its inner surface. Before using the drop-bottle, two or three drops should be allowed to escape from the nozzle so that any foreign matter in it may be washed away.

664. Counter-irritants are local applications used for the relief of pain or the checking of inflammation, some producing mere reddening of the skin, and others actual inflammation.

Mustard-plaster.—Two parts of mustard to one of flour are made into a paste with tepid water. This is spread evenly on a piece of linen cut to a suitable shape and size, and is covered with a single layer of washed muslin ; it is then ready for application.

Mustard-leaves.—These are more convenient to apply than the plaster. They should be moistened in warm water before application, the skin having been previously cleaned.

Application of iodine.—The skin should first be washed, and then the iodine painted on with a camel-hair brush. After the first coat has dried a second should be applied.

When a strong solution of iodine is ordered, the directions as to its application must be minutely observed, as it is very much stronger than the tincture and causes considerable irritation to sensitive skins.

Liniments are very mild counter-irritants, which are rubbed in by the hand after the part has been washed.

Blisters.—These may be applied in the form of a plaster, or painted on the part. When the plaster is used, the part should be well washed with soap and water, and sponged with ether to remove grease from the skin. The plaster is cut to the shape and size required, moistened with warm water, placed in position and secured loosely with a bandage, so as to exert no pressure on the blister when it rises.

When blistering-fluid is used the part to be painted, having been previously washed, should be outlined with vaseline or oil to keep the fluid within the required space. Two or three coats are then painted on and the part covered with wool and a loose bandage.

The plaster should be left on from ten to twelve hours. If the blister has not risen then, a fomentation should be applied. The plaster is then carefully removed, and the blister which has been produced is snipped at its most dependent point with a pair of sharp sterilized scissors, and the fluid gently pressed into absorbent wool. Sometimes the fluid is allowed to be re-absorbed, the blister being left unopened and merely protected with wool and a bandage.

The actual cautery.—As a counter-irritant this may be used—(a) For the relief of pain, in which case the heated point is not brought into contact with the skin, but is moved to and fro just above it so as to produce a reddening of the surface. (b) For the treatment of chronic joint inflammation. Here the point of the instrument which is kept at a dull red, is lightly drawn across the part to be treated, so as to produce a superficial burn, which is dressed in the ordinary way.

665. Leeches are used for the relief of pain and for checking inflammation. Each leech draws from one to three drachms of blood. The smaller pointed end is the head of the animal.

Before applying a leech, the skin should be well washed and thoroughly dried, and when possible briskly rubbed to bring the blood to the surface. It is important to handle the leech as little as possible. A leech will continue sucking for about three-quarters of an hour. It should never be forcibly removed, or its teeth may be left in the skin, which would produce a troublesome wound. A pinch of salt sprinkled on the head will make a leech relax its hold. If the bleeding is to be encouraged, a fomentation should be applied to the bites, otherwise a pad of gauze should be strapped over them. The patient should be carefully watched until the bleeding has ceased, as sometimes this is very troublesome.

666. Ointments may be applied either spread with a spatula on the smooth side of a piece of lint, or they may be rubbed in with the hand, that is to say, by "innunction."

667. Lotions.—Evaporating lotions must be applied on a single thickness of lint, which should be left uncovered. Other lotions are applied by soaking a double thickness of lint in them, squeezing out the excess of moisture but without wringing them dry, and covering with jackonet or oiled silk to prevent evaporation.

668. Poultices are of various kinds, the most common being linseed and mustard.

Linseed-poultice.—Crushed linseed is most commonly used for a poultice.

To make a poultice, a board, a bowl, a kettle, a jug of boiling water, and a large spatula or flat knife are required; also tow or linen on which to spread the poultice. If tow is used it must be pulled out flat and even to the required size.

After the knife and bowl have been heated, a sufficient quantity of boiling water from the kettle is poured into the bowl. The linseed is then added, being quickly sprinkled in with one hand, while the mixture is stirred with the spatula. When sufficient meal has been added the mixture will come away clean from the edge of the bowl and should be turned out on the linen or tow, and spread evenly and quickly with the spatula, the latter being dipped in the jug of boiling water between each stroke. The layer of linseed-meal should be a quarter of an inch thick, and it should be spread to within one inch of the edge of the linen or tow, when the former should be folded and the latter rolled in all round. Care should be taken not to apply the poultice too hot; this can be prevented by first testing it on the back of the hand. When placed in position the poultice should be covered with a thick layer of cotton wool and secured by a bandage.

Mustard-poultice.—This is mustard mixed with linseed, the mustard being mixed separately with luke-warm water and then added to the linseed-poultice. The proportion of mustard to linseed varies with the object of the poultice, being either of equal parts or one of mustard to two of linseed.

669. Fomentations or Stupes.—The best material for a stupe is thick soft flannel. Spongio-piline is sometimes used, also lint and absorbent wool. Boracic wool is used for surgical cases. If used for the relief of pain, a fomentation should be changed every half-hour at least.

The material for the fomentation should be placed inside a towel or wringer and laid across a bowl which has been heated, the ends of the towel or wringer projecting over the sides. Boiling water is then poured over it, after which it is wrung out dry in the towel, taken out, and applied as hot as the patient can bear it. It is then covered with jackonet and wool, and bandaged firmly in position.

Turpentine stupe.—One or two drachms of turpentine are sprinkled carefully on the flannel before being wrung out of the boiling water.

Opium and belladonna are sometimes applied on stupes, half a teaspoonful of the tincture being sprinkled on the flannel after it has been wrung out.

670. Hot bottles may be of tin, earthenware, or india-rubber. For the feet, either tin or earthenware are suitable. For any other part of the body an india-rubber bag is more comfortable and efficacious. All hot bottles should be protected with thick flannel covers. Care must be taken that the bottles do not leak, and that there are no holes in the covers. It must be remembered that the following patients are peculiarly liable to be burnt; those who are unconscious from any cause, the paralysed, those who are suffering from great pain, the dropsical, the very young, and the old.

671. **Ice-bags** are made of various shapes and sizes to suit the part to which they are to be applied. The cup-shaped ice-bag is the one generally used. This should be half-filled with small pieces of ice, with which may be mixed a little common salt to intensify the cold ; sawdust or linseed-meal may be added to soak up the water and so make the ice last longer.

672. **Ice-poultice.**—Crushed ice between thin layers of linseed-meal, is spread to the depth of half an inch between two layers of tissue. The tissue is then sealed up all round with chloroform or turpentine.

CHAPTER L.

BATHS, PACKS, &c.

673. Temperature of baths.—In addition to the ordinary cleansing bath, baths are ordered for a variety of purposes. The temperature of these varies somewhat, but, as a general rule, by a *warm bath* is meant one about the temperature of the body, say 98° F. ; a *tepid bath* is about six degrees less, say 92° ; a *hot bath* is about six degrees more than 98°, say 104°. The bath-thermometer should be used on all occasions.

Before giving any kind of bath, instructions should be obtained as to the temperature of the bath, and the length of time the patient is to be kept in it.

674. Cold bath.—A cold bath is given at about a temperature of 65° F. It is given in cases of hyperpyrexia. In many cases it is not considered advisable to lower the patient directly into the cold water, the temperature to begin with being as high as 85° F., and being cooled down by the addition of iced water.

675. Hot bath.—A hot bath is given to relieve pain in renal colic, to soothe excitement in cholera and delirium, to relieve retention of urine, and to promote perspiration in uræmia.

These baths are usually given at the bedside, the patient being lifted into them from the bed.

676. Hot-air bath.—To give this a special apparatus is necessary. Allen's apparatus without the boiler is generally used.

Blankets are placed over and under the patient, and his shirts removed. A mackintosh must be placed under the lower, and two wicker-work body-cradles over the upper blankets. These are covered with two blankets, over which is placed a mackintosh, and over that again another blanket. The blankets should be well tucked in under the mattress. From the foot of the bed withdraw the blankets covering the patient, insert the spout of the kettle just within the lower cradle and light the lamp, which has several wicks. The spout should be guarded by asbestos, otherwise the blankets, which are pinned round it, will be scorched. A cloth wrung out of iced water should be laid over the patient's forehead and kept cold. He should also be given cold water to sip.

In the absence of any special orders, the duration of a hot-air bath is 20 minutes. At the end of that time the light should be put out, the hot-air pipe withdrawn, and a warm, dry blanket slipped in under the cradles. The temperature may be from 108° F. to 150° F. The latter heat can only be borne when the baths have been in use for some time. The mackintosh and cradles will then be removed and the patient left lying between blankets for an hour until he has done sweating ; he should then be sponged with warm water, and a warm, flannel shirt put on.

If the patient shows signs of exhaustion or faintness during the bath, the lamp must be put out at once and the cradles removed.

677. Vapour-bath.—This is given in the same way, except that the boiler is used in the apparatus, and the steam from the boiling water is introduced into the bed instead of hot, dry air. The water should be boiling when the apparatus is inserted, and the boiler must not be more than half-full. The temperature may be from 105° F. to 110° F.

678. Mercurial vapour-bath.—To give this a patient must be sitting upright in a chair. The same apparatus is used minus the long tube for inserting under the bed-clothes. A small dish containing the amount of calomel prescribed is placed over the spirit-lamp under the chair. The calomel is converted by the heat of the lamp into vapour, which is carried upwards by the steam and deposited upon the patient's body. The patient must not be rubbed down, or the calomel would be wiped off and no benefit follow. He should be put back to bed in a warm, flannel garment.

679. Continuous bath.—This is ordered sometimes for cases of skin-disease, extensive burns, and severe local surgical injuries or disease. The bath may last for some days and should be kept at an even temperature of 100° F. A thermometer should be kept constantly in the bath.

The bath is easily kept hot by removing some of the cooled water from time to time and adding hot water about 200° F., care being taken not to burn the patient in so doing.

680. Arm- and leg-baths are much used for septic cases. They are given in a special, trough-shaped bath. The bath is half-filled with water, to which the prescribed lotion is added. The temperature should be 100° F.

681. Medicated baths :—

Sulphur-bath.—Six ounces of potassa sulphurata are required for thirty gallons of water. The sulphur should be first dissolved in boiling water and then added to the bath.

Iodine-bath.—To every pint of water one drachm of tincture of iodine is added. This is usually given as a local bath.

Bran-baths.—Put four pounds of bran in a muslin bag and pour over it at least one gallon of boiling water. Fill up the bath, squeezing the bag of bran. Temperature 100° F.

Alkaline-baths are prepared by adding six ounces of carbonate of soda, or potash, to a hot bath. This bath is given for rheumatism.

Brine-baths are prepared by adding about six pounds of common salt to an ordinary hot bath.

682. Hot pack.—Prepare the bed by rolling under the patient a long mackintosh with a blanket over it. Cover the patient with a blanket and remove his shirt. Take a large sheet, fold it across into four. Wring it out of water as hot as possible, using a sheet or large bath-towel as a wringer. Lay the patient on his back in the bed, lay the hot sheet over him, moulding it well into him, well into the neck and down the sides. Turn up the sides of the blanket he is lying on. Cover with a mackintosh and plently of blankets.

Hot drinks promote perspiration. The patient should remain in the pack for twenty minutes. Take away the wet sheet, blanket, and mackintosh, and cover up the patient with a hot, dry blanket and leave him for an hour.

683. Cold pack.—Prepare the bed as for a hot pack, wrap the patient in a sheet wrung out of cold water. If the feet become very cold a hot bottle may be put to them. The sheet must be kept cold by being rubbed down with pieces of ice, or by being constantly sprinkled with iced water.

The temperature must be taken every five minutes, and the pulse watched. The duration of the pack depends upon its effect on the temperature.

684. Sponging is employed to reduce the temperature during fever by the evaporation of water applied to the surface of the body. Cold or tepid water is usually used. A blanket should be rolled under the patient and the shirt removed, bath towels being tucked in on each side to catch any water that may run down. The bed-clothes, with the exception of one blanket, are removed. The whole body should not be exposed at one time, only the part to be sponged being uncovered. Sponge the part rapidly, particularly over the great vessels at the root of the neck and in the groin. After sponging, the patient should only be lightly dabbed with a towel. The water should be maintained at the temperature ordered, by adding either iced water, or ice, as required.

CHAPTER LI.

THE NURSING OF HELPLESS PATIENTS.

685. Washing of patients.—When a patient is too ill to go to the bath, he must be washed all over in bed between blankets ; a mackintosh being placed under the bottom blanket. This blanket-bath should be given on admission to all patients who are unable to take an ordinary bath, and, at least once a week, to all patients confined to bed. When giving a bath, any swellings, scars, scratches, or sores should be noted and reported.

Every day each patient confined to bed should be washed as far as the waist, back and front, the shirt being removed. This thorough washing should be done in the morning, and should include the skin over the sacrum, buttocks, and hips. The hands should again be washed in the middle of the day, and the face and hands at night, also the skin over the sacrum, buttocks, and hips. The hair must be combed and brushed, and the patient's brush and comb should be washed at least one a week. The teeth must be washed daily.

686. Cleansing of mouth and teeth.—In acute illness, sordes and mucus collect on the teeth and give them a dirty appearance. When this accumulation of sordes and mucus is rapid, and when the lips and tongue are stiff and dry, attention may be needed every hour, but in ordinary cases twice a day will suffice. The mouth should be kept as moist as possible. The best sponges for washing out the mouth are made of squares of white gauze or lint, which should be burnt directly after use. One of these squares should be wrapped round the index finger, soaked with the wash and inserted into the mouth. The teeth, gums, roof and sides of the mouth should all be gone over. A solution of boracic, or lemon-juice and glycerine may be used. Dressing forceps or small sticks of wood may be used instead of the finger, but the latter is most efficacious. The hands must, of course, be well scrubbed directly after in antiseptic solution.

687. Bed-sores.—To guard against these is one of the most important points to remember with helpless patients. Bed-sores result from continuous pressure on a certain spot or spots, also from friction, moisture, creases in the under-sheet or shirt, and from crumbs in the bed. Bed-sores due to pressure occur most frequently on the hips and lower part of the back, the shoulder, and the heels. Those from friction are apt to come on the ankles, the inner surface of the knees, or on the elbows and back of the head from frequent movements. With patients suffering from paralysis or spinal injuries the utmost care will not always avail, but generally with good nursing, bed-sores can be avoided.

Preventive measures consist in absolute cleanliness, and the removal of pressure. The back and shoulders should be washed

with soap and water and carefully dried night and morning.
After washing, the skin should be treated with spirit in some
form—methylated spirit, brandy, or eau-de-Cologne—which should
be well, but gently, rubbed in, the parts being then dusted with
oxide of zinc and starch powder. In cases where the sphincter
muscles are relaxed the skin should be treated with ointment to
protect it from the irritating effects of the discharges, the patient
being frequently washed.

Water- and air-beds are of the greatest possible value. Rubber
ring-cushions are also very useful. The knees, ankles, and elbows
may be protected by a thick layer of cotton-wool firmly secured
by a bandage. When possible, a patient should never be allowed
to lie more than two hours in one position. He should be turned
first on one side and then on the other, and kept there by an
arrangement of pillows.

The first indication of an on-coming bed-sore should be at once
reported.

688. The moving of helpless patients.—It requires two people,
one on each side, comfortably to move a really helpless patient.
Each passes one hand under the patient's back at the lower part of
the shoulder-blades, the hands being then locked together. The other
hands are passed beneath the patient's thighs close up to the hips,
and also locked together. The patient is then steadily raised and
placed in the sitting position.

If the patient is not too weak, and is able to help himself with the
pulley, one person can raise him in bed by putting the right hand
and arm well behind his back, and the left below the hips, gradually
moving him up the bed, the patient at the same time assisting himself with the pulley.

Should the patient have an injury to the legs, a third person will
be required to support the lower extremities.

To move a patient from one bed to another, the two beds must
be placed side-by-side so that the mattresses are in contact. The
patient is then drawn slowly across by the sheet on which he is
lying, this being afterwards slipped away from under him. If there
are enough assistants, he can be lifted, one taking each corner of
the sheet.

To prevent a patient who is very weak from slipping down into
the bed after being propped up, a bolster is rolled in a draw-sheet
and placed beneath the upper part of the patient's thighs; the
draw-sheet being then tucked firmly in at the side of the bed.

**689. Removal of a helpless patient from a stretcher on to a
bed or operating table.**—To remove a patient from a stretcher
to a bed or operating table, the bearers carrying the stretcher
bring it alongside and raise it to the level of the bed (or table) as
in B of Fig. 157. Two, or preferably three, other bearers standing
on the far side of the stretcher, raise the patient as described in
Stretcher Exercises (Chap. XXII) for lifting wounded. The bearers
carrying the stretcher keep that handle which is nearest to the bed
(or table) steady, and allow the opposite handle to fall like the flap

of a folding table, so that the stretcher assumes the position in C of Fig. 157. The bearers supporting the patient then move forward and lower him on to the bed (or table); the stretcher is then removed.

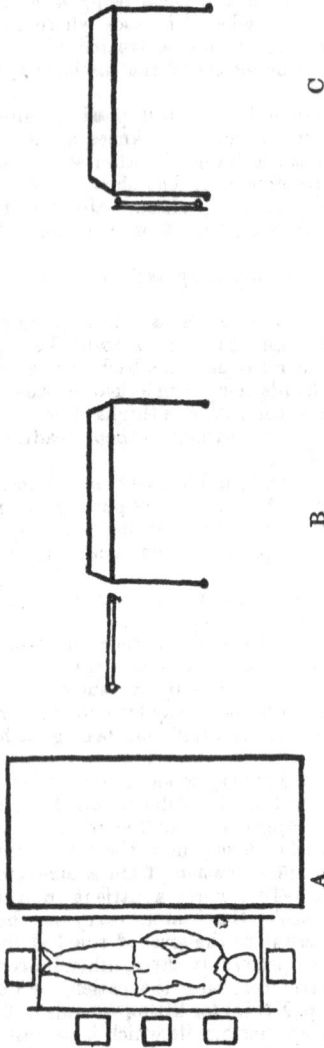

A Patient on stretcher alongside of bed or operating table.
B Transverse diagram showing position of stretcher before lifting patient.
C Transverse diagram showing stretcher after placing patient on bed or table.

FIG. 157.—REMOVING PATIENT FROM STRETCHER TO BED OR OPERATING TABLE.

To remove a patient from a bed or operating table the process is reversed.

690. Changing the sheets.—Unless the patient is very ill, one person can do this easily. Only the upper sheet or a single blanket is to be left over the patient. The lower sheet and draw-sheet to be removed are loosened at the top, bottom, and each side of the bed. On one side they are then folded along their whole length as flatly as possible until they are close up to the patient. The fresh sheets should then be folded lengthwise alternately backward and forward for half their width, and placed on the side of the bed from which the soiled ones have been removed, the loose halves being tucked in at the side. The orderly then moves to the opposite side of the bed, and turns the patient on his side, facing him. The patient can be supported in this position with one hand, while the sheets to be removed are tucked as closely and smoothly as possible up to his back, their place being taken by fresh ones which are made to follow them closely. Using both hands, the orderly now gently turns the patient towards the side of the bed away from him. The soiled sheets and the folds of the clean ones are then drawn through; the former being taken away and the latter smoothed down and tucked in their place, care being taken not to leave the smallest wrinkle. The patient can often assist in this changing by a pulley suspended above the bed, by means of which he can raise himself more or less. If the patient is quite helpless and very heavy, it is advisable to have a second person to assist.

In changing the upper coverings, a fresh sheet and blanket are first spread over, and the others are then slipped away from underneath. It is quite unnecessary to expose any part of the patient in changing the entire bed-clothing.

691. A draw-sheet is used for all patients confined to bed. This is constantly drawn through, thus enabling the patient to lie on a cool spot. When the patient is taking food, the draw-sheet should be drawn after each meal to remove the crumbs, and it should be changed when soiled with discharges. Mackintoshes are used on beds only as a protection to the mattress, and should be withdrawn as soon as they are felt to be unnecessary.

692. Feeding of patient.—Food of a liquid nature should be administered by means of a feeding-cup. If a glass or cup is used it should be only half-filled. Nourishment should be given regularly, in most cases every two hours. If it is necessary to raise the patient's head to administer a drink, one arm should be inserted under the pillow and the head gently raised.

693. Bed-pans and Urinals.—The commonest and most useful shapes of bed-pans are the "Circular" and the "Slipper." The round pan is generally used in hospitals. If the patient is not absolutely helpless, one person can give it. Place one hand almost under the buttocks and help the patient to raise himself, then place the bed-pan in position. The handle should be plugged with a rubber cork. Before attempting to remove it, the patient should be lifted right off it. After use, the bed-pan should be at once covered with a china cover, over which is thrown a cloth wrung out of some disinfectant. It is then straightway removed from the ward, and, unless needed for inspection, at once emptied, the pan being thoroughly flushed with cold water.

Urinals for use in bed are in the shape of bottles. They should be removed from the ward as soon as used. Both bed-pans and urinals should be washed once a day with soap and water. Bed-pans and urinals used by enteric patients, however, must immediately be disinfected by washing with cresol solution ; such utensils must be marked " E." (See Regulations for the Army Medical Service.)

694. Nasal feeding.—In some cases it is necessary to resort to nasal feeding. This is done by means of a tube passed through the nose into the œsophagus. A soft, rubber tube, after being well oiled, is passed into the nostril and straight backwards. The possibility of the tube slipping into the larynx must be borne in mind, but if this accident should happen the patient would at once cough and show signs of urgent dyspnœa. To the end of the tube a glass funnel is attached, and the food, which should be carefully warmed to 100° F. and strained, is poured down in a steady stream, the tube not being allowed to become empty until the entire quantity is given. When the whole of the food has been given, and the funnel is empty, the tube should be withdrawn quickly. It should be compressed by the finger and thumb to prevent the escape of fluid into the larynx on withdrawal.

695. Care of the dead.—After death, before the muscles of the body become stiff and rigid, the eyes should be closed. When necessary, pads of wet wool should be placed over the eyelids. The limbs should be straightened and the mouth closed. The lower jaw is supported either by means of a roller bandage placed under it, or by putting on an ordinary jaw-bandage.

About one hour after death, the body should be washed from head to foot with soap and water, and the rectum plugged with wool. The ankles are tied together with a bandage, fresh dressings are placed on any wound there may be, the hair brushed, and a shroud put on. A clean sheet is placed over all.

CHAPTER LII.

THE OBSERVATION OF THE SICK.

696. Reporting on a patient.—A concise and correct report should be kept, in writing, of all patients seriously ill, noting quantity of nourishment taken, with the times of administration, amount of sleep, urine and stools passed. The temperature, pulse, and respiration must be noted four-hourly, and mention made if any symptom of importance is noticed.

WHAT TO OBSERVE: POSITION, EXPRESSION, &c.

697. Note carefully the appearance of the patient and his position in bed. Does he look ill or in pain? Has he a heavy and listless, or wide-awake and anxious expression? Is he pale or flushed, or is there a bluish tinge about the face? Is he well- or ill-nourished? Which position in bed gives him the most ease, i.e., does he lie on his back or is he obliged to sit up to get ease in breathing? Does he lie with his knees drawn up to relax the abdominal muscles, or does he lie on one side more than the other?

Notice character and duration of any pain the patient may complain of.

THE SKIN, THE EYES, &c.

698. Any scars, ulcers, abrasions, bruises, or discolorations about the skin, any swellings, œdema, jaundice, or any profuse perspiration should be reported. Any rash, redness, or eruption making its appearance on the skin should be carefully noted.

The eyes should be carefully observed and any irregularity in the size of the pupils, or tendency to squint, be reported.

It is important to note pain in or discharge from the ear. In any case of head-injury the escape of blood or clear fluid from the ears should be watched for.

THE DIGESTIVE SYSTEM, &c.

699. The presence of sordes on the lips, teeth, and tongue should be noted.

It should be observed whether the tongue is tremulous or not, whether clean or furred, dry or moist, or if any ulcers are on it.

Any difficulty in swallowing should be noticed, also sore-throat, or symptoms of indigestion, such as flatulence, tightness of the chest, pain at the pit of the stomach or between the shoulders, or nausea after eating, together with the exact relation to food. Quantity and nature of vomit should be noticed.

Blood vomited is known as *hœmatemesis.* When blood has been retained for some time in the stomach it becomes partially digested and resembles coffee-grounds in appearance.

A patient who has vomited blood must be kept in the recumbent position, and all food withheld till he has been seen by the medical officer.

It is important to distinguish between blood brought from the stomach, and blood coughed up from the lungs. Blood from the stomach is generally dark in colour, and sometimes partly clotted. It is also frequently mixed with food or traces of food, and is vomited up. Blood from the lungs is usually coughed up, is bright red in colour, frothy, and rarely clotted. (See also para. 573 (18).)

Any abdominal pain or distension should be noted.

EXCRETORY SYSTEM.

700. Stools.—The points to be noticed are their shape, colour, consistency, amount, and whether they contain blood, mucus, pus, or undigested food ; the frequency of the motion, and whether there is any pain in passing it. Anything unusual should be kept for inspection.

701. Urine.—The colour of the urine should be observed, also if there is any difficulty in passing it. The patient may be unable to pass urine at all, a condition known as " retention of urine." This must not be confused with " suppression of urine " when no urine is excreted by the kidneys.

The quantity of the urine should be noticed, together with the frequency of micturition, remembering that the normal quantity of urine passed in the twenty-four hours should be about fifty ounces.

RESPIRATORY SYSTEM.

702. Respiration.—The points to be observed are the frequency and character of the respirations, the *normal number* being from 15 to 18 per minute. The patient should never know his respirations are being counted. If he is conscious of it he may unintentionally alter their frequency. The best way to manage is, after counting the pulse, and without removing the fingers from the wrist, quietly to count the movements of the chest.

703. Cough.—The points to notice about a cough are its frequency, duration, and character.

Expectoration varies in character in different diseases, and also at different times in the same disease. A specimen of sputum should be kept for inspection, and if the quantity seems excessive it should be measured for the twenty-four hours.

Hæmoptysis or the spitting of blood, if it occurs in any quantity, is almost always due to tubercle of lung.

The patient must be kept quiet, in the semi-recumbent position, and small pieces of ice may be given to him to suck. An ice-bag may be applied to the chest.

THE NERVOUS SYSTEM.

704. Fits most commonly occur in cases of epilepsy, but are a frequent symptom of brain and kidney diseases. The duration and severity of the attack should be carefully noted, and in what part of the body the convulsions begin.

A patient in a convulsion or fit should never be left alone. Care must be taken that he does not injure himself, and that the tongue does not get between the teeth. To prevent this something should be inserted between the teeth to keep them apart.

705. Delirium.—When delirium is present it should be noticed if it is of the low, muttering type, or active and noisy ; also if it is more pronounced during one part of the twenty-four hours than another. It should be observed if the patient picks at the bed-clothes.

706. Sleep.—It should be noticed how long the patient sleeps, and whether his sleep is disturbed, or sound and calm. To encourage sleep, the room should be darkened and the light shaded from the patient's eyes. If a patient does not sleep he may be given a drink of warm milk or some other nourishment if not contrary to instructions, the face and hands may be sponged, the pillows re-arranged, and a hot bottle placed at the feet if required.

THE TEMPERATURE.

707. The temperature is taken by means of a small, glass, self-registering thermometer known as the "Clinical Thermometer." Before taking a patient's temperature, care must be taken that the index is set below 97° F.

The temperature can be taken in the axilla, groin, mouth, or rectum. It should be taken in the morning and evening before the patient is washed. As the thermometer will register slightly higher when the temperature is taken in the mouth than in the axilla or groin, it is necessary always to take it by placing the instrument in the same place, and at the same hour. When taken in the axilla, the part should be wiped dry before inserting the bulb of the thermometer, and the arm folded across the chest. The thermometer should be left in position for five minutes.

When the temperature is taken in the mouth, the bulb of the thermometer is inserted under the tongue, and the patient made to keep his mouth shut, holding the glass with his lips. The patient should not have had anything cold or hot to drink recently.

When taken in the rectum the bulb should be smeared with vaseline and inserted for about one inch, and held in position.

The thermometer should always be washed in tepid, antiseptic solution before giving it to another patient.

708. The *normal temperature* of the body is 98·4° F. In disease, the temperature may be either above or below normal, the former being much the more common. Patients with a temperature above normal are said to be suffering from *pyrexia* ; 102° F. being considered moderate pyrexia, and 104° F. or 105° F. severe pyrexia. If it reaches 106° F. it is called hyper-pyrexia.

Pyrexia varies in character. It may be continuous, remittent, or intermittent. A continuous fever is one in which the fever keeps constantly at a high level. A remittent fever is one in which there is a marked difference between the morning and the evening temperature, but it does not at any time fall to normal. An intermittent fever is one in which for some part of the twenty four hours there is complete absence of fever.

Fever ends either by *crisis or lysis.* If by the former the temperature falls abruptly, reaching normal in from twelve to twenty-four hours ; if by the latter the descent is more gradual, three or four days elapsing before the temperature reaches normal and remains there.

709. Rigors.—A rigor is a most important symptom to take note of. In some cases a rigor marks the onset of an acute illness. The shivering may be only slight, or it may be most severe, with a general shaking and chattering of the teeth, lasting for some minutes. Note should be taken of the duration and severity of the rigor, as well as the time at which it takes place. The temperature of the patient should be taken, and hot bottles, hot blankets, and hot drinks given during the shivering stage.

The Pulse.

710. Taking the pulse needs long and painstaking practice. It is one of the most important guides with regard to the patient's condition. By it one is able to tell whether the patient is gaining or losing strength.

The *pulse-rate* in health varies from 70 to 80 beats per minute. When counting the pulse, three fingers should be placed on the radial artery at the wrist. The pulse of a sleeping patient may be taken by placing the finger on the temporal artery just in front of the ear.

The frequency, size, compressibility, and regularity should all be noted.

A pulse which, with a stationary or falling temperature, gets quicker day by day is a very sure indication of a failing heart.

CHAPTER LIII.

THE SERVING OF PATIENTS' FOOD.

711. Intelligent attention to every detail in connection with the serving of patients' food is a most important part of a nurse's duties. Progress in many cases is much influenced by the amount of nourishment taken and this may often depend largely on the way it is served.

One of the most important points in this connection is scrupulous cleanliness in every detail. The cloth covering the tray or table must be spotless, the glass and plate polished and bright, and the arrangement as dainty as possible.

Notice should be taken that nothing has been spilt in carrying the tray, and that glasses are not filled too full. Food intended to be taken hot should be brought to the patient *hot* and not lukewarm ; covers must always be used. Small portions only should be put before the patient ; a large plateful will often be refused, when a daintily arranged one would have been eaten and enjoyed.

The food must never be kept in the sick-room, but brought freshly to the bedside ; similarly, the tray or table should be removed from the room directly the meal is finished.

Before bringing a patient his meal, the orderly should see that he is quite ready to commence it. If able to feed himself he should be comfortably propped up in bed, and everything he will require put conveniently to hand. If helpless, great patience and care must be taken in feeding him.

Punctuality in serving meals to invalids, and the strictest accuracy in observing and reporting upon the amount of food actually taken are very important points.

As a general rule meals should, as far as possible, come as a surprise and not be discussed beforehand ; some patients, however, have strong likes and dislikes with regard to food, and these when expressed should never be neglected.

CHAPTER LIV.

SURGICAL NURSING.

Two Great Principles.

712. The care of most surgical cases involves the application of two great principles—*cleanliness*, and *rest*.

713. Cleanliness.—By surgical cleanliness is meant something more than ordinary personal cleanliness. It means not only freedom from dirt but freedom from germs. Germs, or microbes as they are called, are present everywhere. They are so small that they are not visible to the naked eye, and can only be seen when highly magnified by the microscope.

To prevent germs from entering a wound, we endeavour to ensure complete freedom from living germs on everything which may be used during an operation or during the dressing of a wound. Articles that cannot be subjected to sterilization by heat are treated by antiseptics.

Two expressions commonly used with reference to the treatment of wounds are *asepsis* and *antisepsis*. By asepsis is meant freedom from germs, while antisepsis refers to the measures employed to destroy the germs which may be present either in the wound or on the skin.

714. *Sterilization and cleaning of instruments.*—Instruments, except knives, are sterilized by boiling. They are put into boiling water to which one per cent. of bicarbonate of soda has been added, and are boiled for ten minutes. Knives should not be boiled, as it blunts their edges. They may be sterilized by being wiped with pure carbolic on a sterilized swab, then placed in ether for 10 minutes, or be sterilized in other ways, according to the instruction of the surgeon.

After boiling or sterilizing, instruments are placed in trays containing carbolic lotion, 1 in 60, by means of a pair of sterilized forceps; on no account must they be touched with the hands. Should an instrument be dropped, or touch anything while being conveyed to the tray, it must be re-sterilized immediately.

After an operation the instrument should be rinsed in tepid water, and then scrubbed with a nail-brush in soap and hot water to which a little bicarbonate of soda has been added, after which they are again rinsed in water to remove the soap, and dipped in methylated spirit.

715. *Ligatures and sutures* are made from silk, linen, silkworm-gut, catgut, kangaroo-tendons, silver-wire, and horse-hair, and they are each sterilized in a special manner. Silk, silkworm gut, and horse-hair can all be boiled.

716. *Bowls and trays* must be sterilized, boiled, or scrubbed before use. If it is impossible to boil them, they should be well scrubbed with soap and hot water, and allowed to stand in 1 in 20 carbolic for twenty-four hours before use.

717. *Towels, gowns, dressings, and swabs* are all lightly packed in tins and sterilized by heating to 212° F., in a steam-sterilizer for twenty minutes. After being sterilized, the tins should be sealed down and not opened till the time of operation. When required, the articles must be lifted by means of a pair of forceps or a sterilized towel, and never touched by the hands. The dressers containing swabs or dressings are only to be opened when required, and their contents conveyed to lotion or to the operator by means of sterilized forceps.

When a tin has been once opened, any of the dressings left over should be re-sterilized.

718. *The hands* of all engaged in surgery require earnest attention ; the nails must be kept short, carefully trimmed and clean, and all tags of skin removed daily. When preparing for an operation, the hands and arms up to the elbows should be very thoroughly scrubbed with soap and water for at least five minutes continuously, special care being taken with the nails and between the fingers. Plenty of soap must be used and the water changed three or four times, or, better still, they should be washed under a running tap. The nail-brush should have been thoroughly sterilized, preferably by boiling. After this thorough washing, the hands should be soaked in biniodide lotion, 1 in 1,000, and left wet, or wiped with a sterilized towel. Rings must on no account be worn.

Having thus cleansed the hands, they must on no account touch anything that is not sterilized ; should this occur the whole process must be gone through again.

719. Rest.—The second great principle is rest, both local and general. Thus, when the stomach has been operated on, it is kept at rest by not giving it any food to digest. General rest is obtained by keeping the patient in bed, and rest in the case of the limbs is carried out by means of splints, bandages, and other mechanical appliances.

It is the duty of the attendant to see that the splints, bandages, and other mechanical appliances are kept as originally applied. In the case of a fracture, if the limb be not kept still, the ends of the bone will constantly rub against one another, so giving rise to continual irritation, and union may be delayed.

OPERATIONS.

720. Preparation of the patient.—Before an operation of any magnitude the patient should go to bed for a day or two, if not already confined there. The day before an operation the patient has a hot bath or is washed all over while in bed, subsequently receiving a change of linen ; his skin is then prepared. While the skin is being cleansed, the patient's bedding should be kept away from the part by means of sterilized towels. Unless orders are given to the contrary, the part should be shaved for ten inches round the place where the incisions will be made, and then gently but thoroughly scrubbed with soap and water, afterwards being rubbed over with ether to remove all grease. A compress is then applied, soaked with some authorized antiseptic, according to the orders of the surgeon. This is firmly bandaged on and left till the time of the operation. On the thoroughness with which this preparation of the skin is done depends very largely the healing of the operation wound.

A purgative is usually given on each of the two nights preceding the operation, and on the morning of the operation enemata should be given till the rectum is empty. Two or three may be necessary. Rectal cases require two days of preparation by purgatives and enemata.

On the morning of the operation a specimen of urine should be saved for examination.

Food in a fluid form, e.g., a pint of beef-tea, should be given four hours previous to the operation, but nothing else unless by special orders.

The patient should be clad in a loose, flannel gown, the legs being covered with long, woollen stockings, which should be sterilized.

False teeth should be removed. The patient should pass water before going into the operation-theatre.

721. After-treatment of operation-cases.—The operation-bed should be made up with clean linen, a draw-sheet and mackintosh placed in position, and the bed-clothes folded over to one side so that the patient can be quickly put back to bed. Hot bottles should be placed in the bed, and a blanket made hot to cover the patient with on return from the theatre.

After any prolonged operation, a hot, saline solution should be prepared and ready at hand in case of need, also blocks to raise the end of the bed.

The patient requires watching carefully until he regains consciousness, and if there is a tendency to vomit, as there frequently is on coming round from a general anæsthetic, the head should be turned to one side. A towel and bowl should be at the bed-head for this reason.

A bed-cradle to support the weight of the clothes is advisable in some cases, and should be at hand in case of need.

After all operations, food is withheld until the anæsthetic-sickness has passed off. Thirst is relieved by drachms of hot water, given slowly. The tongue may be kept moist by allowing the patient to rinse the mouth with a little water or soda-water. Special instructions with regard to the after-feeding of the patient will be given according to the nature of the operation, but to no patient will an ordinary diet be given on the day of the operation. Milk or milk and soda-water would in all probability be the only food allowed.

On the evening of the operation the gown should be changed, the patient's hands and face sponged, and the draw-sheet drawn through. On the morning after operation a specimen of urine is saved for examination.

For the first 24 hours after an operation the dressing should be frequently examined (without in any way disturbing it). Should blood or discharge appear, the dressing will require to be "re-packed" (*i.e.*, a fresh pad of sterilized wool applied outside the original dressing, which must not be disturbed); all antiseptic precautions must be taken. Should this or any other accident happen, such as urine being spilt, the sister or senior N.C.O. should be at once informed, as the dressing may require to be changed.

722. Operating Theatre.—The theatre where the operation is to be performed must be clean and free from dust of a temperature not less than 70° F., and there must be plenty of hot and cold water.

The room and its furniture are kept clean and free from dust by means of wet cloths rung out of antiseptic solution. All brass and metal-work is kept polished. All enamelled metal-work, glass, china, tables, and stools are to be cleaned with soap and water, or boiling water with soda, and 1-40 carbolic; floors, walls, and ceiling being similarly treated.

The table upon which the operation is performed is usually kept warm by means of hot water. It should be thoroughly cleansed before an operation and covered with a sterilized sheet. There are in addition other smaller tables for the instruments, dressings, and bowls of lotion, and one for the anæsthetist's use.

During an operation the surgeon and his assistants wear sterilized aprons or waterproof coats.

723. The after-nursing of cases of abdominal section.—Abdominal section may be performed for a variety of causes, but the nursing of such cases is very similar. If the operation has been prolonged and difficult, the patient may suffer severely from shock. In such a case he must be put back to bed as carefully and quietly as possible, and a pillow placed under the knees, with the head low, one pillow only being used. Hot bottles should be in the bed and the foot of the bed raised. Particular attention must be paid to the pulse. It should be taken and recorded every hour for the first twenty-four hours. The frequency and character of the vomit must be noted. If retching is severe, the wound should be supported by the attendant's hand being placed over the bandage. Note must be taken if urine has been passed or not, if the bowels have acted or not, and whether the patient has passed any flatus by the bowel.

Instructions with regard to the giving of nourishment must be carried out with the strictest accuracy, each feed being recorded on the chart.

Nourishment by the mouth may not be allowed for twenty-four or thirty-six hours, and then probably in very gradually increasing quantities. For allaying the excessive thirst, an enema of normal salt solution, a pint or more, given hot, is frequently ordered; the mouth can be rinsed out with hot water, and the lips moistened from time to time.

Stimulants should be kept near at hand; and if the patient is in an exhausted condition a nutritive enema may be ordered at once.

For uneasiness and pain in the back insert a small, flat pillow. The knee-pillow must be adjusted and changed when necessary.

Abdominal distension must be watched for and reported.

724. Amputations.—After an amputation of either arm or leg has been performed, the stump should, when the patient has been put back to bed, be placed on a small pillow, to which it is secured by a bandage. This helps to restrain the painful muscular startings which sometimes occur in the stump. The stump should be left uncovered by the bed-clothes so that if any hæmorrhage occurs it may be at once detected.

725. Secondary hæmorrhage.—After major operations, hæmorrhage should be watched for during the first twenty-four or forty-eight hours. Indeed, the possibility of such an occurrence should be borne in mind until the wounds have healed perfectly, as "secondary hæmorrhage" may occur several days after the operation. Any bleeding, however slight, should at once be reported. Should the hæmorrhage be profuse, prompt action will be necessary, and unless a tourniquet has been left in position, with instructions how to use it, an endeavour should be made to stop the bleeding by compressing the main artery between the wound and the heart.

726. Shock is a condition of general depression of the whole system. This condition occurs after severe frights, injuries, and operations. Collapse and prostration are words used to express similar conditions. The symptoms to be looked for in shock are a weak, rapid pulse, a sub-normal temperature, pallor, a pinched look on the face and about the lips, cold and clammy skin, and sometimes nausea. The patient must be placed with his head low. If in bed, the foot of the bed should be well raised, and hot-water bottles and hot blankets applied. An enema of hot, saline solution with brandy is often ordered. Ether and strychnine should be ready for the medical officer's use, and stimulants by the mouth will probably be given.

727. Tracheotomy.—This is usually an emergency operation, and consists in making an opening in the trachea, and inserting a tracheotomy-tube through which the patient breathes. A tracheotomy-tube consists of a tube within a tube, made of silver. The outer tube is provided with a shield and is held securely in place by means of two pieces of tape which are passed through holes in the shield and then tied together round the neck. The inner fits into the outer tube and projects for a short distance beyond the lower end.

The after-care consists in the management of the tube, in feeding, and good general nursing. Constant attention to the condition of the inner tube is necessary, as the mucus and membranous deposits are likely to fill it up and thus cut off the air-supply. At first the inner tube should be taken out at least every four hours and cleaned, unless some immediate difficulty arises, when it must be done at once. No attempt must be made to interfere with the outer tube, the surgeon alone touching that. The air the patient breathes must be warm and moist. A steam-kettle may be used, and gauze ordered to be placed over the tube. Immediately any mucus is coughed up it must be wiped away with small, gauze swabs, which should be immediately burnt. If feathers are used for cleansing the tube, they must be sterilized. The gauze over the tube will require constant changing. The dressing which protects the edge of the wound round the outer tube must be changed when soiled. The temperature of the ward should be kept at about 70° F.

Nourishment should be administered regularly. Sometimes this is a matter of some difficulty. Thickening the milk with arrow-root or corn-flour makes it easier to swallow, but in some cases nourishment has to be administered by means of the nasal tube, or by rectal feeding. The patient must never be left alone. A second inner tube, tracheal dilators, pilot, and dissecting forceps should be kept in an authorized antiseptic by the bedside.

728. Skin-grafting is employed when a large area of granu-lation-tissue has to be covered with skin, as after extensive burns. By means of a sharp knife or razor, pieces of skin are pared off the arm or leg of the patient and laid on the granulating surface. The grafts are then covered with prepared tissue to prevent them sticking to the dressing. Those grafts which adhere grow on the granulating surface and become centres from which the skin grows to meet that which is growing from the edges of the wound. The time taken in healing is thus materially shortened.

CHAPTER LV.

MANAGEMENT OF WARDS.

729. Annexes.—To render the condition of a ward wholesome, it is necessary not only to regulate its temperature, but also to provide for the ingress of a supply of fresh air at all times, day and night.

The waste-pipes and sinks in the annexes must be properly cleaned and flushed daily. No soiled or infectious linen and no soiled clothing or dressings should be left standing about in uncovered receptacles. All vessels in use must be kept thoroughly cleansed.

730. Ventilation of wards.*—By ventilation is meant the supply of fresh air to, and the removal of impure air from, an apartment.

Composition of air.—Air consists almost entirely of two gases, oxygen and nitrogen : of the former rather more than one-fifth ; of the latter slightly less than four-fifths. There is, in addition, a minute trace of a poisonous gas called carbonic acid, and a small quantity of watery vapour. In the wards of a hospital the air very soon becomes loaded with impurities.

Every individual in the ward is constantly engaged, during the act of respiration, in removing oxygen from and adding carbonic acid gas to the air. The atmosphere is rendered still more unwholesome by emanations from the patients' bodies, their linen, and excreta ; by any foul wounds or soiled dressings, and by the burning of gas, each jet of which consumes many times as much oxygen as a man.

From these facts it will be at once seen how important it is that the personal cleanliness of patients should be constantly attended to, and that all excreta or soiled dressings be removed from the ward without delay. In addition, in order to counteract this continual fouling of the atmosphere, a frequent and thorough changing of the air is necessary.

731. *Principles of ventilation.*—The principles to be kept in view are :—(i) That the air within the ward shall be kept as nearly as possible as pure as that outside, without chilling the patients. (ii) That the temperature of the ward be maintained at the proper standard, not exceeding 65° F. (iii) That ventilation must be systematic, and sufficiently thorough completely to renew the air in a ward at least three times in an hour.

There are two simple but all-important facts to be remembered in carrying out the principles of ventilation :—(1) Air expands when it is heated : from this it follows that, as the air in a room expands, some of it escapes by the nearest outlet. (2) As a result of its expansion, hot air is lighter than cold air : on this account hot air will rise, and cold air, being heavier, will fall.

732. *Outlets.*—Foul air escapes from a room by (a) the fireplace, (b) the windows, and (c) ventilating-outlets.

---

* *See also* para. 48, Chap. VI

Being lighter than the pure air, foul air will be found in the upper part of the room. Ventilating-outlets are therefore usually placed in the ceiling. For the same reason the windows should be left open at the top to enable the hot, impure air to escape.

The fire-place is a most important aid to ventilation, as when a fire is burning there is a constant current of air leaving the room by the chimney.

733. *Inlets.*—Fresh air enters a room by (*a*) ventilating-inlets, (*b*) the windows.

In hospitals the ventilating-inlets are so arranged that the amount of air entering by them can be regulated and generally diffused over the room, so preventing draughts.

In recently built hospitals the air on entering these ventilators is warmed by coming in contact with hot-water pipes. In the absence of hot pipes the cold air should be introduced above the level of the patients' heads, so that it reaches them after mixing with the warm air of the ward. Windows have already been considered as outlets for foul air ; they also act as inlets for a large quantity of pure air, and should be constantly open at the top. The opening thus caused between the sashes is the inlet. Fresh air will also enter a ward every time the door is opened, and underneath the door even when shut ; but, if this air is from inside the building, the door should not be regarded as a suitable means of ventilation.

Patients frequently complain of draught when the windows are kept open ; the attendant must use consideration and tact as well as firmness, and by the addition of an extra blanket or a hot-water bottle, patients can generally be kept quite warm.

734. *Duty of Attendants.*—Finally, the matter of ventilation requires unremitting attention from attendants on the sick. Neglect of this duty will favour the development or spread of disease, retard the healing of wounds, and generally lower the health of the patients. To test the air of a ward, the attendant should from time to time go into the open air : on re-entering he will at once be able to detect the impurity or otherwise of the atmosphere.

735. Floor of Ward.—The floor of the ward should be swept every morning and again in the middle of the day. In sweeping hospital floors it is important to raise as little dust as possible : by fastening a flannel over the brush or broom this danger can be almost entirely averted.

When the floors are polished they require to be first swept, then the polish used. This must be applied on house-flannel, on hands and knees, and well rubbed on to a section of the floor, which must afterwards be well dry-rubbed by a heavy-weighted, long-handled brush ; the corners being done by hand. Polished floors should be well scrubbed with hot water and soft soap once in six months at least.

736. Dusting.—Dusting should be done twice a day in the wards, with two dusters, a damp and a dry one. The damp one is used first and the dry one for polishing.

787. Walls and Windows.—Walls should be washed down every three months.

The wood-work of windows should be cleaned by washing with warm water and soap. The glass itself is cleaned by sponging with water and methylated spirit and then polishing it with a clean and thoroughly dry duster. This mode of cleaning is not always necessary, for if the glass be wiped over daily with a duster it will generally suffice to keep it in good order. The cloths used should be free from nap or fluff.

738. Stoves.—In cleaning stoves, care must be taken not to soil other things. A good plan to prevent this is to hold a thin strip of wood with one hand against the surrounding wall, while the brush is used with the other hand. The blacklead should be made into a thin paste and applied with the small, round brush over every part that is to be blacked. When the blacklead is dry, the polishing brush should be used briskly until every part of the iron-work shines. The ends of the fire-irons are cleaned in the same way as the stove, and the bright parts rubbed with bathbrick and a piece of leather, or coarse cloth, or burnished.

The best time for cleaning a fire-place is before the fire has been lighted ; but, as this can seldom be done in hospital wards, each morning the fire should be allowed to become low in order that the stove may be cleaned before it becomes too hot.

739. Paint.—The paint-work of a ward should occasionally be scrubbed with hot water and soap. Soda should not be used, as it soon destroys the paint (including enamel).

740. Wood-work and Utensils.—Bedside-tables, the boards over the patients' beds, diet-trays, and all white wood should be scrubbed with hot water and soft soap. Tumblers and all glass articles should be washed separately, first in warm water with soda and then in cold water. Vessels of tin or white metal are best cleaned by washing with hot water to remove the grease, and then polishing with whitening. In washing knives and forks, care must be taken not to put the handles into the hot water. Coal-scuttles and brasses should be polished with a paste made of finely powdered bathbrick and water, unless a patent polish is used, and rubbed with a piece of leather or coarse cloth. When the brasses are very dirty they should be washed with hot water before being polished.

741. Beds.—Beds should be thoroughly aired and the mattress turned every day.

To make the bed, a single blanket is first placed over the mattress ; over this a sheet is laid, leaving enough at the top to roll the bolster in. It is then firmly and tightly tucked in at the sides and foot, the bolster being rolled in the top of the sheet and the pillow placed on top of the bolster. The top sheet, blankets and counterpane are then spread, tucked in round the sides and foot of the mattress, and neatly folded down at the head. A draw-sheet is used for all patients confined to bed. The width of the draw-sheet is usually half the width of an ordinary sheet, but when a mackintosh is used it should be folded so as completely to cover the mackintosh.

742. Air- and water-beds.—Air- and water-beds are used in certain cases. They are a preventative against bed-sores.

The air-bed is laid on the top of an ordinary mattress. There are several patterns, that used in military hospitals having three compartments, the smaller one of which is put to the head. The air is pumped into the three compartments separately. If filled too full, the bed will be hard and uncomfortable. Two under blankets should be placed over the air-bed, and the bed made in the usual way

A water-bed is necessarily much heavier than an air-bed. After being placed in position on the bed, it is filled with water at a temperature of 90° F. It must not be filled too full, and it must be emptied before any attempt is made to move it. To test whether an air- or water-bed is filled sufficiently, lie down on it and try it.

Both air- and water-beds must be thoroughly cleaned after use, and great care taken to avoid damaging them with pins.

The blankets under the patient covering these beds require to be frequently changed, as they become damp from perspiration.

CHAPTER LVI.

FOOD AND COOKERY.

General Instructions.

N.C.Os. and men under training in Military Hospitals as Cooks will be instructed upon the lines laid down in this chapter, as well as in the "Duties of Cooks," as laid down in Standing Orders, R.A.M.C.

743. General remarks.—It is part of a cook's duty to become acquainted with the various cuts or joints into which the carcasses of beef, veal, mutton, and pork, etc., are divided.

He must likewise be able to tell good-quality meat from indifferent or bad meat. In the case of meat, or any other product sent in, which is found to be inferior in quality, or unfit for use, the fact is to be immediately reported to the steward in accordance with the Standing Orders.

744. Meat.—The following hints are for guidance in the matter of detecting good from bad-quality meat :—

Meat may be roughly divided into four classes : (1) Home-bred and killed, including every kind of bull, ox, cow, heifer, sheep, and pig.

(2) Foreign-bred but killed in England, principally beef. This class is generally of good quality, having been well fed. The rigid inspection on arrival in this country is sufficient protection against the importation of diseased animals. There is often a deficiency in fat owing to wasting during the sea-voyage. Occasionally there are signs of bruising or even laceration of the flesh, due to injury from bad weather. Meat in this condition should not be accepted.

(3) Refrigerated meat, chiefly American and Canadian, which is killed and dressed abroad, wrapped in canvas, and hung up in cool chambers, at a temperature of about 36° to 40° Fahrenheit. The meat of this class is generally like that of (2) class, as the animals are killed in prime condition, and the rigid inspection is a guarantee against the importation of unsound meat.

Refrigerated meat differs slightly in appearance from freshly-killed meat ; it can be distinguished by :—(a) The fat of the meat being pink, owing to staining by the juice of the lean which escapes. (b) The outside of the meat presenting a dull, dead colour, when compared with the lustre on the outside of good, fresh meat ; also, occasionally, the marks of the canvas covering being visible   (c) The dressing not being always so clean and neat as in English-dressed meat, and the pizzle and root not being always entirely removed.

If there is the slightest suspicious smell to be discovered on the outside, the flesh should be cut into and examined.

(4) Frozen meat, principally mutton, which is chiefly imported from Australia, and New Zealand in an actually frozen condition.

It can be easily distinguished, before it is thawed, by its hard, cold touch. The fat is not stained as in refrigerated meat. When thawed, it can be distinguished by—(a) The outside having a wet, sometimes greyish or, so-called, parboiled appearance ; there will be oozing and dripping of liquid from the meat. (b) The general colour of the fat is dull-white. (c) The flesh has a uniform pink appearance, owing to the diffusion of the colouring matter of the blood, and is not mottled as in fresh meat.

745. Salted meat.—If there is any doubt as regards salted meats a portion should be tested by cooking, which will often reveal defects otherwise not recognizable.

(1) The salting may be well done, but the parts inferior. Examine those pieces at the bottom of the cask, and compare several pieces to see if there is a fair proportion of good parts of the animal.

(2) The salting may be well done, and the parts good, but the meat old ; here the extreme hardness or toughness and shrivelling is the test. See if the year of salting is on the cask.

(3) The salting may be well done but the meat bad. If the meat has partly putrefied, no salting will entirely remove its softness, and there may be an offensive smell or greenish colour.

(4) The salting may be badly done, either from haste or bad brine. Signs of putrefaction will be present ; the meat is paler than it should be and has a bad odour.

746. Inspecting meat.—When inspecting meat, it should be hung up so that it can be seen on all sides without handling. Twenty-four hours after being killed is the best time for the inspection.

The following points must also be attended to :—(1) Quantity of bone, (2) quantity and character of the fat, (3) condition of the flesh, (4) condition of the marrow, (5) age of the animal, and (6) sex.

Percentage of bone.—In lean animals the bone is relatively in too great a proportion ; 17 to 20 per cent. may be allowed.

Fat.—The fat is a most important item. The interior of a carcass should show bright, healthy-looking fat. In a fat ox it may be as much as one-third of the flesh ; it should be firm, and white or pale-straw colour.

Marrow.—Condition of the marrow. The marrow in the hind-legs should be solid 24 hours after the animal has been killed. The colour should be light rosy-red ; if dark with spots of black, the animal has been sick or putrefaction has commenced. The marrow of the fore-leg bones is more fluid, otherwise it should present the same characteristics.

747. Beef.—Bull-beef may be distinguished from ox-beef by the size of the erector-muscle, pizzle, and pelvic bones, the absence of a plentiful supply of " cod " and " kidney " fat, a general massiveness of the bones and muscles, and almost a total absence of that coating of the fat on the exterior of the carcass which is the characteristic of well-fed ox-beef. The lean will be very coarse and stringy in texture, dark in colour, with an absence of juice and of marbling by fat. The feel to the finger and thumb will convey an indiarubber-like consistency, instead of the smooth and silky touch of ox-beef, which is also marbled, juicy, and florid-coloured in appearance. The fore-quarter of the bull is very large, the collar or crest requires the whole hand to grasp it, whilst in the ox it can be grasped with the fore-finger and thumb. If the neck has been removed suspicion will at once be aroused.

In the fore-quarter of the heifer or young cow the ribs show the pinkness of youth, but in an old cow they will be white and more bleached as age advances, and there is a general want of fat. The meat of a heifer is like that of a young ox, and very difficult to distinguish from it ; whilst that of an old cow is coarse, stringy to the touch, dark in colour, and with an absence of moisture. The fat of a heifer or young ox is plentiful on the exterior, coming right to the shoulder ; in the cow it is yellow in colour and scanty.

748. Mutton.—Good mutton is of deep-red colour when cut, the fat should be white and firm, and should not be coarsely ingrained with the lean. Small-boned mutton is generally the best and most profitable. The greater portion of contract-mutton is too fat, the proportion of fat to lean being so great as frequently to give rise to complaint. The way of detecting the amount of fat on a carcass without cutting it through is to look at the shoulders ; if a bluish tint is discernible the proportion of fat is not too great. Should the contractor refuse to remove the surplus fat, the carcass should be rejected. When joints only are received, if too fat, the butcher should be asked to trim them or to make adequate allowance.

749. Fish.—Fresh fish is firm and stiff, the drooping or not of the tail being a fair criterion on this point. The eyes should be bright and prominent ; the gills a bright-red colour. Flat-fish, like plaice, sole, brill, or turbot, keep better than herring, mackerel, or mullet. All fish should have been cleaned, be unbruised, unbroken, and free from smell, when delivered. Cod-fish is considered better if it is allowed to soak in cold, slightly salted water a few hours before it is cooked, as this makes the flesh firmer.

When small flat-fish, such as plaice or dabs, are tendered, a proper allowance of weight should be made for heads, fins, etc.

Stale fish is not only unwholesome, but sometimes poisonous. Fish with the least unpleasant smell should at once be rejected.

750. Fowls.—Fowls are frequently required for the use of the patients in hospital. They ought to be young, fresh, in good condition, and weigh not less than 1¾ lb. when trussed. Signs of age are shown by stiff, horny feet, long spurs, dark-coloured, hairy thighs, stiff beak and bones.

There should be no smell or discoloration of the skin. The back generally discolours before the breast. The feet should be limp and pliable, not stiff and dry, which is the sure indication of a stale bird. The condition of the flesh should be firm and not flabby, and the bird should be plump ; the breast-bone is sometimes broken across to produce this appearance. There should be some fat, which is a sign of health and good feeding, but there is no advantage in having one excessively fat, as this only wastes away in the cooking and is not always agreeable to a sick person. The flesh is not marbled like that of the ox, but the fat is accumulated in a layer over the body.

From Christmas to April chickens are most difficult to obtain, and consequently during this period of the year greater care and caution should be exercised in inspecting those sent in by contractors.

751. Rabbits.—Young rabbits have smooth and sharp claws. Old ones have the claws blunt and rugged, and the ears dry and tough. Seasonable from September to February.

752. Eggs.—The average hen's egg weighs about 2 oz. avoirdupois. In order to ascertain the freshness of an egg, hold it up to the light; when the centre appears to be the most transparent part, it is a sign of freshness. Stale eggs are more transparent at the larger end. Another method is to make a solution of brine (one part of salt to ten of water) and place the egg in the solution. Good or fresh eggs will sink to the bottom whilst the stale ones will float. Stale or small eggs should be rejected.

In using eggs for cooking purposes, such as adding them to other ingredients, poaching, or frying, each should be broken into a clean cup or basin before being used. In this way, bad ones can best be detected.

753. Milk.—Cow's milk enters very largely into all dietaries; every care must be taken to use it when fresh, as, owing to the action of germs, lactic acid is formed after some hours, and the milk becomes sour. The cleaner the milk the longer it will keep fresh and sweet: therefore great care must be taken that the vessels in which it is kept are perfectly clean, and that it is protected from dust (which always contains germs). The cooler the temperature at which it is kept, the longer will the milk remain sweet.

Genuine milk must contain at the least 8·5 per cent. of non-fatty solids and 3 per cent. of fat; such a milk, though genuine, would be of poor quality; good milk should yield not less than 12·5 per cent. total solids, and 3·5 per cent. fat; and during the winter months these figures should be 12·9 and 3·8 respectively.

The cream should not fall below 6 per cent.: this may be tested by placing the milk in a long glass, marked with graduated divisions, and reading off the amount of cream that has risen after 24 hours: or a strip of paper may be marked in divisions (tenths and hundredths), and gummed to the glass.

The specific gravity ranges between 1·030 and 1·034 at 60° Fahrenheit.

Good milk should be of a full opaque white, or very slightly yellowish tinge; this is best seen by placing it in a glass on a sheet of white paper. It should have a slight, agreeable odour, and characteristic, sweetish taste, without any pronounced taste or smell of any kind.

The chief adulterations are:—(1) the addition of water; (2) the removal of part of the cream, with or without the addition of water ; (3) the addition of starch, gum, dextrine, flour, or glycerine ; (4) the addition of the so-called preservatives, as bicarbonate of soda, borax, boric, salicylic acid, or formalin. The addition of water lowers the specific gravity, and generally speaking there is a loss of three degrees for every ten per cent. of water added. On the other hand, removing the cream (skimming) raises the specific gravity ; so that in milk that has been both creamed and watered the specific gravity may be normal. This test must therefore be used in conjunction with the estimation of the cream present.

On account of the many risks of contamination of the milk, during milking of the cow, during storage, and during distribution to the customer, it is generally desirable to boil, or sterilize, or "pasteurize" it, before use. Milk will be rendered safe for drinking by simply bringing it to the boil for a minute or two, but as many people object to the taste of boiled milk, it is preferable, when possible, not to raise it to the boiling temperature, but to heat it to 160° Fahrenheit for twenty minutes. This is sometimes called "sterilizing" the milk, but it is better called "pasteurization." A special arrangement is provided, consisting of an outer chamber or jacket, to contain boiling water or steam, and an inner vessel in which is placed the milk. The directions accompanying the apparatus must be strictly followed. The milk should be stirred frequently, to prevent the scum forming on the top. Great care must be taken that the milk does not become fouled by dust after it has been heated. All parts of the apparatus must be kept scrupulously clean.

754. Butter.—Butter is obtained by churning, either from the milk directly, or from cream that has previously been separated. It should be of a good, rich-yellow colour, pleasant and characteristic smell and taste; the taste may be slightly salt, but should not be in the least rancid or bitter. The amount of fat in butter ranges between 80 and 90 per cent. : the water should not be more than 16 per cent. : the quantity of salt varies considerably, but nowadays much less (generally 2 or 3 per cent.) is used than formerly, other preservatives, such as boric acid, being used instead ; of this there ought not to be more than 0·5 per cent. Oleo-margarine, which is purified ox-fat, is largely used as a butter-substitute ; but it must be distinctly labelled as such, and must not be used to adulterate butter.

COOKING METHODS.

755. Roasting.—Meat and poultry intended to be roasted, must, after being properly trimmed, or trussed, be hung before a sharp fire, or placed in a very hot oven, for the first fifteen minutes, whereby a thin, brown crust is formed on the outside which prevents the escape of the nutritive juices. This is especially necessary in the case of red meat such as beef and mutton, but it also applies to white meat such as veal, pork, and poultry.

After this the heat must be reduced, or the meat must be drawn back so as to allow it to cook more gently. Veal, lamb and pork should, after the preliminary stage of quick roasting, be cooked by moderate heat, because these take somewhat longer to cook than other meats, and must therefore be cooked more gently. Whether roasted before the fire or in the oven, the basting must be carefully attended, as this renders the meat more juicy and tasty. Either butter or dripping may be used for the purpose, but in the case of poultry, the former is recommended.

756. Time required for cooking meat.—No hard and fast rule can be laid down as to the exact time required for cooking a joint or bird, because this depends greatly upon the size and the age of the animal or bird. As a rule fifteen minutes to the pound in allowed for red meats such as beef and mutton, and twenty minutes to the pound in the case of white meat, such as veal, pork, or lamb. In every case allow fifteen to twenty minutes over and above the specified time.

757. Baking.—The main difference between baking and roasting proper is that in the former case the cooking-process is performed in closed vessels, ovens, or other compartments of that description, in the latter before an open fire.

Baking, like roasting, is cooking by means of dry heat, or dry, heated air. The heat is obtained from close fires, coal or gas, or from steam at a high temperature externally applied, as is sometimes the case in so-called bakers· ovens. As before mentioned, meat can be roasted in ovens, as is mostly the case in large institutions such as hospitals, infirmaries, prisons, etc.; this is known as oven-roasting. Unless the ovens are well ventilated, and are kept clean, the fumes given off by the meat are apt to affect its flavour, and it will not be found so crisp on the outside as that roasted before an open fire. Ovens are chiefly adapted for baking bread, pastry, cakes, and certain puddings.

758. Boiling.—Boiling, or cooking in boiling liquid, is one of the most common forms of preparing food.

There are two distinct objects attained in adopting this process of cooking, which produce different characteristic results; the first being to retain the nourishing juices, and the second to extract the goodness of the materials used, as is the case when preparing stock, soups, or broths.

To retain the nourishing juices when meat or poultry is to be boiled, it must not be put into the pot or vessel until the water, which should be seasoned with salt, and if possible vegetables, is actually boiling. The article thus added must be allowed to boil briskly for at least ten minutes; for here, as in roasting, the heat must be great enough to harden the external portion and so retain the nourishing juices. This hardening-process must not, however, be carried to excess, and after the preliminary stage of actual boiling the heat must be reduced to that of simmering. In all ordinary cooking it must be remembered that simmering heat, which is the middle point of culinary heat, is more effective than violent or fast boiling.

To extract the nourishing juices the materials used must be put into cold water and then be brought slowly to the boil. After removing the scum, the cooking process is continued by slow, *i.e.*, simmering, heat until the preparation is sufficiently cooked in the liquid, which must contain practically all the goodness of the materials used.

The average loss in boiling meat is about 25 per cent. of its weight. About 20 minutes to every pound of meat, and 20 minutes over should be allowed for boiling or steaming. The following parts of meat are the best for boiling, viz., the brisket and round of beef, legs and necks of mutton or lamb. Chops are also suitable for boiling or steaming, and are considered better if so cooked for invalids. Chickens are more digestible when boiled than roasted.

759. Boiling vegetables.—All green vegetables must be boiled fast in slightly salted water. Old potatoes should be put into cold water and allowed to boil slowly till tender ; in other respects the above rules apply equally to the cooking of vegetables.

760. Steaming.—Steaming is cooking in moist heat or heated vapour, *i.e.*, cooking over or surrounded by boiling water. Although in all respects the results of steaming are the same as in boiling, the former process is more gradual (slower) than boiling, and is therefore for many reasons to be recommended. Steaming is regarded as one of the most satisfactory and convenient methods of cooking many articles of food, and is especially recommended in invalid-cookery, and for large institutions where cooking on a large scale has to be daily performed.

Beside being economical, steaming is also a simple process. The best flavour is obtained and the largest proportion of nutritive juices retained by this method of cooking, without loss of substance. The actual loss in weight of meat cooked by steam is slightly less than by boiling. The rules given for boiling are equally applicable to steaming, the preparation of materials being also identically the same as for boiling.

Meat, fish, potatoes, etc., are usually cooked by steam. In all such cases the water or other liquid such as stock, liquor, etc., is to be brought to the boil, and after a period of from 15 to 30 minutes, the steam should be somewhat reduced so as to allow the contents of the steamer to cook more or less slowly till the articles to be steamed, solid or liquid, are quite done and fit for serving. Exception to this rule is made in case of potatoes, full steam being required for these during the whole process.

761. Stewing.—This may be termed an auxiliary of the boiling process. Stewing, in reality, is cooking in a small amount of liquor at a low temperature, and is therefore an improved form of boiling, and forms one of the most popular cookery methods on the Continent. By this method, otherwise coarse or tough parts of meats can be made tender and nourishing, and as the gravy or sauce in which the meat, etc., is stewed is always served up, it naturally contains the good properties of the chief ingredients employed. More nourishment can thus be gained by this mode of cooking than by any other, so that it becomes the most profitable as well as the most useful form of preparing food.

For certain stews, the meat—especially red meat—is par-fried in butter or dripping before being actually stewed, whereby a distinctive development of flavour is obtained. Special care should be taken to avoid the meat being stewed from becoming over-done; it must only be cooked until tender, and not to a rag. This fact is often overlooked by cooks. A little vinegar sprinkled over coarse meat before cooking, considerably aids the process of rendering it tender.

762. **Frying.**—This process of cooking may be divided into two methods :—(a) deep or wet-frying, (b) dry-frying.

(a) *Deep-frying.*—Deep-frying is cooking by immersion in hot fat or oil, at a temperature which must be nearly twice that of boiling water (which is 212° Fah.). There must therefore be enough fat (clarified dripping, lard, suet, or oil) to cover well the articles to be cooked. The fat or oil must be hot enough to produce similar results as in roasting; that is, to encrust or brown the surface of the articles so cooked. Unless the fat is heated to the correct degree of temperature, frying becomes a failure, as anything put into fat or oil which is barely hot becomes sodden, greasy, unpalatable, and often uneatable. It is therefore of very great importance that the frying fat should be of the proper degree of heat before the articles are put in it to fry. When fat or oil is at the right temperature for frying it should be still, not bubbling, and a light-bluish smoke or vapour should rise from it.

Deep-frying is best adapted for fish, croquettes, rissoles, or fritters. With the exception of paste-coated things, or fritters, articles to be fried must be either dipped in batter, coated with flour, or egged and crumbed before being immersed into the hot fat. It is also most essential that anything that is fried should be carefully drained on paper or a cloth before being served in order to free it from excess of fat, which is most objectionable, particularly so in dishes intended for invalids.

The best fat for frying is that obtained from beef-suet, lard, or mutton-suet. The latter is not so good as beef suet. The dripping from roast meat, and the fat from the stock-pot or from stews, should be saved and added to the other bulk of raw or cooked fat when it is being clarified.

(b) *Dry frying.*—Dry-frying, also known as sauté-ing or panfrying, is best adapted for cutlets, fillets, steaks, chops, bacon, kidneys, liver, eggs, etc. Only a small quantity of fat must be used, really only just sufficient to prevent the articles so cooked from burning—just enough barely to cover the bottom of the pan in which the frying is performed. Butter is the most suitable fat to be used for this purpose. It must be allowed to get thoroughly hot, but not burning, before commencing to fry. Frequent turning to prevent hardening or burning, especially in the case of meat, is essential for this mode of cooking. Steak-tongs should be used for turning the articles being cooked, a fork should not be so employed as the punctures made by it allow the juices to escape.

763. **Grilling.**—This is known as the quickest cooking process; it is sometimes called broiling. A clear fire, preferably of

coke or coal, is the great essential to its success. Grilling is to cook in front of or over a fire by the help of a gridiron or grill. Mutton chops, cutlets, kidneys, steaks, fillets, split and skewered pigeons, slices of cod, haddock, whiting, and soles, etc., can be cooked in this manner. Fish must always be well done. The gridiron must be kept clean, and well greased every time it is used. The articles to be grilled must be placed between or over the grill. Frequent turning is most necessary. From ten to fifteen minutes are required to cook a moderate-sized chop or steak. They should be juicy when grilled and not allowed to cook dry.

764. Directions for carving.—All meat, whether roast, boiled, or steamed, should be carved as economically as possible. Joints of meat, such as a leg of mutton or lamb, shoulder of mutton or lamb, ribs of beef, or sirloin of beef, should invariably be cut through to the bone, so that the richer juices which lie near the bone may be served to the best advantage. Neatness in carving must at all times be aimed at, for a joint which is mutilated and hacked to pieces instead of being cut into neat slices, is not only wasteful, but spoils the appearance as well as the enjoyment of an otherwise well-cooked and wholesome meal.

A carving knife and fork, and a steel wherewith to sharpen the knife, are all the tools needed. If the knife and fork are properly handled, there is no need to touch the meat with the fingers, as is too often the case.

(a) *Beef.*—In small hospitals the parts sent for roasting are generally the middle and chuck ribs (the middle has four, and the chuck three ribs), or part of them. In this description of joint the bones should be cut out, broken and placed in the soup, and the meat then rolled, skewered, and tied with a strong string. If baked, the meat should have a piece of greased paper placed over it. In carving for distribution, the meat should be cut in slices ; if, however, the joint is roasted with the bone, the meat should be removed in one piece from the bone by inserting the knife under it, close to the bone ; the bones should be used for soup.

When the buttock and mouse-buttock are supplied for boiling, the meat should be cut when raw from the bone and then cut across in pieces two inches thick.

(b) *Mutton.*—Mutton should be carved into rather thicker slices than beef, but not too thick.

Fat, both here and in beef, should be evenly distributed, allowing a small piece or slice for each diet or ration.

In carving a leg of mutton, the leg should be held in position with a carving fork, rounded side uppermost. The knife should be carried sharply down across the centre of the joint, and slices taken from either side. The fat should be sought near the tail-end and distributed as required. The better done part of the joint is the knuckle-end, and slices should be taken from here and apportioned as necessary.

In a shoulder of mutton, the meat, before being cut up into diet-portions, should be removed from the bone in the following way :—Cut the meat off in one piece from the under part of the blade-bone by running the knife close to the bone ; then turn the joint over and cut down on each side of the ridge-bone ; then run the knife up under the meat close to the blade-bone ; there will only remain a few pieces round the shank-bone, which should be cut up and distributed among the diet-portions. The meat should be cut in slices across the grain.

If a neck of mutton is roasted, it should be trimmed and a great part of the fat removed. The scrag-end should be boned, rolled, and tied round, the bones being put into the soup. For broth, the neck of mutton should be divided into chops ; for convalescent diet, they should be skewered and tied up, and boiled in the broth.

RECIPES AND DIRECTIONS FOR COOKING.

765. Stock and stock-pot.—It is most important that a stock-pot should be kept going daily in every kitchen. The object of a stock-pot is to produce a nourishing broth or liquor, which is used for various purposes instead of water, but mainly for gravies and soups. A large boiling-pot, a copper boiler, or steam vessel can be used for this purpose, and it should be provided with a tap.

Into it are put all kinds of bones from meat (provided they are fresh), and trimmings of meat. The bones must be chopped small before they are put in the stock-pot or cooking-vessel ; either cooked or raw bones and meat can be used. To these the necessary quantity of cold water is added (average quantity being three pints of water to one pound of bones and meat). The whole must then be allowed to come slowly to the boil, when the scum which rises to the surface must be carefully removed. Fresh soup-vegetables (not potatoes), such as onions, carrots, turnips, and also a small cabbage if possible, previously washed, cleaned, and cut up, are next added. Allow about four hours of gentle boiling. During the process of boiling the scum must be removed occasionally, but the fat rising to the surface must not be removed until the stock is finished. A little salt should be added with the bones, etc., as this will help to bring up the scum and other impurities more quickly. After this the stock should be strained and used as directed.

NOTE.—*In warm weather, stock should be made without vegetables, or it will turn sour. Vegetable flavouring can be added as required.*

766. Fish-stock.—Put the skin, bones, and trimmings of fish in a saucepan, and cover it with milk and water in equal quantities ; add pepper and salt to taste, also a slice of onion and carrot, a sprig of parsley, and a blade of mace. Simmer for about half an hour and strain ; it is then ready for use.

767. To clarify fat.—Ingredients in the following proportions should be used, viz., 7 lb. fat (beef-suet or mutton-fat) to 1 pint water. Cut the fat in small pieces of even size, and remove the skin or sinews ; put the fat into a large stew-pan with the cold water. Boil it, stirring occasionally until the liquid is quite clear and the pieces of fat appear crisp. Allow it to cool a little, and then strain it into a basin containing a little cold water.

768. Beef-tea.—1 pint water (cold), 1 lb. lean beef, ½ teaspoonful salt.

(*a*) *Quick method.*—Remove all fat, sinews, and skin from the meat, then shred the meat finely, put it in a saucepan with the water and salt, and let it soak for 15 minutes ; put the saucepan over a very moderate heat, and stir with a fork for half an hour ; strain through a fine strainer, add more salt if necessary, and serve hot.

(*b*) *Slow method.*—Remove all fat, sinews, and skin, and shred the meat finely, put it in a jar with the water and salt, stand the jar in a saucepan of simmering water, or put it in a cool oven for two or three hours. Strain ; remove any fat with kitchen-paper, and serve.

(*c*) *Raw beef-tea.*—1 oz. finely-shredded, lean beef, 1 tablespoonful water. Put the meat and water into a jar, and stand the jar in a warm place for one hour ; strain and serve in a coloured glass or cup.

769. Iced beef-tea.—Beef-tea made by either the slow or quick method can be iced. Allow the beef-tea to get cold and put it in a pewter pot or earthenware basin. Place this in a pail surrounded with crushed ice and salt, and let it stand for about 40 minutes. At the end of that time stir up the beef-tea and beat up for several minutes ; allow it to stand for another 10 minutes and repeat this operation two or three times until it appears to be frozen and is quite smooth.

770. Beef-tea with oatmeal.—Mix a tablespoonful of well-cooked oatmeal with two of boiling water ; add a cupful of strong beef-tea, and bring to the boiling point. Rice may be used instead of oatmeal. Add salt and pepper to taste, and serve with toasted bread.

771. Beef-tea jelly.—Soak half an ounce of gelatine in water, heat up nearly a pint of strong beef-tea, or mix a small 1 oz. pot of essence of beef or extractum carnis with three-quarters of a pint of hot water. Drain the gelatine, melt in a small stew-pan and add to the beef-tea when quite dissolved. Strain into a wetted mould and stand in a cool place till firm. Un-mould and serve as required.

772. Beef-juice.—Place half a pound of lean, juicy beefsteak on a griller over a clear, hot fire ; heat it through without actually browning ; cut it into strips ; press out the juice with a lemon-squeezer into a hot cup, add a little salt, and serve with toasted slices of bread.

773. Mutton-broth.—One lb. scrag-end of mutton, 1 quart of water, 1 dessert-spoonful of pearl barley or sago, 1 clove, 6 pepper-corns, 1 teaspoonful of chopped parsley, salt to taste.

Take the meat off the bones and cut into dice. Trim off the fat and put the meat and bones into a saucepan with the water ; add the salt and bring slowly to the boil. Skim well. Add the rest of ingredients. Simmer gently for about three hours, skim again, then add the parsley. When cooked remove the bones.

Note.—If vegetable flavouring is allowed, cut up a small onion half a small carrot, and a turnip, and cook them in the broth. Blanch the barley before using; chop finely about 1 teaspoonful of the cooked meat, and add it to the broth before serving.

774. Chicken-broth.—One small chicken, 1 quart of water, 6 peppercorns, 2 cloves, 1 onion, 1 dessert-spoonful of chopped meat, 1 teaspoonful of parsley, 1 ounce of blanched barley, pepper and salt to taste.

Cut the chicken into small pieces, put it into a saucepan with the cold water; simmer gently for about three hours; season and strain. If liked, an ounce of barley or tapioca may be cooked with it. A small, chopped onion would also make it more savoury.

775. Filleted fish.—Fish should, if possible, be filleted from the bone. This is done by first removing both skins, cutting off the head, making a cut down each side of the backbone, and then running the knife under the flesh close to the bone. Each sole will make four fillets, which should be placed in a previously buttered baking-dish. A piece of buttered paper is then placed over the fish, which is baked in the oven from 10 to 15 minutes. Small haddocks and large whiting are best filleted and cooked in the same way as soles. Slices of cod can also be cooked in this way. (See also other methods.)

776. Boiled fish.—When cod, haddock, ling, etc., are to be boiled they should be cut into slices when raw, and each slice rolled and tied round with string, which is removed when the fish is dished up. This should be served with a plain white or parsley-sauce.

777. Boiled whiting.—Put the whiting into a saucepan of hot water flavoured with vinegar and salt. Cook gently for about six minutes. Do not allow the water to boil, or the fish will break. Try with a skewer to see if it is cooked. Drain and serve on a hot plate.

778. Fried fish.—Fish to be fried is best filleted (except cod which can be fried if cut into slices); the fish must be dried as far as possible in a cloth, and then be dipped into batter (frying batter) or else be egged and crumbed. There must be sufficient fat in the frying-pan well to cover the fish during the whole process of frying, and the fat must be boiling-hot before the fish is put into it (see instructions for Frying).

779. Fried sole.—Wash, wipe, skin, and trim the sole. Dip it lightly into flour, and season with very little pepper and salt. Egg and crumb the sole. Fry in boiling-hot fat. Drain it carefully and serve hot.

Note.—A more simple way to fry a sole is to dip it into milk and then into flour; then fry to a golden-brown in hot fat.

780. Fried filleted plaice.—Fillet the plaice (remove the black skin), put a little salt, pepper, and lemon-juice on each fillet; roll up or leave them flat, then brush over with beaten egg and cover with bread-crumbs, fry in boiling fat, drain on a cloth or paper, and serve.

781. To steam fish.—Skin the fish (sole or whiting), point the tail, remove the eyes, and cut off the fins ; then sprinkle over the fish a little salt and a few drops of lemon-juice.

Have a steamer or saucepan of boiling water ready ; put the fish in the steamer or on a plate or colander over the saucepan, and steam until the flesh will come easily from the bone (about 20 minutes is usually sufficient) ; put the fish on a hot plate, pour over it enough white sauce to cover the fish, and serve hot.

Note.—Slices of cod are also suitable for steaming, and are prepared in the same way as above directed.

782. Fish-cakes.—Half pound of cooked fish (cod, whiting, haddock, or other white fish), 2 oz. mashed potatoes, ½ oz. of butter, one yolk of egg, pepper, and salt.

Free the fish from skin and bones, and chop the meat finely. Melt the butter in a saucepan ; stir in the fish and potato, and bind with the yolk of an egg. Season to taste. Form into small, round, flat cakes. Egg and crumb them. Fry in very hot fat, drain carefully and serve on a hot dish.

783. Fricassee of fish.—First cook the fish in salted water flavoured with a blade of mace and a sprig of parsley. Remove the skin and bones and divide it into small portions. Make a white fish-sauce. Season it with lemon-juice, nutmeg, pepper, and salt. Put in the pieces of fish and heat up. Serve with plain boiled rice. If cooked fish is used, put the bones and skin into the water and simmer for ten minutes with the spices, then make the sauce as directed.

784. White fish-pudding.—6 oz. of cooked fish, 1 oz. soft bread-crumbs, one egg, mace, nutmeg, salt, pepper, and 2 oz. of butter.

Chop or mash the fish and warm it up in the butter, add the bread-crumbs, previously soaked in half a gill of milk or cold stock. Season with salt, pepper, a pinch of ground mace, and a grate of nutmeg, then add the beaten-up egg and mix well. Steam in a buttered mould one hour, or bake in a tin buttered and coated with bread-crumbs for half an hour.

785. Chops and Steaks.—Both chops and steaks are best if broiled on or between a griller in front of or over a good fire (coal, coke, or gas). When this is not possible, they should be broiled, *i.e.*, dry-fried in frying-pans, adopting the following method :—Slightly trim the chops from superfluous fat, and flatten a little with a bat : the same applies to steaks. Use a clean and dry pan ; heat it over the fire and put in a little dripping or butter (barely enough to cover the bottom of the pan) ; when hot, put in the meat and let it cook, *i.e.*, broil, rather quickly so as to brown the surface of the meat ; then turn it (avoid piercing the meat with a fork or knife, or the juices will escape) and let the other side get browned likewise. After this, allow the meat to cook somewhat slower till done. Chops and steaks of moderate thickness require from fifteen to twenty minutes to cook—they must not be over-done and every care must be taken that the meat is juicy when served.

786. Steamed chop.—Loin-chops are best : trim off the fat and roll up the end, which may be skewered. Place it on a small plate and put it in a stew-pan containing stock or seasoned water, also a sprig of thyme and a little parsley. Cover the pan, and cook thus for half an hour or longer till the meat is tender. Serve it with mashed potatoes.

787. Minced mutton.—Remove the bone and fat from a mutton chop, and mince the remainder very finely. Melt ½ oz. of butter in a small stew-pan ; when hot put in the meat and cook very gently for 10 minutes. Season very lightly with salt and pepper, and serve with small fingers of toasted bread or dry biscuits.

788. Beefsteak-balls.—Scrape the required quantity of lean beef with a sharp knife, so that there is nothing left but the tough fibres ; to each half pound of meat add the yolk of one egg, season with salt and pepper, and mix well. Shape into balls of even size. Use a little flour or bread-crumbs for shaping. Melt some butter for dripping in a frying pan ; when hot put in the meat-balls, and fry to a golden brown. Serve with a little thin, brown sauce.

789. Roast and baked fowl.—Previous to cooking, the fowl must be plucked, singed, and drawn. To draw the fowl, lay it back-downwards on the table ; cut a slit in the skin of the neck, leaving enough to form a flap; through this opening insert the middle finger and loosen the entrails, doing this carefully and thoroughly so that less trouble may afterwards be met in drawing the bird. Next, cut off the vent and draw the fowl carefully, taking out all the entrails. Special care must be taken to avoid breaking the gall-bladder as this may ruin the bird by imparting a very bitter taste to the flesh. The inside must then be carefully wiped out, as also the flap of skin at the neck. Lastly, dip the legs in boiling water, scrape them, and cut off the claws, also the tips of the pinions.

A fowl to produce 1 lb. of meat (or two diets) should weigh, when dressed and drawn and ready for cooking, not less than 1¼ lb. and not more than 1¾ lb. in its raw state. (*Note :* The foregoing specification is for Great Britain, it may vary at other stations.) It should be roasted whole, and afterwards divided. But if one portion of a fowl only is required, it should be cut from the raw fowl, covered with buttered paper, and either baked or roasted. In baking fowls, the oven should be hotter than for meat. If a fowl has been once cooked, to make it hot again place it on a plate in a basin, with very little water under the plate ; it should be covered over with a little utter and heated in the oven for 20 minutes.

790. Gravy.—A little hot gravy should always be poured round each portion of roast or baked meat and poultry. To make gravy, proceed as follows :—Pour off the fat from the pan in which the roast-joint or fowl was cooked ; strain this fat (the excess should be kept for further use) ; then add the required quantity of stock or bone-liquor, stir over the fire so as to blend the whole, season lightly with salt and pepper, boil for 5 minutes, then skim and strain.

791. Boiled chicken.—Draw the chicken for boiling in the same way as for roasting. To truss, cut off the legs at the knee-joint ; then loosen the skin over the legs, and force the lower part of the leg under the skin ; put a skewer through the wing, upper part of leg, body, other leg, and wing; tie a piece of string round the "parson's nose," then round the lower part of the chicken so as completely to close the opening. Put the chicken into rapidly boiling stock, boil it for five minutes; then let it simmer for 20 minutes to each pound and 20 minutes over; lift the chicken out of the stock, drain it well, put it on a hot dish, and remove skewer and string. Cut it up into portions and serve with plain, white sauce, or with egg-sauce, as may be ordered. If served plain, a little of the stock or liquor should be poured over each portion.

792. Rabbit, boiled and roast.—Same as for chicken.

793. Stewed rabbit.—It should be well washed to remove any congealed blood, then wiped clean and cut into pieces. An onion should be added for flavouring, and a little dried herbs. Place the pieces of rabbit in a stew-pan with sufficient cold water to cover; add the onion cut up small, a few herbs, pepper and salt to taste, and let it simmer gently from one to one-and-a-half hours according to size. About fifteen minutes before serving, skim off all the fat, make a little thickening of flour and water, pour in and stir till it boils. A small piece of fat bacon or salt pork will greatly improve the flavour.

794. Stewed tripe.—One lb. of tripe, 1 onion, ½ pint of milk, ⅓ oz. of flour, pepper, and salt.

Blanch the tripe and remove all fat, and cut into square pieces. Put the tripe, the onion (chopped), and the milk into a saucepan. Season with pepper and salt. Simmer gently for two hours. Blend the flour smoothly with a little cold milk and pour it in. Stir until it boils up, let the whole simmer for ¼ hour and serve very hot.

795. Savoury suet-dumplings.—To each ½ lb. of flour, take 4 oz. finely-chopped beef-suet, 2 eggs, ½ teaspoonful of baking-powder, ½ teaspoonful sweet herbs, 1 tablespoonful of chopped parsley, salt and pepper to taste. Mix the dry ingredients in a basin, and moisten with the egg previously beaten up and mixed with a little milk or stock into a fairly stiff paste. Make up into small balls, and boil or steam them for about ¾ hour in stock or water These dumplings can be served with gravy or white sauce.

Sauces, &c.

796. Plain fish-sauce.—A plain sauce can be made of the skin, bones, and trimmings by boiling them in a little water with a slice of onion, a sprig of parsley, and salt, and then straining.

797. White fish-sauce.—To be served with baked, steamed, or boiled fish. 1 oz. of butter, ½ oz. of flour, 1½ gills of milk or fish-stock, pepper and salt, 1 teaspoonful of lemon-juice.

Rub the butter into the flour until quite smooth, put it into a saucepan with the milk and stir until it boils. Season with pepper, salt, and lemon-juice, cook for at least ten minutes and strain. Pour this over the fish with which it is served.

798. Anchovy-sauce.—Take a pint of white sauce, or of melted-butter sauce, and mix whilst hot with an ounce of essence of anchovy. (A few drops of lemon-juice may also be added.) This sauce is served with boiled or fried fish, and should always be sent to table in a sauce-boat and not poured over the fish.

799. Melted-butter sauce.—Two oz. of butter, 1½ oz. of flour, about 1¼ pints of cold water, salt.

Melt the butter in the saucepan, stir in the flour, add the water gradually (if it is to be served with fish, use fish-stock in place of water), stir, bring it gently to the boil, and season with salt.

This sauce is served usually with boiled vegetables or with boiled fish.

800. White sauce.—1½ pints of milk, ½ pint of ordinary stock, 1 onion, 1 clove, 2 oz. of butter, 3 oz. of flour, 6 peppercorns, 1 bay-leaf, a pinch of salt, nutmeg.

Boil the milk in a saucepan, peel the onion and stick the clove in it, put it into the milk with the bay-leaf and peppercorns. Stir the flour into the butter previously melted in a saucepan. Cook without browning for a few minutes, then moisten with the stock and boil up, then add the milk, etc. Let all boil until the flour is thoroughly cooked, this will take about ten to fifteen minutes. Take out the onion, bay-leaf, and peppercorns. Add a pinch of nutmeg, if desired, and one of salt. If it is not smooth, pass it through a sieve. Should a richer sauce be desired, a small piece of fresh butter or a little cream may be worked in after the sauce is strained, but it must not boil again. This sauce is suitable for boiled mutton, chicken or rabbit.

Another white sauce which is commonly used for boiled vegetables, such as cauliflowers, artichokes, onions, etc., is made as follows :— Melt a piece of butter, the size of a walnut, in a saucepan ; when melted add a spoonful of flour and thoroughly mix a mixture of half stock and half milk to make it of a consistency of cream. If too thick add a little milk or stock gradually to thin it : the sauce should be of a consistency to cling to the article of food. Then add sufficient milk and boil, and pour over vegetable and serve.

801. Caper-sauce.—Make ½ a pint of melted-butter sauce as directed, chop coarsely 3 tablespoonsful of capers, add these with a tablespoonful of vinegar to the sauce, boil for five minutes and serve. This sauce is usually served with boiled mutton or with boiled fish.

802. Parsley-sauce.—Heat up a pint of white sauce. When quite hot, stir in the chopped parsley (add one teaspoonful of lemon-juice if liked), boil for five minutes and serve.

N.B.—The parsley after being chopped should be put in the corner of a cloth and washed under the cold-water tap, and squeezed dry before it is put into the sauce.

803. Egg-sauce.—One pint of white sauce or melted-butter sauce, 2 eggs, a few drops of lemon-juice.

Boil the eggs for fifteen minutes, put them into a basin of cold water to cool, take off the shells and chop the whites of the eggs not too finely. Heat up the sauce, and when ready stir in the chopped whites. A few drops of lemon-juice or vinegar may be added if desired.

804. Brown-sauce.—1¼ pints of gravy or rich stock, one onion, one carrot, 2 oz. of butter or dripping, 1½ oz. flour, ½ oz. of mushroom-ketchup, ⅓ oz. of vinegar, salt, and pepper.

Peel the onion, scrape the carrot, cut up both into small pieces ; melt the butter or dripping in a saucepan and when hot add the vegetables and flour, stir over the fire until brown, put in the vinegar, ketchup, and gravy, and continue stirring up until it boils, then skim well, and allow it to simmer for twenty minutes. Strain and season to taste, re-heat and skim, and serve as required.

805. Fried potatoes.—Wash and scrub the potatoes, peel them thinly, cut them lengthwise into slices, then cut the slices into long, thin strips, keep them in cold water until ready to fry. Have a frying-pan with sufficient hot fat (lard, dripping, or oil) to cover the potatoes. Drain the potatoes carefully and fry in the hot fat until they are a light-brown colour ; lift them out and drain them well on a cloth or paper and serve. Frying is one of the best methods by which to cook potatoes.

806. Brussels sprouts.—Trim the sprouts by removing the outer leaves, and wash them in cold water. Add a tablespoonful of salt to the boiling water, put in the sprouts, and keep them boiling rapidly, without a cover, until the stems are soft (usually about twenty minutes); then melt 1 oz. butter in a saucepan for each pound of sprouts, add the sprouts to it, strain, season with salt and pepper, then shake them well, dish them up and serve hot.

NOTE.—*Soda is often added to preserve the colour of vegetables ; this is quite unnecessary if vegetables are boiled rapidly and served at once. Soda may cause indigestion and therefore should never be added in invalid-cooking.*

807. Baked tomatoes.—Cut the tomatoes in halves, crossways, scoop out a little of the pulp, and mix in with bread-crumbs, grated cheese, chopped parsley and a little butter. When these ingredients have been well mixed, fill the tomatoes with them, place them on a buttered tin, season with a little pepper and salt, and bake in a hot oven from fifteen to twenty minutes.

808. Spinach.—For each 1 lb. of spinach take ½ oz. of butter or dripping, salt, and pepper.

Pick all the stalks off the spinach, wash it well in several waters and put it into a stew-pan with the drops of water that hang to the leaves ; let it boil till thoroughly tender, then rub it through a wire-sieve. Put it back in the stew-pan with the butter and a tablespoonful of cream, pepper and salt, mix well until it is thoroughly hot, then serve with pieces of toast around it.

Note.—Additional water is not necessary to cook spinach if it is properly washed and picked, and the leaves put in the stew-pan with the water hanging to them.

809. Cauliflower.—Select a cauliflower with a firm, close head, wash it and trim off nearly all the leaves (a few left will be a protection to the flower), soak in salted water for one hour in order to displace any insects, etc., put it into boiling water and cook till quite tender, which will take from 20 to 30 minutes. When it is plainly boiled for table, split the stem across in opposite directions, so that it will cook as quickly as the flower, place it in the saucepan with the head downwards so that if any scum arises it may be removed easier from the surface of the water, and at the same time the flower will be kept much cleaner. To test if it is sufficiently cooked, press a little of the leaf with the fingers, and if soft take it out on a hair-strainer or cloth, trim off all the stalk, reverse it upon the dish so that it is in the same position as when growing and serve up covered with the white sauce referred to in paragraph 800.

810. Carrots.—Should be washed clean, scraped, and cut into quarters of as nearly the same size as possible. Place in cold water until required for cooking. To boil, place in boiling water with a little salt (for every half gallon of water, 1 tablespoonful of salt), boil until tender (young carrots will cook in 15 minutes), strain through a wire-sieve, place on a vegetable-dish and serve hot.

811. Parsnips.—Wash thoroughly, and scrape well, removing any black specks with the knife, and if very large, cut the thick part into quarters. Place them in a vessel of boiling water, salted as for carrots, and boil rapidly until tender. Take them up, drain, and serve on a vegetable-dish.

812. Turnips.—Pare them and if large divide into quarters, otherwise cook whole. Place in saucepan of boiling water salted as described above and boil gently until tender, generally requiring half an hour. Turnips are frequently served mashed. After being well boiled, drain through a wire-sieve or colander and squeeze them as dry as possible by pressing them with the back of a plate. When dry place in a clean saucepan and add butter, salt, and pepper to taste. Keep stirring them over a fire till butter is well mixed, dish and serve hot.

813. Beetroot.—Remove leaves one inch from the crown. Rub off as much dirt as is possible with the hand. Place in boiling water and allow to boil from one to one and a half hours according to size; then strain off the water and allow to cool. When cold, peel them, cut into thin slices, place in vinegar, adding pepper and salt to taste. The great object in cooking beetroot is not to prick or break the skin before they are cooked, otherwise they will loose the rich, red colour. A good method of cooking them is to place them in nets first, so that they can be more easily removed from the cooking vessel.

814. Scrambled eggs.—Two eggs, ½ oz. butter, 1 tablespoonful milk, pepper and salt, 1 slice of hot, buttered toast.

Beat up the eggs, add to it the milk, pepper, and salt, melt the butter in a saucepan, pour in the egg-mixture, and stir until the egg is just set, spread it on the prepared toast, and serve hot.

815. Poached egg.—Break the egg into a cup to make sure it is fresh. Take a frying-pan and fill it three parts full of clean water (if only one egg is required, a small saucepan will be more suitable), add a little salt and a few drops of vinegar or lemon-juice, place it on the fire and as soon as it boils, turn the egg into it. Be careful not to let it boil too fast; keep the yolk of the egg covered with the albumen by the aid of an egg-slice; allow to boil for 3 to 3½ minutes;

take it out, trim the edges, and serve hot on a small piece of buttered toast.

816. Savoury omelet.—Two eggs, $\frac{1}{2}$ ounce of butter, 2 teaspoonsful of chopped parsley, 2 drachms of milk, pepper and salt.

Break the eggs into a basin, beat them well with a fork, add milk and parsley, season with pepper and salt. Dissolve the butter in a frying or an omelet pan. When quite hot, pour in the mixture, stir slowly with a fork over a quick fire and shake the pan. When the eggs begin to set, shape and roll the omelet on one side of the pan, allow it to take colour, then turn quickly on to a hot dish and serve.

817. Sweet, or jam omelet.—Two eggs, 2 drachms of milk, $\frac{1}{2}$ oz. of sugar, $\frac{1}{2}$ oz. butter, $\frac{1}{2}$ to 1 oz. of jam, a pinch of salt.

Break the eggs into a basin, beat them well, add the milk, half the sugar, and the salt. Melt the butter in an omelet-pan, and when this is hot, pour in the other mixed ingredients, and stir over a quick fire. When the eggs begin to set, shape and roll the omelet towards the edge of the pan, allow it to take colour, put the jam previously warmed in the centre, fold in the edges, turn the omelet on to a dish, sprinkling over it the remainder of the sugar, and serve hot.

Puddings.

818. Rice-pudding.—One oz. Patna or Carolina rice, $\frac{3}{4}$ pint of milk, $\frac{1}{2}$ oz. sugar, 1 egg.

Wash the rice, put it in a saucepan with the milk, and let them simmer until the milk is thick, add the sugar and flavouring and well-beaten egg, pour the mixture into a slightly greased pie-dish or pudding-tin and bake in a moderate oven from 20 minutes to half an hour, dredge with sugar and serve.

Note.—Lemon, cinnamon, nutmeg, cloves, and other spices may be issued as flavouring. When flavouring is used, it should be put in the pudding just before it is baked. A thin piece of lemon-rind boiled in the milk and removed before baking is found excellent.

Other farinaceous foods which can be used and suitable for milk-puddings are tapioca, sago, barley, cornflour, semolina, etc.

819. Tapioca-pudding.—Three-quarters of a pint of milk, 1 oz. of tapioca, $\frac{1}{2}$ oz. of sugar, 1 egg, flavouring-essence.

Put the tapioca to soak in the milk for a few minutes, then cook over the fire until the tapioca is quite tender. When it is cooked let it cool slightly, then add sugar and beaten egg and a few drops of flavouring essence. Butter a pie-dish, pour the pudding into it, and bake for about twenty minutes.

820. Custard-pudding.—One pint of milk, 2 eggs, 1 oz. sugar flavouring.

Beat the eggs, add to them the milk and sugar and flavouring, pour the custard into a pie-dish, and bake in a moderate oven for twenty minutes; sprinkle sugar over, and serve either hot or cold. The same ingredients can be put in a greased basin and steamed, or they can be put in a double saucepan or jar and boiled.

821. Savoury custard-pudding.—A savoury custard can be made by substituting herbs, chopped meat, and pepper and salt for sugar and flavouring.

822. Suet-pudding.—One oz. beef suet, 1 oz. flour, ⅛ oz. baking-powder, and ₁⁄₁₆ oz. of salt.

Remove the skin from the suet and chop it very finely. Put it in a basin with the flour, baking-powder and salt, and stir. Work into a smooth paste and fill into small, well-greased moulds. Cover each with greased paper and steam for forty-five to sixty minutes. Turn out and serve.

823. Sago-pudding.—One oz. sago, ⅔ pint milk, 1 egg, ½ oz. sugar. Proceed the same as for rice-pudding.

Jellies.

824. Calves'-foot jelly.—Two calves' feet, half-pound of loaf-sugar, the shells and whites of five eggs, the rind and juice of two lemons, ½ oz. isinglass, 1 glass of sherry, and 6 pints of cold water (to make one quart of jelly). Scald the feet well to remove all hair, split them in two, remove fat, wash well in hot water, and put in a clean saucepan with the whole of the water. Place on fire and allow to simmer for 6 hours. Then strain through a sieve into a large basin, and put in a cold place to set. After the liquor is strained off, measure it to ascertain that the requisite quantity remains, *i.e.,* 2 pints, 6 ounces (the six ounces is allowed for fat and sediment); if more than this quantity, return to saucepan and let it simmer down to the above amount. If there is a less quantity, make it up with boiling water. When cold, carefully remove any fat from the surface and wash well with warm water to remove any traces of fat. Turn jelly out of the basin and remove any sediment from below. Wipe the jelly with a clean cloth and break into small pieces. Whisk well the shells and whites of the eggs with the sugar, then stir the whole of the ingredients together. Place the saucepan on the fire with the jelly and all ingredients in it. Let it gently come to the boil, but do not stir after it begins to get warm. Allow to simmer for 5 minutes, then pour in half a cup of cold water, and withdraw the saucepan from the fire carefully so as not to shake the jelly. Cover and allow it to stand for half an hour near the fire. Meanwhile prepare the jelly-bag from some fine flannel, wash it well with hot water (without soap or soda), wring dry and fasten on top of a rimmed basin. Pour the jelly carefully through it near the fire to prevent it setting. Now dip the moulds into cold water for a few seconds and pour the jelly into them, and place in a cool spot to set; or ice may be packed around the moulds. When required for table, dip the moulds into hot water and wipe outside with a cloth. Lay a dish on top of the mould and turn it quickly over. It is sometimes also served in broken square pieces Earthenware or glass moulds are preferable to those made of tin or pewter. Cow-heels can be used instead of calves' feet, but the preparation takes longer.

825. Milk-jelly.—Half-pint of milk, ¼ oz. gelatine, rind of ½ lemon, 1 oz. sugar.

Put the gelatine in the saucepan with as small a quantity as possible of water to melt it; add the milk, sugar, and lemon-peel cut very thin, and stir over very moderate heat until all is well blended; then strain it into a basin and stir occasionally until it is cool. Pour it into small moulds and put in a cool place to set.

826. Lemon-jelly.—Half-pint of lemon-juice, 1½ pints of water, 6 oz. of sugar, 1 inch of cinnamon, 4 cloves, 2½ oz. gelatine, the rind of 4 lemons thinly cut, 2 whites of eggs and the shells.

Put all these ingredients into a saucepan together. Whisk until it boils. Let it stand for five minutes. Strain through a clean cloth previously scalded. When firm turn out into jelly-moulds.

827. Wine-jelly.—If wine is allowed, add one gill of sherry to the above, in which case use that amount of water less.

828. Egg-jelly.—Two lemons, 6 oz. sugar, 2 eggs, ½ oz. gelatine.

Put the gelatine into a saucepan, add to it the sugar and lemon-rind, strain on to this the lemon-juice, and make up to 1 pint with water, to this add the eggs previously beaten, then stir over the fire until the gelatine is melted and the eggs are well blended; the mixture must not boil. Strain into small moulds, and put them in a cool place to set, and turn out when required.

The chief points in preparing egg-jelly are, firstly, that the jelly must not be allowed to boil (if it does boil, the albumen of the eggs become hardened and indigestible), and, secondly, that the lemons must be very thinly peeled, or the jelly will be bitter.

Beverages, etc.

829. Lemonade.—Two large lemons, 1½ oz. sugar to every 2 pints of boiling water.

Put the thinly-peeled lemon-rind, the lemon-juice, and sugar into a jug, and pour over this the boiling water. Cover and let cool, then strain and serve. A little more sugar may be added if needed. Great care must be taken to peel the lemon very thinly and to remove the white skin afterwards, otherwise the lemonade will be bitter.

830. Toast-water.—Toast three slices of stale bread to a very dark brown, *but do not burn them;* put them into a jug, pour over a quart of boiling water, cover closely, and allow to stand on ice or in a cool place until cold; strain. A little wine and sugar may be added if allowed.

831. Oatmeal-tea.—Three oz. of coarse oatmeal, 1 quart boiling water, the thin rind and juice of half a lemon, 1 oz. sugar.

Put the oatmeal into a jug. Pour on to it the boiling water and add the thin rind of half a lemon and the sugar. Cover the jug and let it stand near the fire for an hour or more. Then strain off the tea and serve it.

832. Tea.—In making tea the vessel must be quite clean. It should be heated and rinsed with hot water, the dry tea put in and boiling water poured over it, and the pot then closed for four or five minutes to allow the tea to brew. It should then be strained, and the leaves well rinsed with the additional boiling water required before adding the sugar and milk. When making large quantities of tea, it will be found better to put the dry tea into thin muslin bags, loosely tied so as to allow sufficient space for the leaves to expand and give out their full flavour. Place them in the vessel, pour on the boiling water, and allow to remain in a warm place closely covered for four or five minutes; then withdraw the bags and add the necessary milk and sugar and serve as hot as possible. Tea should never be made in a boiler that has contained broth or soup.

833. Coffee.—To prevent adulteration, coffee should be bought in the bean and ground. Care should be taken that only sufficient coffee is ground for the day's consumption, as when the bean is broken the aroma quickly escapes. Coffee of an inferior quality may be improved by the addition of chicory, but not more than 2 oz. of it to 1 lb. of coffee. Beans and chicory are used in the adulteration of coffee. Chicory may be detected by sprinkling a little of the mixture on some water in a glass. The chicory at once sinks to the bottom, whilst coffee will float for a while. If a little is shaken with water, the coffee will rise and the chicory sink. Coffee should not be allowed to boil, as by doing so its aroma is dissipated. It should if possible, be first warmed, which causes each grain of the powder to separate, then the amount of boiling water required should be poured on it. The cans should be well rinsed with hot water, the dry coffee placed in them and the boiling water added gradually, so as thoroughly to extract its strength. Coffee should be made immediately before being required for consumption and served up as hot as possible, and the required amount of hot milk and sugar added.

834. Cocoa.—This should always be made into a paste in the first place. Boiling water is then poured over, and sugar and milk added. Then boil the whole for two or three minutes in order to cook the starch which it contains. Stir well and serve. One tea-spoonful of cocoa for each half-pint will be found sufficient; milk and sugar in the same proportion as for tea.

835. Rice-water.—Carolina rice 2 oz., sugar 2 oz. to every 5 pints.

Wash the rice thoroughly in cold water, then soften by steeping it for three hours in a quart of water kept at tepid heat; afterwards boil slowly for an hour and strain. This may be flavoured with lemon-rind or clove. The sugar may also be added if liked.

836. Barley-water.—Two oz. barley, 2 oz. sugar, for every five pints.

(1) *Clear.*—Blanch the barley by covering it with cold water bringing to the boil and straining; then put it back into the sauce-pan and add five pints of cold water. Bring it to the boil and let it simmer for half an hour. Strain, and add the sugar. Allow to cool.

(2) *Thick.*—Proceed as above, only instead of boiling for half an hour, boil down to two-thirds of liquid. Strain, and add sugar.

As barley-water will only keep a few hours, it should stand in a cool place and should never be heated to boiling point again.

837. Barley-milk.—Quarter of a pound patent barley, 1 pint of milk, ½ pint of water, 1 oz. of sugar.

Boil the barley in the milk and water for two hours, sweeten with the sugar and serve while it is just warm.

838. Egg-flip.—Two eggs, ½ oz. sugar, 1 small glass of wine or lemon if allowed.

Put the yolks of the eggs and the sugar in a tumbler, and stir until creamy. Beat the whites of the eggs to a stiff froth and stir it lightly in. Serve. Half the juice of a lemon or a little wine (sherry or Marsala) can be used to flavour if allowed.

839. Junket.—Half a pint of milk, 1 teaspoonful sugar, teaspoonful rennet, 2 drops of flavouring essence.

Dissolve the sugar in the milk. Warm the milk to 98° F. Add the rennet and flavouring. Allow it to cool, and when firm place it on the ice for about an hour. Serve with sugar, and cream if allowed.

840. Gruel.—Two oz. of oatmeal, 1¼ oz. sugar to make 2 pints.

Mix the oatmeal with a little cold milk or water ; boil the remainder and pour it, when boiling, on the oatmeal ; return the mixture to the saucepan and boil for ten minutes. Add the sugar and serve very hot.

841. Flour-gruel.—Mix a teaspoonful of flour with enough milk to make a smooth paste, and stir into it 1 quart of boiling milk. Boil for half an hour and be careful not to let it burn. Salt and strain.

842. Arrowroot-gruel.—Mix one teaspoonful of arrowroot with four of cold milk ; stir it slowly into half a pint of boiling milk and then let it simmer for five minutes. The mixture must be stirred all the time. Add a half-teaspoonful of sugar, a pinch of salt, one of cinnamon (or in place of cinnamon use a little brandy or a dozen large raisins).

A corn-starch, or rice-flour gruel can be made in the same way.

843. Oatmeal-porridge.—Two oz. of oatmeal with 8 oz. milk.

Stir the oatmeal gradually into a pint of boiling water, and let it come to the boil whilst stirring. Cook gently for about an hour. Add a pinch of salt and serve with cold milk. The porridge must be stirred occasionally whilst cooking.

844. Milk-porridge.—One oz. of flour, 1 pint of milk, ¼ teaspoonful of salt.

Heat the milk in a clean saucepan, saving enough cold milk to mix the flour to a smooth batter. Add this gradually to the hot milk and cook for half an hour, stirring frequently. Add a pinch of salt and serve.

845. Bread-and-milk.—Rub bread-crumbs through a fine sieve, put them in a cup and cover with boiling water, then place a saucer on the top of the cup ; allow the crumbs to steep for fifteen minutes, drain off the water and in its place pour on some warm milk. Beat the whole well up, and then put the bread and milk into an enamelled saucepan and boil gently for a minute or two, stand it aside to cool a little, and, before giving it to the patient, stir it, and see that it is nice and smooth, adding a little sugar and more milk if liked.

846. The Aymard Milk-sterilizer.—Directions for sterilizing milk with the Six-gallon Tin Sterilizer :—

The water is placed in the outer pan to such a height that it will run out of the tap. The tap is turned off, and the fire is lighted. The two lids are now removed, and the required quantity of milk is poured into the milk-chamber (it is best to strain the milk previously). Now replace the two lids and insert the thermometer through them. In about twenty minutes the milk will indicate upon the thermometer a temperature of 195° F. The furnace-door must now be opened and the milk kept at this temperature for five minutes ; then rake the fire out. The milk is now sterilized. In order to cool the milk, remove the thermometer and the outer lid, but on no account the inner lid, for if the inner lid is removed even momentarily a scum forms. Introduce a hose-pipe into the outer pan, or in case no constant supply is available, pour water in with a bucket, at the same time turning on the tap. Place a thermometer again in the inner lid in position. The cooling process must be continued until the temperature falls to 100° F. After this the thermometer may be removed, cleaned, and placed in a position of safety. The milk is now ready to be served out, and should be ladled into vessels for distribution ; or if intended to be kept in the canteen should be transferred to a separate vessel. It should not be stored in the sterilizer. The vessel the milk is transferred to should be covered with a clean cloth to prevent unnecessary exposure to the air. The milk should be stirred every three or four minutes during heating and cooling by drawing the handle of the stirrer up and down once or twice. In order to get all the milk out of the sterilizer, lift it bodily out of the pan and pour it out through the spout. The sterilizer should be cleaned by filling the milk-chamber with cold water, allow it to stand for a short time, then wipe out and dry. The water in the outer pan will be ready for use without re-filling. Always leave the lid off the sterilizer until required for use again. No sand should be used in the milk-chamber, and soda is unnecessary. If the thermometer gets broken the following means may be adopted, viz. :—In about twenty minutes from the commencement of heating, steam will issue freely from the lid and spout. This does not occur until the temperature of the milk has reached 195° F., as previous to this the milk-chamber acts as a condenser.

847. Preserved provisions.—As a rule in most cases it is only necessary to remove the lid of the tin and place the latter in a stew-pan of boiling water. The pan should be kept on the fire or in the oven until the contents are thoroughly warmed, then remove the fat from the top and serve hot. In making a stew of beef or mutton, the vegetables should be cooked first, after which the meat cut up into squares should be added. Season according to taste. Preserved meat may also be used to make curries, pies, etc., and so form an agreeable change on service or in camp.

848. Peptonized foods.—For patients whose digestive organs are extremely weak, this kind of food is of the utmost value, because part of the digestion is thereby accomplished, and the digestive functions of the stomach are relieved. Peptonized food must be administered with every precaution and care, and only under medical directions.

To peptonize any liquid food or stimulant, a certain quantity of liquor pancreaticus and bicarbonate of soda is employed in the form of an infusion. The quantity used varies according to the degree of peptonization. To one pint of liquid the average quantity used is one tablespoonful of liquor pancreaticus, and a salt-spoonful (25 grains) of the bicarbonate. As soon as the liquid has reached the degree needed it must be served immediately ; or it must be boiled up at once so as to prevent any further action of the liquor pancreaticus ; otherwise, if left standing too long, a bitter and objectionable flavour will be imparted. If peptonized milk is consumed as soon as the process is carried far enough, that is, to the degree needed by the patient, the actual boiling need not take place.

Note.—Liquor pancreaticus is a chemical preparation, produced from beef-pancreas (pancreatine), which acts similarly to pepsine, possessing the power of digesting albumen and turning it into a soluble form.

INDEX.

A.

C.

D.

F.

440

(B 10977) 2 F 2

T.

U.

V.

Page.

W.